Psychoenvironmental Forces in Substance Abuse Prevention

COGNITION AND LANGUAGE
A Series in Psycholinguistics • Series Editor: R. W. RIEBER

Psychoenvironmental Forces in Substance Abuse Prevention

Lorand B. Szalay and
Jean Bryson Strohl
Institute of Comparative Social and Cultural Studies, Inc.
Chevy Chase, Maryland

and

Kathleen T. Doherty
Gettysburg College
Gettysburg, Pennsylvania

Kluwer Academic / Plenum Publishers
New York, Boston, Dordrecht, London, Moscow

Library of Congress Cataloging-in-Publication Data

Szalay, Lorand B.
    Psychoenvironmental forces in substance abuse prevention /
Lorand B. Szalay and Jean Bryson Strohl and Kathleen T. Doherty.
      p. cm. -- (Cognition and language)
    Includes bibliographical references and index.
    ISBN 0-306-45963-9
    1. Substance abuse--Psychological aspects. 2. Students--Substance
use--Psychological aspects. 3. Substance abuse--Prevention. 4.
Social perception. I. Strohl, Jean Bryson. II. Doherty, Kathleen T.
III. Title. IV. Series.
    HV4998 .S93 1999
    362.29'17--dc21
                                                          99-17262
                                                              CIP

ISBN: 0-306-45963-9

© 1999 Kluwer Academic / Plenum Publishers
233 Spring Street, New York, N.Y. 10013

10 9 8 7 6 5 4 3 2 1

Printed in the United States of America

Preface

The three major causes of death in the US are all drug related . . . If we could reduce substance abuse, we could save lives, save money and enjoy a better and less expensive health care system. . . . The answer to recent increases in teen drug use is renewed prevention efforts that have at their core a no-use message; such programs cut drug use in half in the 1980s.

——Joseph Califano, President
Center on Addiction and Substance Abuse, Columbia University

Is Drug Prevention Possible?

In a world alarmed and bewildered by the pandemic growth and devastation caused by drug abuse, drug prevention is certainly an appealing idea. Yet, as attractive as it is, there is much professional skepticism and little evidence that drug prevention works, or that it is realistically feasible. If one can view drug abuse as unpredictable and determined by the substance chosen, and that the person is outside of the equation, it is no wonder that prevention has been called a pipe dream.

The investigations discussed in this volume have been built on the premise that systematic prevention focused on the human factor is a viable and realistic option. What it requires is to refocus attention and resources on the people who are making the choice to use drugs or to reject them.

A New Approach

Our research, conducted with 30,000 college students and a diversity of elementary and middle schools nationwide, has produced massive new findings that support prevention as a realistic possibility. It also offers new and effective tools to pursue prevention systematically, solidly based on research findings. The work was conducted under the sponsorship of the National Institute of Drug Abuse, the U.S. Department of Education, and the National Institute of Juvenile Justice, and in cooperation with over 60 schools since the late 1980s.

A Window on Internal Dispositions

Based on an advanced, computer-assisted method of noninvasive imaging and mapping, our research is producing new insights into internal and external influences previously beyond the reach of empirical assessment. This technology offers insights into behavioral dispositions that are elusive to direct questioning partially because they involve decisions related to substance use below people's conscious awareness. These dispositions and their influences are at the center of our presentations throughout this volume.

Prevention Built on Research

The strategy of systematic prevention builds on the new research findings and their natural relationship:

- Substance abuse is promoted by internal dispositions, dominant perceptions, attitudes, and environmental influences that are identifiable.
- These dispositions, which vary from person to person and from group to group, are identified through comparative imaging and mapping.
- A systematic targeting of programs on the dominant dispositions and influences is the key to successful prevention.

The dominant psychological dispositions revealed by comparative imaging can work in two opposing directions. Certain dispositions support substance abuse: The tendency to ignore the consequences, harms, and risks associated with alcohol or other drugs, or the preoccupation with pleasure, joy, and instant gratification form aggregate propensities for use, identified as *vulnerabilities*. The opposing trends in perceptions and attitudes, such as concern with harms and risks and the desire to maintain control over one's life and future, reveal propensities that build *resistance*.

We have organized the book into six parts. Each part addresses a different aspect of measuring psychological and environmental factors relevant to substance abuse and its prevention.

The Assessment of Internal Dispositions through Comparative Imaging (Part I)

The reconstruction of the images of drug users and nonusers offers previously un-suspected opportunities to identify perceptions and attitudes that are the sources of their differences in behavior. The importance of these insights into factors leading to substance abuse will be particularly appreciated by those familiar with contemporary practices based mostly on conflicting, unverifiable assumptions. Differences in images in the domains of Alcohol and Drugs were found to be the most dominant sources of perceptual and attitudinal dispositions shaping the students' behavior related to the use of harmful substances. These images reflect remarkably similar perceptual and motivational dispositions for heavy users, and reflect contrasting dispositions for nonusers. Comparisons of their dominant perceptions and attitudes reveal characteristic differences of high consistency. The next most influential domain, Entertainment and Friends, is presented and discussed. Four additional domains are analyzed: Self, Family, Problems, and Fears, along a rank order of decreasing influences. The findings consistently reveal analogous differences in images and domains reflecting two different worlds, two different systems of representation and cognitive organization.

The Assessment of Vulnerability / Resistance through Cognitive Mapping (Part II)

The dominant perceptions and motivations in the images used in the investigations revealed contrasting trends of vulnerabilities and resistance; that is, contrasting propensities to use or not use harmful substances. These dispositions can be identified based on imaging technology. The Vulnerability/Resistance scores, measured independently from the self-reported use of particular substances, as well as other categories of behavior, were found to be accurate indicators of usage behavior. Their predictive accuracy increased with the frequency of substance use reported.

Tracing the Effects of Background and Lifestyle on the Use of Harmful Substances (Part III)

With their accuracy tested on large populations of frequent users and of non-users, the Vulnerability/Resistance measures are valid indicators revealing the effects of various lifestyles ranging from school achievement and skipping classes to sports participation and attendance at religious services. Similarly, they provide information on how sociodemographic background, age, gender, and ethnicity affect propensities for substance use. Of similar importance to substance abuse prevention, the vulnerability/resistance measures have proven to be sensitive measures of environmental influences on increasing or decreasing propensities for using harmful substances.

Tracing Environmental Influences, Cultural and Social (Part IV)

Based on broadly tested applications gauging the effects of high-use and low-use college environments on the propensity to use harmful substances, the results demonstrated new and sensitive capabilities. These capabilities measure culture change, cultural distance, and acculturation, that is, the influence of particularly subtle but elusive change processes relevant to the spread of substance abuse. A culturally relevant application developed and extensively used is illustrated through the experiences of the Center for the Improvement of Child Caring headed by Kerby Alvy. He has been using the AGA methodology in cultural training since the late 1970s.

Applications: Diagnostics, Program Planning, and Evaluation (Part V)

The findings and the research technologies support three main applications, each important individually, but particularly effective in combination. The first is the diagnostic use of imaging and cognitive mapping to identify dominant psychological dispositions, including their aggregates indicating vulnerabilities or resistance. Secondly, the new technologies offer research-based information for developing and targeting programs on the psychological dispositions characteristic of particular populations. Finally, they offer feedback and program evaluation useful to assess impact in the psychological dimension critical to program success.

The Latest Developments and Future Perspectives (Part VI)

A brief review is offered of some of the best known approaches in the field of substance abuse prevention. Unfortunately, little is known about their actual success. The methods of imaging and mapping affect most closely recent developments in the cognitive sciences and neurosciences. In cognitive psychology, the latest results on implicit cognitions and representations are of direct relevance. From neurobiology, the role of neural images, their integrated functioning as a system of neural representations, and the key parameters of this system as described by Antonio Damasio are of direct relevance. They provide the background for placing the present results and their potential applications in broad perspective.

Contents

Contents

Acknowledgments

The Associative Group Analysis methodology for measuring psychological dispositions has a long history that spans thirty years of research and collaboration with colleagues in many disciplines. We would like to acknowledge the federal agencies which sponsored much of the research reported here, including the National Institute on Drug Abuse, the Department of Education (especially FIPSE, the Fund for Improvement of Postsecondary Education), and the Office of Juvenile Justice and Delinquency Prevention. Although there are far too many individuals to be mentioned by name, we would like to extend our personal gratitude to Dr. Andres Inn, a psychometrician, who was instrumental in developing the extensive software system that made indepth data analysis of 30,000 students possible; to Shelly Vilov who for almost ten years worked closely with the college prevention community throughout the data collection, training, and evaluation process; to Dr. Joel Aronson, whose professional and editorial input strengthened the bridge-building between researchers and practitioners; to Audrey Maisel for her continued enthusiasm and untiring efforts in analysis, editing, and assembly of the manuscript; and to our families without whose sustaining support we would not have had the energy to carry this work out into the world to practical applications.

Introduction

Tracing Dispositions Affecting the Use of Harmful Substances

The new insights offered in this volume—the assessment of internal dispositions that shape people's decisions without their awareness the capability to trace changes and influences previously beyond the reach of empirical assessment—come from an advanced technology called Associative Group Analysis (AGA). This technology is used to reconstruct people's images and to map their internal world. When the respondents give their spontaneous reactions to strategically selected themes (or pictures), they are unaware of the clues they are offering about the dominant perceptions, attitudes, and implicit cognitions that guide their behavior. Use of this technology in domestic and overseas applications related to culture and communication, education, and mental health illustrates certain characteristics of this assessment relevant to the identification of behavioral dispositions leading to substance abuse.

Changes Shown by the Surveys of the University of Michigan

For more than 20 years, the Institute for Social Research (ISR) at the University of Michigan has been monitoring marijuana use among high school seniors nationwide, and it is widely considered the most authoritative research on adolescent behavior and attitudes regarding drug use. An ISR publication in the *Journal of Health and Social Behavior* noted a downturn in marijuana use (Bachman, Johnston, O'Malley, & Humphrey, 1988). The authors, seeking factors which might explain the decline, identified two main factors: the shift toward more "conservative," less "trouble-prone" behavior on the part of young people and a shift in their perception toward greater "harmfulness."

More recently, their report has shown a sharp increase in marijuana and other drug use over the past few years, more than doubling since 1992 (Johnston,

O'Malley, & Bachman, 1996). The authors observed a downward shift in the number of young people who said they perceived drugs as dangerous as an important part of the explanation of the subsequent change in behavior. The ISR survey was designed to reflect current behavior and shifts in behavior over time.

The results of the longitudinal ISR surveys are of considerable interest. They show an inverse relationship between an important perception and the resulting behavior: the students' disposition to perceive drugs as harmful, and the students' behavior, that is, their use of drugs. The ISR results show that an increasing tendency to perceive drugs as harmful resulted in a decreasing frequency of use. In turn, a decrease in perceived harmfulness was accompanied by an increase in the frequency of use. The surveys, repeated periodically, have a broad nationwide foundation on representative samples. The relationship between perceived harm and substance abuse is consistent and significant.

Comparable Findings from Comparative Imaging

The findings presented throughout this volume illustrate that the students' choices to use or not to use harmful substances are intimately related to perceived harm, as well as to a host of other perceptual and attitudinal trends. Our extensive research offers timely and useful knowledge of perceptual and attitudinal dispositions that shape people's decisions and behavior with regard to the use of harmful substances. It provides a way to support prevention by promoting the realization that the critical choice to use drugs comes from people's behavioral dispositions, shaped by similarly invisible environmental influences.

Our results show clearly that substance use has its foundation in psychological dispositions, which lead some people to use drugs and others to remain resistant. From the angle of successful prevention, it is of critical importance that the dispositions promoting the use of harmful substances are identifiable. Once these dispositions are identified, they can be addressed in programs and activities that challenge the dispositions toward substance use and reinforce the dispositions that support resistance to substance abuse. This new system of prevention focuses on existing psychological dispositions in order to address the problem of substance abuse before it has actually developed. It goes to the hidden underlying causes and main contributing factors, and allows us to work with a genuine sense of prevention.

With the methodology described in this volume, the psychological factors mediating drug involvement, such as the perception that drugs are dangerous, can be investigated and quantified in a rigorous way. Now we can go well beyond the general association made by the ISR between perceived harmfulness and drug involvement. We can assess the *degree* of perceived harm felt by people and the consequences they expect from engaging in drug use. At last, we have a handle on how people are predisposed to recognize the nature and consequences of drugs *before* they get involved. The information obtained about the relevant psychological dispositions can be used to develop a variety of fresh prevention activities and better focus those we already have. For example, drug information curricula can be designed for specific age groups, cultural groups, and living conditions.

As it turns out, the degree of danger people associate with drugs is an important factor regarding whether they will get involved with them, but it is not the only factor and none of them operate in a void. As we describe, our research shows conclusively that whether an individual will engage in substance abuse depends on the net push–pull of several kinds of psychological dispositions within the individual *and* aspects of the environment in which the individual operates. It is the interaction between the cluster of dispositions, which we can measure, and the cluster of relevant environmental factors, which we also can measure, that is reflected in the Vulnerability score introduced in this volume.

EARLY WORK ON IMAGES, MEANINGS, AND CULTURAL DIFFERENCES

The early development of the techniques for comparative imaging and cognitive mapping began in the 1960s as an outgrowth of Lorand Szalay's studies with psychologist Charles Osgood. Osgood's Semantic Differential is well known as an instrument for measuring the subjective meaning from its rating scales. The AGA method was the result of the authors' interest in assessing people's subjective worlds more comprehensively and in greater depth. As described in greater detail in the appendix, the AGA strategy is to identify and to reconstruct key images and then to map their relation to other images in the system of cognitive–semantic representations. Comparison and contrast between groups are integral to this approach, that is, two or more cultures, males and females, or drug users and nonusers. Subjective meanings and images fall into the broad category of *psychological dispositions,* which Campbell (1963) defined as also including perceptions, attitudes, and beliefs.

Improving Communication between People of Different Cultural Backgrounds

We originally applied comparative imaging and mapping to the in-depth comparative study of cultures, their subjective worlds built on their systems of cognitive–semantic representations. We developed "communication lexica" and other materials for use in cultural training to enhance mutual understanding of members of foreign cultures by considering their psychological dispositions, images, meanings, and characteristic frames of reference. We also developed a series of communication lexica to support language instruction and cross-cultural communication and to bridge differences between the U.S. frame of reference and the frames of reference of specific overseas cultures.

The resource materials for improving cross-cultural communication and understanding included Hispanic (Mexico, Colombia), Middle Eastern (Jordan, Iran), and Far Eastern (China, Korea) cultures. The underlying research for most of these applications involved comparisons of American students with students in the foreign cultures. In some instances, intracultural comparisons revealed differences in the cultural perspectives, such as the ones found among Mexican farmers, students, and workers. That information was disseminated through commercial publishers, as well as through the ERIC system, and became a standard stock-in-trade for language instruction oriented toward increasing cultural sensitivity and effective communication with members of foreign cultures.

The Iranian–American communication lexicon is a characteristic prototype in this cross-cultural series. The U.S. Department of Education Language and Area Studies Program funded the project at the time when the Shah of Iran was in full power and then President Carter characterized Iran as a showcase of democratic development and stability. The completion of the data collection and analysis happened to coincide with the collapse of the Shah's regime. How poorly based our nation's judgment was of the Iranian democracy became evident through the events that occurred just at the time our volume was published.

Based on our contrastive analysis of American and Iranian perceptions and attitudes, our in-depth psychological assessment showed the heavy influence of ideology and religious fanaticism on the Iranian public. This was a critical factor that was not evident in the conventional surveys conducted by the United States Information Agency (USIA) with Iranian emigres in the United States, which suggested that Iran was secularized and oriented toward Western democracy. Our findings showed that the Iranian way of political thinking was permeated by religious contexts, that the USIA conclusions about secularized political thinking were erroneous, and that in the Iranian frame of reference, politics and religion were still closely intertwined during the Shah's regime. Our assessment was on target and historical events confirmed our conclusions.

Cultural Factors in Minority Mental Health

In the 1970s and 1980s, most of our work conducted within the context of American society involved cultural factors in domestic problems of minorities (African-Americans and Hispanic-Americans). The National Institute of Mental Health (NIMH) sponsored our comparative studies of Hispanic-Americans from different parts of the United States (Mexican-Americans, Puerto Ricans, and Cubans). The concern was that Hispanic-Americans did not utilize the services of mental health facilities to the same extent as the American mainstream. It was obvious that this underutilization was not a result of a lesser need; in addition to common mental health problems, there were also the stresses of poverty and cultural change. Their lack of reliance on these services was generally attributed to cultural factors, but what these cultural factors were and what to do about them remained a puzzle.

Our in-depth cultural analysis using the AGA imaging and mapping technology included a large number of key themes for which Americans and Hispanic-Americans had different meanings. In particular, we found fundamental differences between the two groups regarding the concepts of mental health and mental illness. For Hispanic-Americans, "mental health" had practically no meaning, but "mental illness" was seen as strongly negative: it was incurable, a stigma on the family, a punishment of God, and a sin. These and other such beliefs prevented Hispanic-Americans from taking advantage of the mental health services, even though they were free and readily available.

One of our primary recommendations to mental health professionals was to avoid labels which could be misleading for Hispanic-Americans. Speaking of mental health when it did not mean anything positive to them or speaking of mental illness when it meant only something incurable and hopeless would not appeal to them. We suggested using other labels, such as "community services," "educational services," or "health services," which for Hispanic-Americans were positive, meaningful, and attractive and did not elicit negative reactions. Unfortunately these recommendations were not always welcomed by mainstream mental health professionals. Time has shown that changing certain critical labels in the field of mental health services has helped to enhance the use of mental health services by Hispanics-Americans

Stresses of Cultural Adaptation Increase Risk of Substance Abuse

Another application of the imaging and mapping technology was dealing with some of the problems of Puerto Rican acculturation. In the early 1980s, statistics showed that Puerto Ricans living in rural Puerto Rico had a very low rate of substance abuse—about one-tenth of the average rate among mainstream Americans for crack and other hard drugs. However, after moving to the large Eastern cities of the United States, their substance abuse increased dramatically. In the Bronx and in other cities, their use of drugs became ten times *heavier* than the use by the surrounding Americans.

Our studies of several hundred Puerto Ricans—those who never came to the United States and those who moved to the United States and stayed for various lengths of time—provided a solid framework for a systematic assessment of changes related to migration to the United States. Comparison of Puerto Ricans both in and out of the United States with Anglo-Americans of similar age and living conditions

gave us a means of measuring shifts from the original Puerto Rican cultural perceptions and attitudes to American cultural perceptions and attitudes.

Our comparisons showed that Puerto Ricans who moved to the United States
fell into two subcategories: those who did make systematic adaptation to American cultural values and norms, and those for whom this process of acculturation
had been suspended and delayed. We found that Puerto Ricans who more readily
adopted American cultural perceptions and attitudes had developed coping mechanisms which made them resistant to substance abuse and helped them remain
drug free. On the other hand, Puerto Ricans who moved to the United States and
failed to adapt also failed to develop such protective mechanisms although they
were losing their native cultural anchors. This was the group that became highly
susceptible to substance abuse.

Our identification of these differences enabled us to address the simplistic
generalization that Puerto Rican acculturation compellingly leads to the development of vulnerability and eventually to substance abuse. Puerto Ricans who do
adopt American cultural values in shifting their own cultural perspectives are acquiring protective factors that can shield them from increased risk of substance
abuse. This topic is explored in greater depth and detail in chapter 11.

Mapping the Psychological and Environmental Forces of Change

Our work with acculturation showed that the imaging and mapping process could
trace even the gradual adaptation to a new cultural environment. Perhaps the single most important feature of this new approach is that it encompasses both *psychological forces* related to culture, personal belief systems, and attitudes, and
environmental forces, such as the social climate and peer influences that work in
various ways to change and support the individual. In the drug context we can say
that the measurement of changes, from language learning to cultural adaptation,
have distinct and clear implications in the area of substance abuse. People who
adapt slowly to the American culture but quickly give up their own original cultural perceptions and values become increasingly vulnerable to the dangers in the
new environment in which they live. For those people, the negative social influences can produce both high vulnerability and low resistance to substance abuse.
For Puerto Ricans, or anyone else, who adapt to the new environment relatively
quickly and acquire the protective mechanisms (e.g., independence, internal locus of control) from their new environment faster than they give up their native
protective mechanisms (e.g., parental authority, external locus of control), the acculturation process is not likely to have a negative effect. If they do not give up
their native protective factors before they have picked up the new protective capacity, they can apparently withstand the stresses of change involved in the acculturation process.

Another implication of our results is that internal changes picked up by the x-ray nature of our comparative imaging approach involve psychological dispositions as they are gradually shaped by the influences of the social environment. To register these changes and to trace the interaction between dispositions and environment is a particularly challenging task because the changes are usually gradual and cannot be identified through surveys that do not tap the internal processes that occur below people's awareness. These exceptional characteristics of the AGA method explain its potential for dealing with psychological and social–environmental factors that are beyond the reach of traditional direct approaches that involve questions or scaling.

APPLYING IMAGING TO THE PROBLEM OF SUBSTANCE ABUSE

Since the late 1980s, we have used the imaging and cognitive mapping approach in drug-related research and we have developed capabilities specifically related to the special needs of evaluating treatment effects and planning drug prevention. In all of these applications, the measurement of internal changes and the assessment of social influences have been characteristic features of the analysis. Our first activities involved the evaluation of treatment programs. We found that treatment, justifiably focused on chemical dependency, can progress with various degrees of success in producing changes in the perceptions and attitudes of the people undergoing treatment. Our evaluations of several treatment projects showed clearly that changes in their dominant perceptions and attitudes are related to the capability of the treatment process to achieve the changes necessary for them to become drug free.

With prevention, the focus must be on reaching people before chemical dependency develops and we must focus on factors that contribute to vulnerability and lead to experimentation with harmful substances. Our research has shown that these possibilities exist. Once dominant contributing factors are clearly identified, we can design methods, plan activities, and target programs in such a way that they take these key factors into account, and then we can monitor progress in terms of those same factors. The program has to start by identifying the dominant perceptual and attitudinal dispositions characteristic of specific groups, and once they have been identified, it needs to focus on those that emerge as most influential in promoting vulnerability or reducing resistance in the specific population at hand.

The results from our imaging and mapping studies showed that substance use is a behavior promoted and shaped by powerful psychological dispositions that influence people's choices mostly without their conscious awareness. Choices to use or not to use are influenced by attitudes, values, belief systems, goals, and experiences that can be measured via AGA. We showed, furthermore, that substance use is also promoted and shaped by environmental influences about that people are unaware and that are generally beyond the reach of conventional assessment. In the following chapters, we demonstrate in detail that users and nonusers differ in identifiable ways in their attitudes and perceptions regarding not only alcohol and drugs but also other various domains of life, such as social relationships and what they view as entertainment, and that these dispositional differences clearly affect the differences in their behavior.

PREVENTION—THE PROBLEM BEHIND THE PROBLEM OF SUBSTANCE ABUSE

In treatment, the focus of attention is on helping the client become free of his or her dependence on a particular substance. In prevention, with its primary focus on protecting young people who are not addicts, the central requirement is to find effective ways to help them avoid experimentation or involvement with alcohol and other drugs. We cannot adequately understand use unless we understand the psychological dispositions behind it. Our research supports positive and promising conclusions that alcohol and drug abuse prevention is a realistic and feasible goal, granted that its basic requirements are recognized and effectively pursued. Furthermore, the results suggest alternative solutions that take into consideration the dominant characteristics of particular populations and of environmental conditions.

Requirements for Effective Prevention in Light of Findings

What differentiates scientific prevention from a fishing expedition is that it is systematically designed to address the causes of the problem it was designed to prevent. Scientific prevention is a systematic activity designed to cope with those main contributing factors responsible for the development of the problem it aims to avoid. This is true of all prevention efforts, ranging from the prevention of a particular disease, to forest fires, to substance abuse.

It is true that the prevention of substance abuse represents a particularly complex and difficult task. In certain ways addiction is a disease, but there are some important differences that cannot be ignored. With common diseases caused by germs and viruses, once the causative agent has been identified, it has been relatively straightforward to find a way to control it and to develop effective methods of prevention. But with substance abuse, there are no germs or viruses; the source of the problem is deeper and it involves psychological and environmental factors in addition to the biochemical dimension of causation and consequences. Until now, there had been limited ability to identify and address these hidden factors and that has delayed progress in proactive prevention.

This means that effective protection of students from involvement with harmful substances depends on valid information about the psychological and environmental forces that shape their decisions to use or not to use harmful substances. The psychological dispositions that shape such decisions have been beyond the reach of empirical assessment, but now we can identify them clearly through the assessment technology of cognitive mapping. This new knowledge bears directly on the question of causation. It tells us the extent to which individual students or particular social cohorts have the psychological propensity to use harmful substances, that is, to what extent they tend to be vulnerable or resistant to substance abuse. The assessment shows the foundation of the general vulnerability or resistance in terms of dominant perceptions and attitudes and in terms of dominant psychological dispositions.

Information on the dominant perceptual and attitudinal dispositions reveals the dominant forces shaping vulnerability and resistance. Their clear identification makes it possible to develop prevention programs systematically targeted on the key variables that make the difference. We expect that this information will open new vistas on substance abuse prevention.

Debunking Old Myths and Correcting Fallacies That Have Been Barriers to Progress

The studies of perceptual and attitudinal dispositions described in this volume have helped to identify several fallacious assumptions and myths about substance abuse. They explain why the field of prevention, rich in programs and activities, has failed to achieve a major breakthrough.

"Addiction is Random and Unpredictable." Random events cannot be prevented. To view substance abuse as an unpredictable random event promotes skepticism about prevention as a realistic objective. Our results demonstrate that there are clearly identifiable behavioral dispositions shaping substance abuse.

"Knowing the Nature of the Chemical Substance is the Key." The disastrous effects of drugs explain why people interested in prevention tend to focus on the particular harmful substances and their observable dramatic effects. Yet, as the following results indicate, the unseen problems behind the visible problems really represent the key to effective prevention. The findings show what these hidden forces are and how to cope with them. An understanding of psychological dispositions is indispensable for developing successful programs.

"The Illusion: There May Be a Universal Solution." The belief that there may be stock formulas or a single universal solution for prevention is a myth. It ignores the fact that people differ in their dispositions and in their vulnerabilities. Addressing and targeting their dispositions require different solutions.

"Responses to Direct Questions Represent the Reality." The assumption that program effects can be objectively assessed from answers to direct questions about the popularity of a particular program is frequently fallacious.

"Answers to Why People Use Drugs Can Be Identified Through Epidemiological Surveys on Reported Use." Another fallacious assumption is that survey data that show the increase or decrease in the level of substance abuse or the popularity of specific substances provide sufficient information to address etiological questions—for example, What are the reasons for the changes observed? As much as the identification of psychological dispositions promoting substance abuse is essential, the answers are beyond the reach of direct survey questions.

Some of these assumptions come from the field of treatment, but they are misplaced in application to prevention. Medical treatment of the addict has a long-standing history and builds on rich experiences. In comparison, drug prevention is a new field. Drug prevention became an issue only in the last few decades when the scope of substance abuse, particularly in the United States, assumed such proportions that it no longer could be seen as an isolated personal problem. Thus, prevention has developed under the influence of the original interests of treatment to reduce chemical dependency rather than finding ways to avoid it. The natural opportunities to avoid substance use become secondary or are altogether ignored.

PREVENTION REQUIRES A FUNDAMENTAL PARADIGM SHIFT

The findings do more than suggest a shift from preoccupation with alcohol and other drugs to a focus on human choices and decisions that lead to experimentation with drugs in the short or long period that precedes addiction. The shift requires looking at the problems behind the problem and examining the psychological and environmental forces at the depth necessary to be informative regarding factors that shape substance abuse. As the following findings demonstrate, the assumption that the relevant psychological factors are beyond the reach of empirical assessment is outdated in light of the information produced by the new technology of comparative imaging and cognitive mapping. The results presented in this volume help to refute the myths that have paralyzed progress in the field of prevention. They promise the knowledge needed for developing prevention programs targeting psychological factors and environmental influences shaping decisions related to the use of alcohol and other drugs.

The New Focus: Who Starts to Experiment with Drugs and Why?

Successful prevention depends to a large extent on finding out why and how students start to experiment with alcohol and other drugs. Substance abuse is not an automatic, unconditioned response to harmful substances. For those who get involved with these substances, the process usually begins with a period of early experimentation. In this period, each use involves an independent and relatively free choice. Our results show that those who do not get involved differ from those who do in certain characteristic ways. The approach we followed in our investigations is based on the assumption that decisions to use or not to use substances largely depend on people's behavioral dispositions, which are by their dominant perceptions and attitudes toward alcohol, drugs and other aspects of life.

As involvement progresses, the addictive qualities of the substance and the user's genetic predispositions can make a great deal of difference, but in the early stages there must be other explanations for continuation. In the past these latter explanations were ignored because they were beyond the reach of the analytic capabilities available. In the following chapters, we show in detail that users and nonusers differ reliably in identifiable ways and that those differences are consistent with respect to perceptions and evaluations related to alcohol and drugs, as well as to a number of social values and human problems.

The novelty and utility of this information goes far beyond the obvious conclusion that users like alcohol and that nonusers reject it. What is new and useful is the ability to reconstruct people's images—the composition of their images in their true proportion. By understanding how they are thinking and what their subjective experience has been, we can grasp what matters to one group as compared with another.

As the following chapters show, perceptions and attitudes combine to form propensities, such as vulnerability and resistance to substance abuse, and reveal aspects of the users' and nonusers' subjective worlds. When we know what matters to them and how to approach and more meaningfully communicate with them, prevention programs can become more effective by targeting variables that are likely to make the most difference in promoting desired program objectives.

Revisiting Prevention with New Tools

The ability to trace dominant psychological dispositions that promote substance abuse offers new opportunities for systematic substance abuse prevention. As the following findings demonstrate based on solid research evidence, substance abuse is not merely a chemical dependency without a history and antecedents. There are psychological dispositions which play a powerful and identifiable role in determining who will experiment with harmful substances and who will not.

The successful identification of dominant dispositions offers the opportunity to identify which psychological dispositions and environmental influences are causative or contributing factors in substance abuse. These invisible forces do exert powerful influences on people's choices and decisions to experiment with the use of harmful substances.

Diagnostic tools sensitive enough to identify the relevant behavioral dispositions and to trace their influences on behavior offer useful opportunities for successful substance abuse prevention systematically targeting variables that influence decisions related to use. Much of this new information comes from the results of comparative imaging.

TRACING PSYCHOLOGICAL DISPOSITIONS THROUGH COMPARATIVE IMAGING

Our approach to identifying the psychological dispositions that lead to substance abuse relies on an advanced technology that offers quantitative, research-based insights about variables believed to be inaccessible. Our findings are based on two fundamental assumptions. First, drug use is promoted by perceptual and attitudinal dispositions toward alcohol, drugs, and a variety of related subjects; similarly, the avoidance of drugs is supported by a contrasting set of perceptions and attitudes that support no use.

The second assumption is based on the experience that behavioral dispositions leading to drug use can be traced through comparative imaging that uses multiple-response free associations. As our extensive investigations conducted with free associations have demonstrated, they offer insights of unexpected depth and practical utility regarding the foundation of people's behavior on their internal behavioral dispositions. These insights become particularly informative as they emerge from the responses of people who are similar in background but differ in behavior in the area relevant to the research interest.

Free associations are one of oldest and least understood subjects of psychology. There are several contrasting schools that use changing terminologies, presenting a disappointingly confusing situation. To simplify the situation we are relying on a commonsense description of the procedure we are using. Additional details can be found in the technical discussion of the AGA method in the appendix. Basically, we ask the respondents to give as many responses as they can think of in 1 minute for each theme presented. The responses offer mosaic elements of their subjective images or meanings in proportionate representation.

Since the late 1960s, we have used the AGA method to identify the dominant perceptions and attitudes that differentiate members of one group from those of another. Research results have been published in numerous articles and monographs since that time. AGA does not involve asking direct questions of the respondents (although following the AGA data collection, we do use questionnaires to gather background information). The respondents, when listing their related thoughts and ideas, are spontaneous in revealing their world, unhampered by fears of expressing their beliefs and opinions. A strategic selection of words and pictures serves as the basis for reconstructing the respondents' world in select domains relevant to the research interest.

Contrasting Users and Nonusers

The analysis uses medium-sized groups of 100 to 400 people who produce from hundreds to thousands of spontaneous responses. We use analytic software to first cluster all the responses related to a specific image and then to map the groups' results in a way that sharply demonstrates their differences. The instructions used in the administration of the multiple free-response tasks, as well as the several analytic procedures used in the analysis of the responses are discussed in the appendix. Our contrastive analysis is designed to show that the images of people who behave differently (e.g., drinkers and nondrinkers) reflect differences in their perceptions and evaluations of alcohol. To the extent that this assumption is true, the comparison of their images offers us insights into those dominant perceptions and attitudes that are behind their differences in behavior.

Most of the findings presented here along our interest to identify differences in images and in the dominant perceptions and attitudes reflected by these images rely on the comparison of 400 frequent users and 400 nonusers. The groups were drawn from a composite data base of 6,212 students tested at 17 colleges at an intermediate stage of our continuing student research, which currently includes more than 57 campuses. The selection criteria for these groups were determined by the respondents' self-reported use of alcohol and various other substances. Our group of users ($n = 400$) includes both heavy alcohol users (daily or almost daily) and frequent alcohol users (1–3 times/week) who have used any illicit substance. We selected the group of nonusers ($n = 400$) from among those who indicated they never use alcohol and never use drugs. To the extent possible, we matched nonusers and users with respect to sociodemographic background factors. Most of the students were White (94% of users, 81% of nonusers) and unmarried (95% of users, 86% of nonusers). There were more males in the user group (64%) than in the nonuser group (53%). The average age of the students in both groups was 20.6 years.

The AGA uses 24 standardized stimulus words (the most productive ones from an original list of 140 words we explored in 1989) that are categorized into six "domains," each concerned with an important aspect of life. They are as follows: Self and Family, Social Institutions, Friends and Entertainment, Social

Self and Family	Social Values
ME	AUTHORITY
I AM	DISCIPLINE
FAMILY	RESPONSIBILITY
FATHER	RELIGION
Social Institutions	**Alcohol and Drugs**
SCHOOL	ALCOHOL
CAMPUS	DRUGS
SOCIETY	MARIJUANA
GOVERNMENT	DRUNK
Friends and Entertainment	**Problems**
FRIENDS	PROBLEMS
FUN	HOOKED
PARTY	SMOKING
GETTING HIGH	FEAR

FIGURE I.1. The 24 stimulus words used in the campus studies arranged by domain.

Values, Alcohol and Drugs, and Problems. The set of stimulus words is listed in Figure I.1.

Reconstruction of Mental Images That Reveal Contrasting Dispositions

We have included most of the details of how we obtained and scored the responses in the appendix. What matters here is that, over the years, we have demonstrated repeatedly that responses that occur with a higher frequency reflect more important, more influential elements than responses that occur less often. To illustrate, we will step through our analysis of the stimulus word DRUNK.

First, we tally all the responses, from users and from nonusers, to a given theme. Then, we tabulate the weighted frequencies of each response and present them in a form like Figure I.2, which we have designed to summarize a large amount of immediately useful information. Generally, the responses resolve into a dozen or so main components (alcohol, beer, liquor) and each component is made up of a number of frequently given responses, which we call *mosaic elements*.

Figure I.2 shows the main components of the mental image of DRUNK derived from both the users' (dark bars) and the nonusers' (shaded bars) responses. The bars are arranged so that they start with the highest scoring component or response cluster for the users (alcohol, beer, liquor). This reflects their most salient set of perceptions and attitudes surrounding the term DRUNK. At the bottom of the figure,

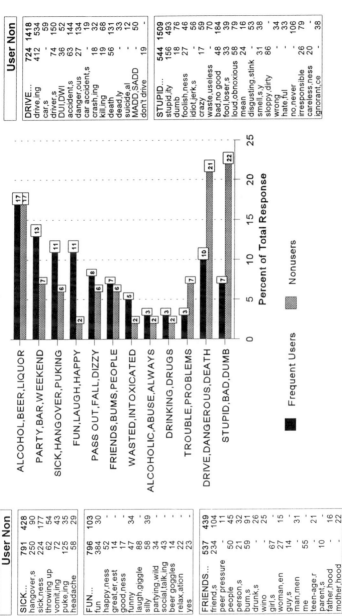

FIGURE I.2. The elements of an image: Perceptions and attitudes, of DRUNK by frequent users and nonusers of alcohol.

the last bar represents the highest scoring response cluster for the nonusers (stupid, bad, dumb). The length of each bar represents the proportion (%) of all responses that fall into that component for that group. Comparisons show similarities as well as differences in the images of the users and of the nonusers.

The lists in the boxes along both sides of the central figure provide more specific detail about the underlying content of each main component. For example, the third main component, "sick, hangover, puking" incorporates all responses to the stimulus word DRUNK that relate to the negative physical reactions of being drunk. The small box in the top left corner of the figure lists the user and nonuser responses, which were *hangover* or *hangovers; sick* or *sickness; throwing up;* and so forth. Similarly, the other boxes show detailed response scores for other components. We refer to this underlying detail as the "mosaic." Each mosaic carries a score value and, taken together, they form a surprisingly revealing picture of the subjective reaction to various ideas, concepts, and situations.

As you consider the line pairs for the several components, note that the component "fun, laugh, happy" is much more salient (i.e., has a larger proportion of the total number of responses) in the users' image of what it means to be drunk, whereas in the nonusers' image it is much less so. At this level of analysis, where the focus is on general conclusions from the user–nonuser comparisons, the 11% to 2% ratio is a rough indicator of the relative importance of fun and happiness within the image of being drunk of the users and of the nonusers.

In a similar way, we can make within-group comparisons based on the relative frequency of a response. For the users, the relative importance of the "fun, laugh, happy" component exceeds the importance of the "stupid, bad, dumb" component by a ratio of 11% to 7%, indicating that, for them, the fun and happiness aspect of being drunk outweighs the negative qualities. For the nonusers, the corresponding ratio from their responses is 2% to 22%, indicating an attitude about being drunk that incorporates negative evaluation and rejection much more than any acceptance that being drunk is fun.

We gain still more understanding from the mosaics. For instance, within the "fun, laugh, happy" component, there is a sharp contrast between users and nonusers with respect to both the scope and the nature of the responses. All 16 response mosaics of the users express distinctly positive sentiments conveying high mood and spirit. There are only 3 comparable mosaic elements from the nonusers: *fun, funny,* and *silly.* Each of those has a far lower score for nonusers than for users, and the overall number of responses for nonusers within this component is about one-eighth of that for users.

Why analyze images in such detail? Because the identification of the dominant components of perceptions and attitudes yields concise trends, it could be argued that the detailed information from the mosaics is superfluous. This might be true if our only objective was to provide information about psychological dispositions. However, our second objective is to offer practical information about the dispositions that emerge from the comparative imaging data so that they can be targeted by new prevention programs. For this application, the results of the second level of analysis are of special importance. Here, the user–nonuser differences can be seen in broader perspective within the frames of reference of the users and of nonusers. A familiarity with this background and an understanding of the dominant influences are essential for the effective use of the new information.

Trends across Themes

Behavior results from the net impact of many attitudes, beliefs, and expectations, and is never unidimensional. Our global analysis shows that virtually all of the 24 stimulus words elicit strikingly divergent sets of responses from the two student groups. We found users to be loaded with emotional ambivalence about family, friends, and self. They crave love, respect, and support and complain about pain, distrust, and problems. They are more entertainment oriented and preoccupied with having a good time, particularly at parties and at bars. At school, they focus more on campus life and social contacts. They give low priority to the importance of education and express boredom with classes. They think of using alcohol and drugs as a way to have fun and to relax, and they pay less attention to the negative health or legal consequences. Although they recognize the need for controls and limits, they also are negative toward authority and discipline. Users are extremely skeptical and cynical about society, government, and religion.

The nonusers' data present an entirely different picture. They are strongly oriented toward positive personal qualities, such as being honest, responsible, and good, and these are important both for their own self-images and for their images of family and of friends. Nonusers are more concerned than users with intimacy in relationships. Caring, trust, love, sharing, listening, and talking are important elements in their lives. Nonusers express a more positive view of social institutions than do users. For nonusers, parties and having fun are tradition oriented and family oriented. They express strong disapproval of getting drunk and using drugs based on their concern with the human and social consequences.

We began this demonstration with the main components of our analysis because they provide an immediate outline of the composition of the mental image. However, the logical sequence of analysis really begins with the specifics represented by the mosaic elements, which lead to the identification of the components. The mosaics of the images provide a useful resource for addressing the dominant psychological dispositions that offer the most leverage and the most potential to change existing dispositions into desired directions.

The perceptual and attitudinal components of the mental images offer insights into dispositions that are the keys to differences observed in the behavior of the groups compared. This information is helpful in identifying the sources of differences in choice making with regard to experimentation with harmful substances.

The reconstruction of psychological dispositions behind alcohol and other drug use and nonuse has produced findings consistent with common sense experience; nonetheless, the real value of this approach lies in its solid quantitative foundation and its diagnostic relevance. The chapters in Part I will carry the contrastive analysis forward. The results emerging across themes and domains are informative in promoting the recognition that substance abuse has its foundation in a diversity of images and their interrelationship within the broad system of representation.

Part I

The Assessment of Internal Dispositions
through Comparative Imaging

Alcohol, Drugs: Images That Help to Identify Sources of Differences between Use and Non-Use

We have just illustrated how imaging can be used to identify dominant perceptions and attitudes at the source of differences between use and no use. Next we apply the same approach to trace analogous differences in perceptions and in attitudes revealed by comparing users and nonusers in the domain of alcohol and drugs. It is interesting to see how this strategy, based on the comparison of the images of users and those of nonusers, works in tracing hidden behavioral dispositions that are at the foundation of behavior. Because the domain of Alcohol and Drugs emerged as the most prominent, the trends observed across this domain are of special interest.

Using the image of DRUNK as an example, we found clear and consistent differences in responses between the group of users and the group of nonusers. At the same time, the members in each group showed a high level of consistency. That is, respondents with similar behavior revealed similar psychological dispositions in their responses to the stimulus word DRUNK.

Based on the image of DRUNK, we found that users have a strong tendency to view being drunk as an appealing state and a source of fun and joy, whereas the nonusers view it as an objectionable state replete with harm and dangers. It is naturally questionable how far we may go to draw conclusions from a single image. Therefore, in this chapter we extend our analysis to include two alcohol images and two drug-related images.

To what extent are the images derived from the four stimuli different for students with different alcohol and drug behavior and to what extent are they similar for students with the same behavior? We examine the images of DRUNK and ALCOHOL for data regarding psychological dispositions related to alcohol use by users and nonusers, and we review the images of MARIJUANA and DRUGS to offer comparable insights on drug-related themes.

IMAGES OF ALCOHOL AND DRINKING

Figure 1.1 is the same image of DRUNK we used in the last chapter and Figure 1.2 shows comparable information for the image of ALCOHOL. We should point out that when the AGA is administered, the 24 primary stimulus words are randomly presented to the participants so that the results for each concept are independent of the others. By comparing the two images, we can see how general trends and observations emerge.

Being Drunk Has a Positive Appeal to Users

As can be seen in Figure 1.1, the users focused on the choices of alcoholic beverages (*beer, wine, liquor*), particularly hard liquor, that may lead to drunkenness. They described physical effects of excessive alcohol consumption (*stumbling, pass out, wasted, hangover*), suggestive of more personal experience than is evident in the nonusers' perceptions. The users focuses on positive feelings of enjoyment (*fun, laughter, happy*) and on the social aspects of drinking (*parties, bars, dancing*). They also thought of *sex* in relation to being drunk. Some identified themselves (*me*) as drunk. An ambivalence was exhibited in their references to *problems, stupidity, and fighting* as well as to the euphoric effects. Compared to nonusers, they showed strikingly little concern with alcohol-related accidents and possible death.

The nonusers expressed strong disapproval of getting drunk as *stupid, bad, irresponsible* and *disgusting*. Although users and nonusers placed about equal attention on alcoholic beverages, nonusers strongly anticipated the physical dangers involved (*driving, dangerous, death, accidents*). The nonusers appeared to be concerned with the loss of control inherent in getting drunk. Although they did not refer to themselves as drunk, the nonusers showed concern about the drinking habits of other people, including some *family* members and *friends*. However, the people that came most to mind for nonusers were *bums* and *winos* whereas users are more likely to think of friends.

Alcohol as a Pathway to Pleasure or Pain

The users' image of ALCOHOL is dominated by specific varieties of alcohol, beer, and hard liquor. The attention given to specific types appears to be proportionate to their popularity in the college student population. They think of parties and bars as favorite places where they drink and socialize. Users have a strong tendency to

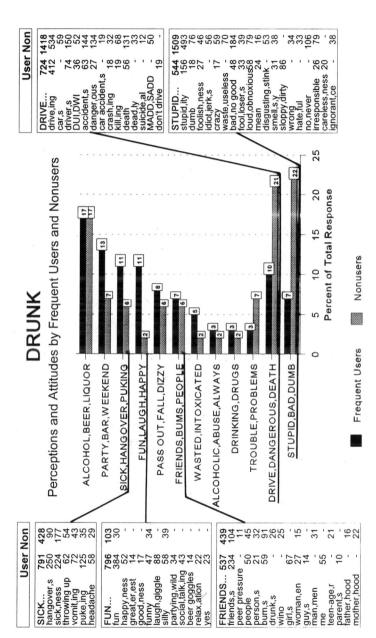

FIGURE 1.1. The image of DRUNK for users and nonusers.

view alcohol in predominantly positive terms, and to identify it as an important source of fun, enjoyment, and relaxation. A distinct element in this process is opportunity for sex and social connections. This strong orientation toward entertainment helps to explain users' interest in alcohol.

The nonusers' image of ALCOHOL reflects contrasting perspectives and evaluations. The most salient group of nonuser reactions suggests rejection and disapproval (*bad, stupid, smell*). The main reasons behind this pervasive negative attitude toward alcohol are evident: Alcohol is perceived by the nonusers as *unhealthy* and *dangerous,* leading to *car accidents* and even *death.* Also, they see ALCOHOL much more as a *drug* and relate it less to friends and relatives than to people with various human *problems.* For them, alcohol use is closely linked to *abuse* and *addiction.* They see it as an illegal, harmful substance and as a source of major personal and social problems.

Perhaps the most striking result of the comparison is that the two different themes (DRUNK and ALCOHOL) relate to remarkably similar behavioral dispositions for each of the two subgroups. Whether they respond to the image of ALCOHOL or to that of a DRUNK person, users tend to think of beer and hard liquor, parties and bars, fun and happiness, entertainment, social events, sex, and so forth. Nonusers' predominant reactions are expressions of highly critical attitudes based on aesthetic, moral, and social considerations, and concerns about harmful consequences, bodily harm, addiction, illegality, and traffic accidents. Within both sets of data, the differences between users and nonusers are large and consistent.

The mosaics enrich the detail of the similarities and differences in the perceptual and attitudinal elements of the images of DRUNK and ALCOHOL. In the mosaic elements surrounding the bar graphs in Figures 1.1 and 1.2, we can see that the frequencies of the specific responses:

- *Are quite consistent across images*—For example, the user/nonuser ratio for the component "fun" is 7.7 to 1 for the stimulus DRUNK and 7.6 to 1 for the stimulus ALCOHOL.
- *"Make sense" across images*—Users associate "bad, stupid" with DRUNK about four times as much as they associate those negatives with ALCOHOL by itself; nonusers also are more critical of DRUNK than they are of ALCOHOL.

Although we have explored just two of the images from the domain of Alcohol and Drugs, the results suggest that, at least within this domain, the choice of the specific image makes little difference. Whether using DRUNK or ALCOHOL, the perceptual and attitudinal dispositions we have identified through comparative imaging based on sizable samples are consistently similar within the group of users and within the group of nonusers.

Some of our comparative research has included a group of occasional drinkers, and their results offer some additional insights into self-protective factors. As might be expected, the results showes that occasional drinkers fall between the users and the nonusers in their perceptions of alcohol use. They are attracted by the social

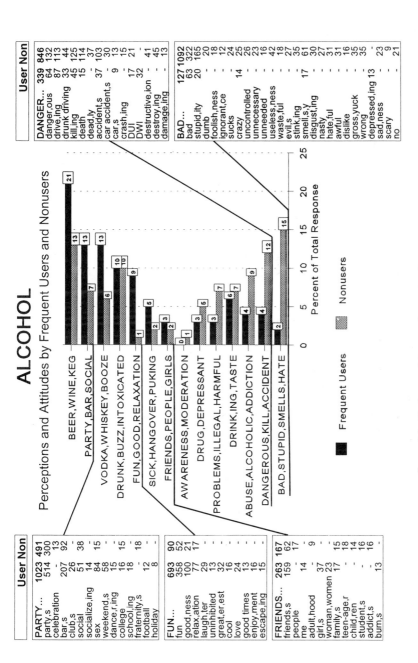

FIGURE 1.2. The image of ALCOHOL for users and nonusers.

settings and the fun/enjoyment, but at the same time they show awareness of the dangers and the need for moderation: drinking is okay, getting drunk is not.

IMAGES OF DRUGS

In order to add detail to the picture of the differences between the perceptions and psychological dispositions of users and of nonusers, we review results derived from two drug-related images: MARIJUANA and DRUGS. The users' and the nonusers' subjective image of MARIJUANA is presented in Figure 1.3 and their subjective image of DRUGS is shown in Figure 1.4.

Is Marijuana Perceived as a Harmful Drug?

The users' familiarity with marijuana is evident in their knowledge of slang terms (*pot, weed, ganja*). They focus on the process and paraphernalia of *smoking* (*bong, bowl, pipe*) and show particular interest in marijuana's mind-altering effects (*high, stoned, euphoria*). In contrast to nonusers, they do not tend to connect marijuana with alcohol or other drugs. Users view MARIJUANA positively as a source of *relaxation, fun, good times,* and *laughter,* and they expect to find it at *parties* and with their *friends.* The main thing that sets the users apart from the nonusers is their positive attitude toward MARIJUANA and their lack of concern with its potential harm. The fact that they connect marijuana with pleasant experiences and that they see little risk in its use adds to their vulnerability to substance abuse.

Nonusers have a negative image of MARIJUANA, categorically rejecting it as *bad, stupid,* and *wrong.* Furthermore, they see its use is *dangerous* with potentially fatal consequences (*death, killing*). Unlike the users, nonusers consider marijuana to be *addictive* and *habit-forming.* Nonusers clearly define MARIJUANA as a *drug.* They do not show the diverse vocabulary or personal knowledge revealed by the users. The *illegality* of marijuana also weighs heavy on the minds of the nonusers. They do not share the users' expectation of finding marijuana at parties or its acceptance among their friends. In general, they focus on the personal and social harm that can result from using marijuana and have almost nothing positive to say about it. The strong disapproval and perceived harm represent protective factors against use, creating strong psychological resistance among nonusers.

Drugs as a Source of Fun and Social Connection

Within their image of DRUGS, users think of a diversity of substances: *marijuana, cocaine, heroin, acid, mushrooms,* and *ecstasy. Marijuana* appears to be the most popular drug of choice. While they do think of *getting high, stoned* and *escaping,*

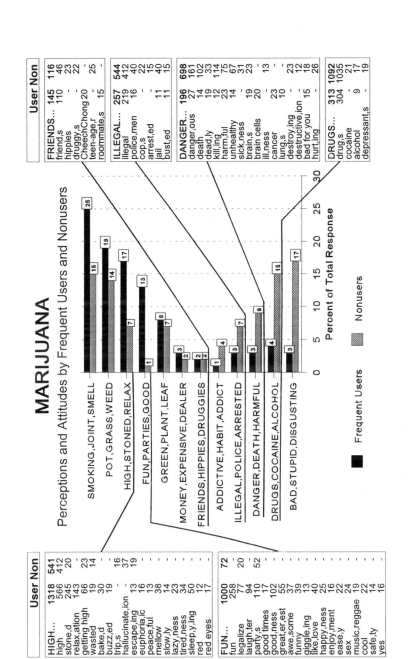

FIGURE 1.3. The image of MARIJUANA for users and nonusers.

it is not with the same intensity as was noted in the image of MARIJUANA. Compared to marijuana, users are also more inclined to view DRUGS as *bad,* which may help explain why they do not tend to link marijuana to other drugs. They are not nearly as disapproving as the nonusers. The users see DRUGS as a source of *fun* and social connection (*parties, friends*). In contrast to nonusers, users show a great deal of interest in *marijuana* and a number of other specific drugs. The largest contrasts with nonusers are the users' perception of drugs as fun and good and as a means of getting high in social settings.

The nonusers view drugs as socially unacceptable (*bad, stupid, wrong*). They also judge drug use as *stupid, crazy, disgusting,* and *irresponsible.* Drugs are viewed as *dangerous, harmful,* and *deadly;* they believe that drugs *kill.* They acknowledge the *addictive* nature of drugs but pay little attention to their euphoric effects. Compared to users, the nonusers are more aware of the legal consequences of illicit drug use and the drug trade. However, drugs are also recognized for their medicinal value for the *sick* and in *hospitals.* Many think of *alcohol* in the context of drugs. For nonusers, drugs do not serve the social function that they do for the users.

The images of DRUGS and MARIJUANA have a high degree of within-group similarity. When the two groups are compared, they reflect the same type of differences on both of these images. When we examine these themes, together, we see that users respond with more specific harmful substances, from alcohol to cocaine. In both contexts, they think very much of fun, sex, and various types of entertainment, and they think of being with people, especially friends. In contrast, nonusers think more about people who are harmed by the substance: *junkies, druggies, users, bums,* and *teenagers* and *children.* They reflect intense awareness of *harm, danger, killing, death, destruction,* and other possible consequences and of the general danger of addiction. They express strong condemnation and rejection (*bad, stupid*) as well as moral reservations (*wrong, evil*).

As will be true consistently, the content and weight of the specific responses provides the rich detail underlying the different perspectives. Much of that information is relevant to the more effective targeting of prevention programs to specific behavioral dispositions and to program planning more generally.

USER VERSUS NONUSER DISPOSITIONS ACROSS THE DOMAIN
OF ALCOHOL AND DRUGS

The findings across the four images (Figures 1.1 to 1.4) are clear, have a high degree of internal consistency, and provide a good basis for focusing on some of the more global aspects of the data regarding the psychological dispositions, perceptions, and attitudinal trends of users and of nonusers.

The images of DRUNK, ALCOHOL, MARIJUANA, and DRUGS show a remarkably high degree of similarity for users and for nonusers, respectively. For the users, the

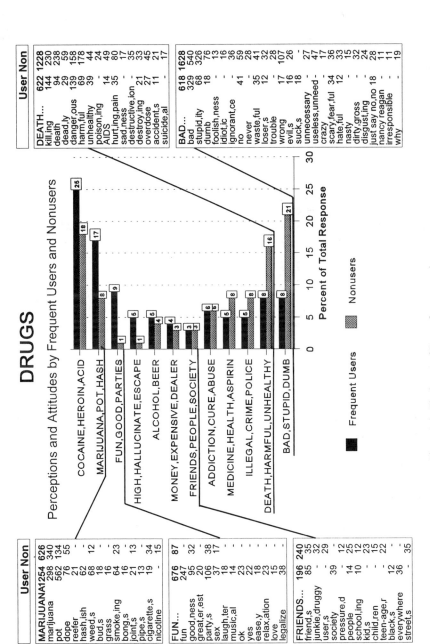

Figure 1.4. The image of DRUGS for users and nonusers.

main difference among these images is that ALCOHOL evokes more references to specific types of alcohol, particularly beer and hard liquor, and DRUGS elicits responses that reflect more intensive involvement with specific narcotic and harmful substances as well as alcohol. For the nonusers, ALCOHOL is seen as much more dangerous to others, especially due to dangerous driving and accidents, whereas DRUGS are also perceived as dangerous, but primarily to the individuals involved rather than to the general public.

Entertainment and Friends

Users focus on the social aspects of drinking and drug use and the fun and enjoyment they bring. These substances are a means of relaxing and having fun in the company of friends and others. In their images of being DRUNK, users think of humor and laughter and accept that they may feel dizzy and sick. In their view, there is a close relationship to friends and parties. The nonusers do not share this view at all.

The nonusers do not see the fun, good feelings, and social connections that the users do. Their concern is for the impact that involvement with alcohol and drugs has on others and on themselves.

Disapproval and Concern for Dangers

Nonusers express extreme disapproval of alcohol and drugs and are especially concerned about the dangers of use to self and others. They see drug and alcohol use as potentially fatal and they have much greater awareness of the illegality of drugs and marijuana and their connection to crime. They are also preoccupied with the potential loss of control.

Users understand that there is a certain amount of danger involved, and that there are some negative physical and psychological effects, but for them death is only a remote possibility, overshadowed in the context of ALCOHOL by concerns about car accidents and being arrested for drunk driving. For users, the positive elements of fun and parties take precedence over their concerns for well-being.

QUANTIFYING COMMON SENSE

What is really new and useful in these research findings? Despite the elaborate assessment, many of the results appear to be just plain common sense: Drinkers like beer, abstainers reject it. Although our data certainly do not conflict with common sense, they go much further. Even quantifying common sense can inform prevention. For example, our research tells us that "scare tactics" may bolster resistance in nonusers, but may not lower vulnerability in users. Because users are so entertainment oriented, prevention focussed on alternative entertainment might be more effective. What we offer is a quantification of how strong various dominant psychological dispositions are and how likely it is that people with given dispositions will either use or not use alcohol and other drugs. Our research shows clearly that AGA comparative imaging technology can identify those perceptual and attitudinal dispositions that make the difference between use and no use. The findings are encouraging and supportive of using the imaging technology to obtain useful information on the groups' psychological dispositions.

Although some may feel it is safe to assume that attitudes and perceptions regarding alcohol and other drugs are the most influential elements driving behavior in that domain without further assessment, we want to be more certain. And, although these may indeed be the primary dispositions influencing differences in drug-related behavior, they may not be the only important dispositions.

We are looking for a solution that uses the imaging technology systematically by focusing on a strategically selected number of images that must meet two main requirements. First, the selection must provide optimal opportunities to identify dominant perceptual and attitudinal differences between groups (users and nonusers) in domains of life influential in shaping a particular behavior (e.g., substance abuse). Second, it should involve the smallest number of images that can provide the widest possible coverage of domains necessary so as to assure generalizable conclusions.

The results from the alcohol and drug-related images, though they are encouraging, offer an incomplete answer. To follow the rationale further, we will turn our attention to the domain of Friends and Entertainment.

Additional Images (Friends, Fun) Useful in Tracing Psychological Dispositions to Use Alcohol and Drugs

Next to Alcohol and Drugs, the Friends and Entertainment domain emerged as the most influential in shaping substance abuse. The images of alcohol and drugs, for the users, are closely related to entertainment. An extension of comparative imaging to include additional domains (Self and Family, Problems, School, etc.) reveals additional insights about the dominant perceptions, attitudes, and other internal dispositions that shape young people's behavior in regard to experimentation and use of harmful substances.

IMAGES OF FRIENDS AND HAVING FUN

Using the same approach as in Chapter 1, we introduce four new images and look at the common perceptual and evaluative trends that emerge. Figure 2.1 presents the users' and the nonusers' images of FRIENDS, Figure 2.2 shows their perceptions of and attitudes toward FUN, Figure 2.3 contrasts their images of PARTIES, and Figure 2.4 shows users' and nonusers' conflicting views about GETTING HIGH.

Nonusers Seek Deeper Relationships with Friends

Users focus on the entertainment aspects of having friends, namely, *parties, fraternities,* and *hanging out.* For them, friends are associated with *fun, laughter,* and *good times.* An admirable, popular quality of friends is being *cool.* They tend to

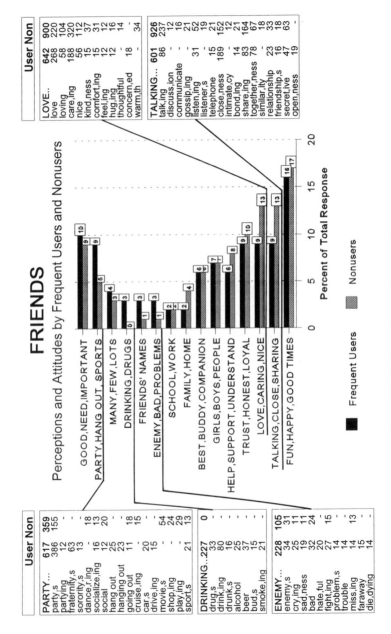

FIGURE 2.1. The image of FRIENDS for users and nonusers.

think about the quantity of friends and list them by name. One of the most noticeable differences between the users and the nonusers is that the users link *drinking, alcohol,* and *drugs* to friends, whereas this does not even occur to the nonusers. Users and nonusers place similar weight on character qualities in friendships—the *trust, honesty,* and *loyalty* among friends. However, users think of friends less as nurturing (*caring, nice, kind*). They tend to think in opposing terms of friends and *enemies* and indicate having problems with their friends (*crying, hate, trouble*). There is also some expression of loss (*miss, faraway, dying*).

Nonusers think warmly about friends as bringing *fun, laughter,* and *happiness* into their lives. The nonusers emphasize *talking, sharing, listening,* and *secrets,* all suggesting more intimate connections. Along this same idea, friends are viewed as an important source of *help, understanding,* and *support.* Although users do speak of *close* friends, they do not stress the give and take in friendships as do nonusers. Nonusers describe friends as having positive, nurturing qualities (*caring, loving, nice*). They do not show the ambivalence of the users, who think of friends in both positive and negative terms. Nonusers also see a closer link between family and friends than do the users, with the implication that family members can also be friends. In their social connections, nonusers are less interested in parties and describe sharing a broader part of their daily activities with friends, such as *shopping, playing,* and going to the *movies.*

The users' reactions reflect some strained relationships with friends, which, along with the drinking and drug use among friends, can be contributing factors to vulnerability to substance abuse. The nonusers' image reflects a deeper appreciation of and commitment among friends and also the importance of mutual communication—someone with whom to talk and to whom to listen. Strong social connections that provide emotional intimacy provide a protection regarding vulnerability to substance abuse. Activities that help build deeper friendships that serve more than an entertainment function can help strengthen resistance along the natural inclinations of the nonuser.

What Do Users and Nonusers Do for Fun?

Users envision fun as *parties* with *music* and *dancing* in the company of *friends.* A salient and distinctive component of their image of fun involves *drinking, beer, bars, drugs,* and *getting high.* It is this component that most distinguishes them from the nonusers, who barely mention drinking as a source of fun. For users, associating "fun" with the image of ALCOHOL is conceptually different from associating "alcohol" with the image of FUN. The first refers to their subjective perception of alcohol—they expect to have fun by using it. The latter refers to the perception of fun—for example, "I want to have fun tonight. What should I do?" Alcohol is one of the first things that comes to mind. Users also consider *going out* and *sex* as

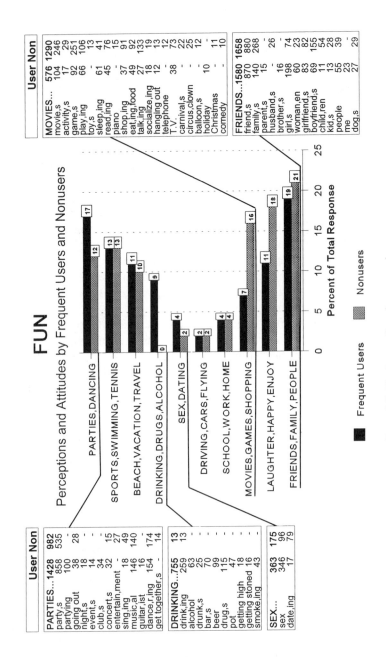

FIGURE 2.2. The image of FUN for users and nonusers.

sources of fun, and the male users think frequently about girls and women. Having fun with other people, particularly *friends,* is important. Users also identify themselves as fun. Compared to nonusers, their focus seems to be more on external stimuli—*parties, dancing, sports* and outdoor activities—and less on inner cues of pleasure, such as *laughter* and feelings of *happiness* and *enjoyment* expressed by the nonusers.

Nonusers are most interested in the people involved in having fun. *Family, friends, boyfriends,* and *girlfriends* are important sources of fun. Their focus on *family* distinguishes them from users. Whereas users look more to special occasions like *parties* and *concerts* for fun, the nonusers tend to view a broader range of daily life activities as fun, such as *games, movies, t.v., playing,* and *shopping.* Nonusers enjoy communicating with others (*talking, socializing, telephone*) as well as solitary activities such as *reading.* Pleasurable emotional feelings are linked to fun, such as: *laughter, happiness, enjoyment* and *relaxation.* Regarding their environment, both users and nonusers think of *school* as a place to have fun, but only the nonusers think of *church,* and only the users speak specifically of *fraternities* and *sororities.*

The close linkage between fun, friends, and alcohol and other drugs is clearly demonstrated here in the proportion of attention given to them by users as compared to nonusers. Interest in sex is also noted among the users. The prevalence of these dispositions among users places them at higher risk regarding their vulnerability to substance abuse. The counterbalancing components evident in the nonusers' image of FUN include family connections, committed relationships (girlfriend/boyfriend), and a wider range of alternate activities that are considered fun. Each of these dispositions contributes to the students' resistance to substance abuse.

Is It a Party without Alcohol?

Users view a party first and foremost as an opportunity to *drink* (*alcohol, beer*), with the expectation of getting *drunk.* Included in their image of parties are the effects of excessive drinking (*puke, pass out, hangovers*). The presence of *drugs* is familiar to the users, and not unknown to the nonusers in their perception of parties, but only the users think of *pot* and getting *high.* They show little interest in the food or other party trappings. Parties are a popular form of entertainment where one can *socialize* and find *friends* and other people. As in their image of FUN, the users are more preoccupied with *girls* and *women,* and see parties as an opportunity for *sex.* The users wonder about when the next party will be (*weekends, all the time, often*).

Nonusers have a traditional view of PARTIES. They think of specific times of *celebration* (*birthdays, weddings, Christmas*). Much attention is given to the party setting and the accompanying *food, cake, candles, balloons,* and *hats.* They expect

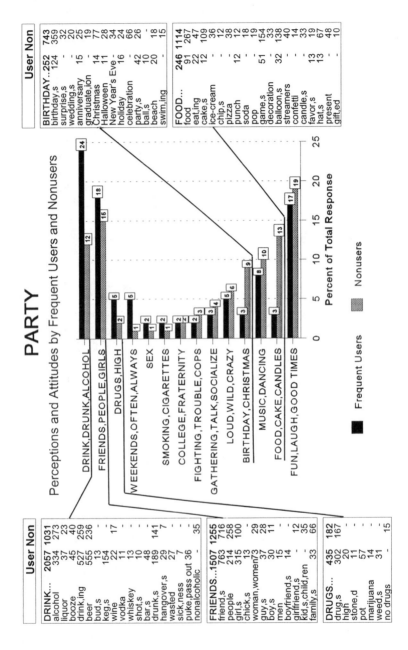

FIGURE 2.3. The image of PARTY for users and nonusers.

parties to be *loud, noisy,* and *crowded,* with *music* and *dancing.* Unlike the users' focus on *sex* at parties, nonusers tend to include *family* and *children* in their notion of parties much more than do the users. For nonusers, parties bring good feelings of *fun, laughter,* and *happiness,* but they are somewhat ambivalent and are more likely than the users to see parties as *boring, bad, stupid,* or *uncomfortable.* Although the nonusers recognize that parties may offer *alcohol* and *drugs,* they also think of alternates (*nonalcoholic, no drugs*). As in other themes examined, the nonusers are attracted to more intimate social interaction such as *talking* and *togetherness.*

The users' strong entertainment orientation is clearly evidenced here, along with their high expectations for finding alcohol and drugs at parties that they attend. As usual, they show interest in having people around them and in friends, and, for the male users, girls, although they are less inclined to view parties as an opportunity to get to know people better through talking together. It is interesting to note that users think of girls but not girlfriends. The nonusers' image is again much broader than that of the users, who are preoccupied with drinking and drugs. Prevention activities that appeal to the users' entertainment needs and that incorporate the nonusers' diversity of reasons for gathering and celebration may help to build dispositions that provide more resistance to substance abuse.

Getting High on Drugs and on Life

Users think predominantly of *pot* and *marijuana* as a means of getting high and cite various methods of use (*smoking, joint, bong*). They also think of *drugs* in general and, to a lesser extent, of other illicit substances (*cocaine, acid*). The users express familiarity with the physical sensations and psychological effects of getting high (*stoned, flying, buzz*). One of their most dominant perceptions is that getting high is a source of *fun, relaxation, laughter* and *good times.* The users' view of getting high is even more positive than their views on MARIJUANA or DRUGS. *Friends* appear to play an important role in drug use. Their view of getting high as fun far outweighs any negative or harmful consequences they perceive. Users show interest in timely opportunities to get high (*now, sometimes, everyday*).

Nonusers focus not so much on the means and methods of getting high as on its undesirability and harmfulness. They overwhelmingly reject it as *stupid, bad, wrong,* and *crazy.* The *dangerous* and *harmful* consequences of getting high are emphasized. They view it as *unhealthy, destructive,* possibly *addictive,* and even a cause of *death.* The nonusers think more of *drugs* in general, though *pot* and *cocaine* are mentioned to a limited extent. The nonusers appear to be unfamiliar with the variety of physical and mental effects of getting high, reflecting their lack of personal experience with drugs. It apparently has little appeal for them as *fun* or *enjoyment.* Nonusers, much more than users, express the expanded meaning of

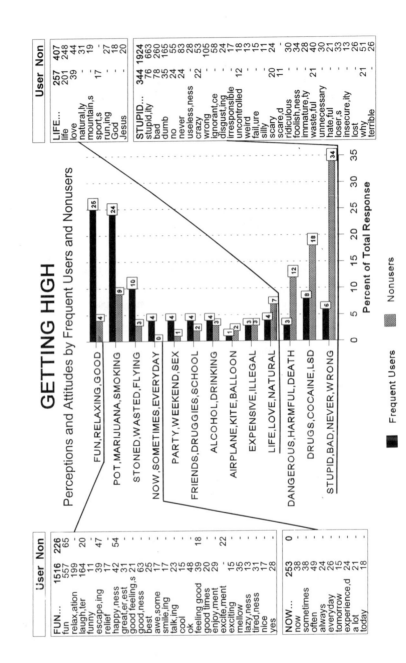

FIGURE 2.4. The image of GETTING HIGH for users and nonusers.

getting high on *life*, referring to the natural highs accompanying life experiences in nature (*mountains*), sports (*running*), and religion (*God, Jesus*).

The users' priorities on entertainment and feeling good are illustrated here in this general context of getting high. Their disposition to view getting high on drugs as fun and relaxing with little risk involved adds to their vulnerability to substance abuse. The perceived harmfulness of getting high for nonusers and their strong disapproval demonstrate their strong resistance to substance abuse.

User versus Nonuser Dispositions within the Domain of Friends and Entertainment

Expectations Regarding Alcohol and Drugs

Within the domain of Friends and Entertainment, the four stimulus words elicited similar responses. For the users, alcohol and drugs are an integral part of their images of FUN, PARTIES, and of course, of GETTING HIGH. Drinking and drugs are also linked to FRIENDS. In each of these contexts, the users think of drinking and getting drunk, with the most frequent image being beer. They associate a greater variety of beverages (including *whiskey, vodka,* and *wine*) with PARTIES.

Nonusers do not consider alcohol and drugs as fun. Although they relate alcohol to parties, it is not the pervasive expectation we found among users. Nonusers do not think in terms of the variety of alcoholic beverages nor of the details of excessive drinking (*getting sick, passing out, hangovers*) common among the users. The alcohol and drug results offer probably the strongest contrasting trend we observed in the domain of Friends and Entertainment.

Social Life and Entertainment

The nonusers' views of PARTIES and FUN are more traditional and family oriented (e.g., *birthday parties, celebrations*). Whereas the users go into detail about the specifics of alcohol and drugs, the nonusers react with detail about the foods available at social gatherings (*pizza, ice cream*), the surroundings (*balloons, decorations*), the locale (*school, home, work*), and the types of activities that are fun. The nonusers focus on a much wider range of activities involving friends, such as *shopping* and *movies*. Although nonusers take an extremely negative view of getting high because of its close linkage to drugs, even in this context they think of other alternates such as getting high on *life, nature, running,* and *God*.

In their images of FUN, PARTIES, and FRIENDS, the users focus more narrowly on drinking and partying with friends. They are much more outgoing and action oriented in their ideas of fun, preferring parties and dancing to movies and games.

The users also express their strongest positive feelings (*fun, relaxation, laughter*) in the context of GETTING HIGH, whereas that concept evokes almost no such feelings from the nonusers.

Interpersonal Relationships and Friendships

Regarding interpersonal relationships and human interaction, we found that users do not look far beyond the superficial level in their relationships with others. They do not see as close ties between family and friends as do the nonusers. They consistently express more interest in *sex, girls,* and *women,* not only when thinking of PARTIES, FUN, and GETTING HIGH, but also regarding FRIENDS, where they make more gender distinction.

Nonusers are much more strongly attuned to the affective dimension of *love* and *caring* and *laughter* and *happiness* while having fun at parties and among friends. In all of these contexts, the nonusers think about the quality of relationships and are interested in making connections through *talking, listening,* and *supporting.* Unlike the users, they regard talking as fun and they see it as an essential part of friendship.

CONSISTENT TRENDS IN TWO DOMAINS OF LIFE

Across the group images involving FRIENDS and FUN and other images related to entertainment, the user versus nonuser comparisons have revealed distinctive differences. As was true of the Alcohol and Drugs domain, in the Friends and Entertainment domain the users reflected their preoccupation with drinking and drug use in every image to a varying extent. They had strong expectations of drinking, drug use, and getting high as elements of social entertainment, of fun with friends, and of parties. Again in this domain, as in the Alcohol and Drugs domain, their interest in sex and women is high, but their interpersonal relationships have been revealed as being somewhat superficial.

Nonusers, on the other hand, revealed as their concern with the negative consequences of alcohol and drugs most strongly in the context of GETTING HIGH and their responses revealed that those substances have little to do with their social life. Nonusers consistently emphasize the importance of nurturing human relationships through personal exchange—*talking, listening, helping,* and *supporting.* Their social life has a wider range of alternates: parties are not just associated with drinking, but with birthdays and with seasonal celebrations as well; fun is not had just by going to parties but also by going to the movies, by going shopping, and by playing games; friends are not just drinking buddies but also supportive companions in everyday life. Family and friends are more intertwined for nonusers.

These trends affirm and reinforce the results we reported in the previous chapter. Taking the results of both the Alcohol and Drugs domain and the Friends and Entertainment domain together (and including some underlying details from our research that we have not presented in these pages), we can sketch a more comprehensive picture of users and of nonusers:

- Users associate strongly positive expectations with all of the alcohol- and drug-related images, while seeing the potential problems or negative consequences as possible but very unlikely. They link alcohol and drugs with *fun, sex,* and various types of entertainment involving friends. They tend to be interested in concrete specifics such as the names and number of friends (*many, a lot*), when the parties will occur (*weekends, often*), and where the fun is (*party, beach, school*).
- Nonusers also are interested in fun and entertainment, but they tend to anticipate possible problems such as fighting and trouble at parties, harmfulness and possible loss of control in getting high, and occasional sadness and tears among friends. In the domain of Alcohol and Drugs especially, nonusers focus on the real possibilities of risk and danger to health and property that can lead to accidents, addiction, and personal failure (*junkies, druggies, bums*).

By considering the images in combination, we can identify general psychological dispositions that are characteristic of users and of nonusers and that set them apart from one another. It is true that each of the 24 stimulus images generates dozens of individual, seemingly separate mosaic pieces, but those myriad details combine naturally into a few major perspectives. Once we recognize the perspectives, the underlying mosaic details help us to recognize how those perspectives lead to different choices regarding alcohol and drug use. With that understanding, practitioners can plan empirically based programs that take students' psychological dispositions into account and then retest them to acquire feedback on effectiveness.

Users' and Nonusers' Perceptions of Problems

The students' perceptions and evaluations of certain problems provide clues regarding how they may be inclined to deal with them. In addition to PROBLEMS (Figure 2.5) and FEAR (Figure 2.6), two other images were reconstructed in exploring the domain of Problems—SMOKING and HOOKED.

Who Looks for Solutions to Problems?

The users think of friends and relationships as their biggest problems, followed by problems at school and at home. They identified *drugs, alcohol,* and *drinking* as more salient problems than did nonusers, even though users did not seem worried

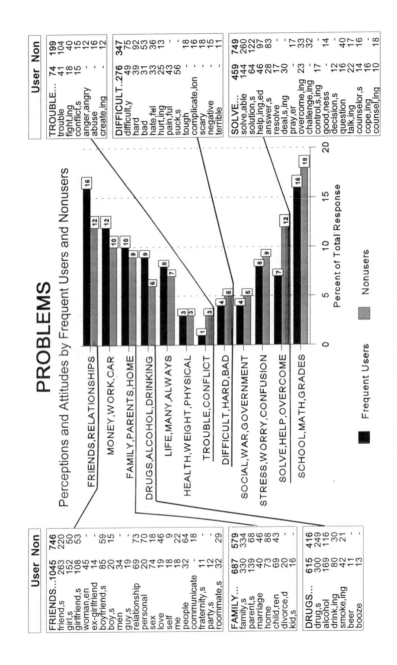

FIGURE 2.5. The image of PROBLEMS for users and nonusers.

about the harmful effects of the substances themselves (Chapter 1). The users revealed friends and interpersonal relationships—*girlfriend, boyfriend, men,* and *women* and *sex*—as even greater sources of problems. They paid more attention to *money, jobs,* and *cars,* possibly indicating a greater interest in the material dimension of life, although the differences between the two groups are relatively small. *Family* problems, particularly *parents,* are a priority in the users' image. Their emphasis on family, friends, and the opposite sex suggests that users experience relationships that are more strained than those of nonusers. As in their image of FRIENDS, the users showed a strong need for social connection; here they mentioned emotion problems of feeling *alone* and *sad.* Users tended to think of the number of problems (*many, lots, few, none*).

Nonusers have a distinctly stronger disposition toward solving problems. They think more about the *solutions, questions,* and *answers.* The nonusers' hopefulness in finding solutions is reflected in their describing problems as *good* and *challenging. School* is a big problem for both the users and the nonusers, and their interest in math may partially explain their emphasis on problem solving or their academic orientation. Compared to users, nonusers indicated somewhat more *stress, worry,* and *confusion* in facing problems with which they struggle. This is further reinforced by the perceived *difficulty* and *complications* that problems bring. nonusers are more sensitive to *conflict* and *trouble.* There are problems common to Nonusers and users (e.g., physical, social, emotional, etc.) with only slightly greater attention from one group or the other.

What Do Users and Nonusers Fear?

In relation to problems in general and FEAR in particular, the users expressed less worry and anxiety than the nonusers, but the nonusers showed much more optimism about overcoming their problems and finding solutions. Users expressed greater fear of *failure,* fear of *death,* fear of *violence,* and financial concerns. Their responses indicate a fear of being *alone* or *lonely* and a fear of *love.* Users appear to be slightly more worried about *failure* and *loss* in their lives than the nonusers.

Nonusers expressed more fear of the *unknown* than did the users, and thought more of *anxiety, phobias,* and *panic.* They expressed more discomfort with *insecurity* and *doubt* and indicated a stronger physical response to FEAR (*running, shaking, crying*).

Users and Nonusers Differ in Their Views of Smoking and Getting Hooked

Users showed greater familiarity with SMOKING and link it equally to smoking cigarettes and to smoking marijuana, yet they were much less concerned than are nonusers with the possibility of smoking becoming a habit or addiction. As in their

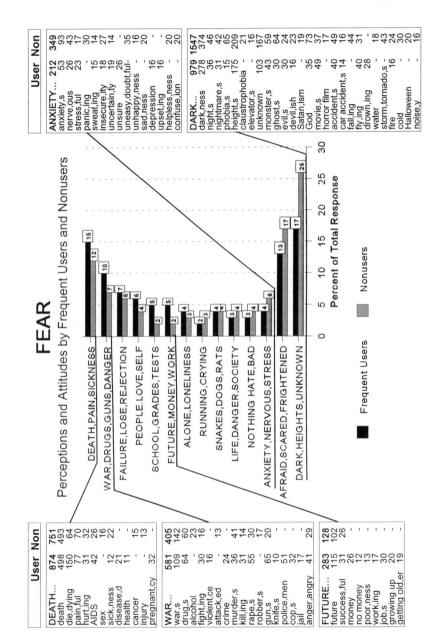

Figure 2.6. The image of FEAR for users and nonusers.

images of DRUNK, MARIJUANA, ALCOHOL, DRUNK and GETTING HIGH, the users saw SMOKING as another way to relax and have fun in social settings such as parties and bars. The nonusers were extremely negative toward SMOKING, just as much as they were toward MARIJUANA or DRUGS. They viewed smoking as a serious health hazard and tended to connect it with drugs. The users generalize and destigmatize the idea of being HOOKED by thinking not only of drugs, but also of being hooked on *girls,* on *sex,* on *sports,* and on *smoking.*

The nonusers are far more likely to be concerned about the issues of control and of losing control. In fact, the nonusers' concern with control over their own destiny is a recurrent theme in all of the research. Not surprisingly, nonusers think more often about loss of control from drinking, drug use, and fear, as well as about the need to maintain control through rules and order.

DIFFERING VIEWS OF AUTHORITY, DISCIPLINE, AND OTHER VALUES

Comparison of users' and nonusers' social values has revealed perceptual and attitudinal differences that directly impact the students' vulnerability to substance abuse. In the original study, AUTHORITY, DISCIPLINE, RESPONSIBILITY, and RELIGION were included to represent the domain of Social Values. From the two images presented in Figures 2.7 and 2.8, we show how the motivational dispositions in this domain are likely to impact behavior.

The users, as might be anticipated, are more negative toward DISCIPLINE and AUTHORITY than the nonusers. Not only did they judge DISCIPLINE and AUTHORITY as *bad* and *wrong* (except when they relate to sports and exercise), they also suspected that they are improperly used (e.g., *abuse, misuse*). Users are concerned about the "appropriate" amount of responsibility, discipline, and authority—neither *too much* nor *too little. Trouble* and *problems* are recognized as situations where discipline is required. There is some ambiguity in the negative responses— for example, *bad* meaning a negative attitude toward DISCIPLINE or *bad* meaning bad behavior calling for discipline. The users emphasized various settings where discipline is needed (*school, work, home*); they also think of *sports, football,* and *exercise.*

Nonusers, on the other hand, expressed strong approval of discipline and authority and emphasize the rules and expectations for proper behavior. They emphasized personal *responsibility,* personal *authority,* and self-*discipline.* They are concerned about the punishment that is tied to infractions of the rules. (This general concern also emerged in relation to other areas of life, such as their view of SOCIETY and GOVERNMENT, where they pay attention to the standards, laws, and rules set by higher authorities.) The nonusers appear more inclined to *behave* and *obey. Rules* and *control* had higher salience for them than for the users and only the nonusers spoke specifically of *self-control.*

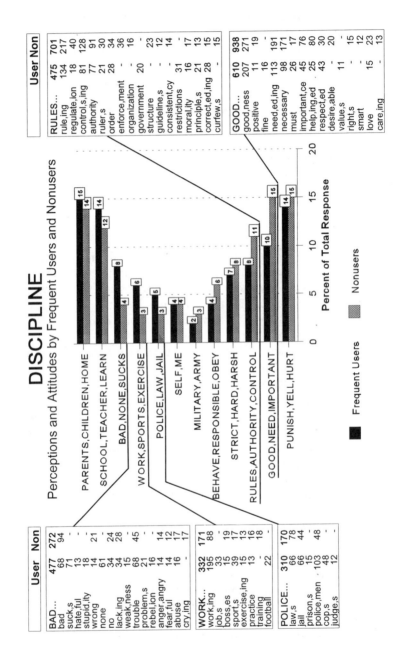

FIGURE 2.7. The image of DISCIPLINE for users and nonusers.

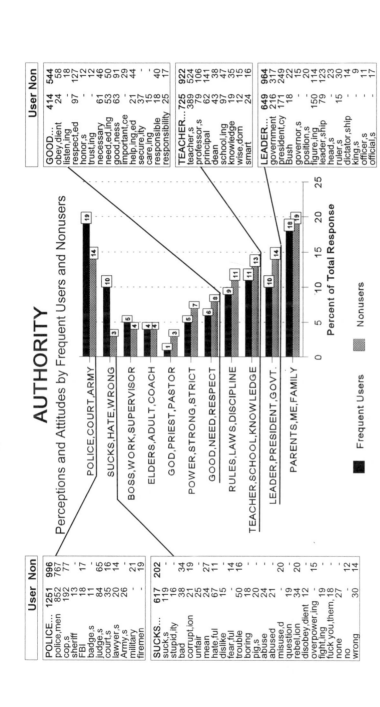

FIGURE 2.8. The image of AUTHORITY for users and nonusers.

Users and nonusers differed in whom they view as authority and discipline figures. Nonusers spoke more of *parents, teachers,* and leaders in general, whereas users thought of the *police* and legal authorities. Similarly, there was a general tendency for the nonusers to express more approval and acceptance of social values and social institutions, whereas the users tended to be skeptical about authority and somewhat critical about its authenticity.

RELIGION, another theme in this domain, appears to be much more important to the nonusers than to the users. This is supported by their self-reports of their frequency of attending religious services. Nonusers expressed more positive attitudes toward RELIGION and its role in teaching the values of *love, hope,* and *peace,* whereas users' evaluations were negative, viewing it as *confusing, boring, stupid,* and *false.*

SELF-IMAGE AND THE MEANING OF FAMILY

Self-esteem and self-image have been found to be strong psychosocial correlates of substance abuse (Braucht, Brakarsh, Follingstad, & Berry, 1973; Kaplan, 1982). Botvin (1983) stressed the importance of enhancing self-esteem, a sense of personal control, and the ability to cope with anxiety in order to increase students' resistance to social influences that encourage drinking and experimentation with drugs. Many aspects of the family situation from which the student is emerging also can impact personal coping style. Our own studies have shown that students' perceptions and attitudes toward FATHER are linked to drug behavior (Szalay, Strohl, & Wilson, 1991). To tap these two important personal dimensions, we tested two themes related to self-image (ME, I AM) and two related to family (FAMILY, FATHER). We found the following trends in the comparative analysis of users' and nonusers' responses to this domain.

In their self-image, nonusers are preoccupied with being *nice, good, loving, responsible* and *honest.* Social approval and harmonious relationships are important to this group of students. They tend to take their role as student seriously, describing themselves as *smart, intelligent,* and *hardworking.* Users express more emotional ambivalence toward themselves as well as toward their family. They see themselves as *happy, fun,* and *friendly* on the one hand and as *confused, stupid, tired,* and *bored* on the other. They express stronger negative feelings in general than do the nonusers. Users appear to be much more pleasure seeking, outgoing, and extroverted than the nonusers. They are more interested in group social settings, such as parties and sports events, and in their family's social atmosphere of fun and leisure activities.

The nonusers' perceptions and evaluations of FAMILY indicate a stronger and broader support base of brothers and sisters as well as of extended family (*aunts, uncles, grandparents*). Although love and caring were important to all of the students, the nonusers identified these qualities in closer relationship to FAMILY as well as to SELF. Users expressed stronger feelings and judgements toward FAMILY and FATHER, thinking not only of the *fun* but also of the pain and hurt of problems, of fighting, and of the father's physical and emotional distance.

PERCEPTIONS OF, AND ATTITUDES TOWARD, SOCIAL INSTITUTIONS

We expected the perceptions of and attitudes toward large social institutions to differ for students who use illicit substances and for those who live within the limitations set by contemporary societal standards. To explore this hypothesis, our study of college populations included the themes of SCHOOL, CAMPUS, SOCIETY, and GOVERNMENT. Although the differences between users and nonusers in this domain were not as large as those we had found in the domain of Alcohol and Drugs, they point to some contrasting psychological dispositions that could be helpful in substance abuse prevention.

In their perceptions of SCHOOL and CAMPUS, the users distinguished themselves from nonusers in their preoccupation with having fun, going to parties, and having friends. In this context, as in others, it was the users for whom the entertainment aspect is very important: "Is it fun?" "Will my friends be there?" In contrast, nonusers tended to define SCHOOL and CAMPUS in terms of physical elements and structures, and as places of learning and of study for intelligent students. This is consistent with their interest in structure in general, and in attending to the rules and boundaries set by those in authority. Users are not only more negative about many aspects of campus life than the nonusers, they are also more positive about other aspects. This is similar to what we have seen in other domains: the users have both strong emotional evaluations about the world around them and ambivalent feelings toward it.

Users expressed overwhelmingly negative judgements and skepticism about SOCIETY and GOVERNMENT. They suspected corruption and deceit in government and in society at large, and were concerned about problems of racism, drugs, debts, and taxes. Nonusers expressed some skepticism, but this view was counterbalanced by their recognition of the positive aspects of society and government, that is, that they are good and necessary structures.

THE INNER WORLDS REVEALED BY COMPARATIVE IMAGING

We have been comparing the world of users and the world of nonusers from the practical perspective of identifying psychological factors that can explain why some students are drawn to experiment with drugs and others are not. In pursuing this interest, we found that perceptions and attitudes are among the powerful influences shaping the subjective world of users and that of nonusers. Recognition of the processes and mechanisms through which these influences are promoted and mediated is of fundamental importance not only in understanding the etiology of substance abuse but also in developing programs that can use the processes effectively to promote a drug-free lifestyle. We have demonstrated that we can trace these hidden but powerful influences on substance abuse.

Our main conclusion is that users and nonusers look at the world differently—that they live in two different subjective worlds. These worlds are made up of contrasting combinations of psychological dispositions related to alcohol, drugs, entertainment, human problems, and values. The results of our comparative imaging procedures provide solid empirical evidence of the role of these dispositions in shaping behavior. The evidence is important because the combined effects of these perceptual and attitudinal forces, particularly on factors affecting substance abuse, have not been measured or recognized for their broader implications. The differences registered by imaging in the dominant perceptions and attitudes of users and of nonusers help to explain the differences in behavior as well as the processes by which the differences develop.

Understanding how the users' world influences their behavior requires a recognition that they are predisposed by a host of converging perceptual and attitudinal trends to experiment with and to use harmful substances. Their images of alcohol and drugs show how harmful substances are seen as attractive and favorable and how their hedonistic emphasis on fun and parties strengthens the appeal of alcohol and drugs and their promise for desired fun and relaxation, together with sex and other social rewards and benefits.

Similarly, the many perceptions and attitudes of the nonusers—their strong gut-level rejection of alcohol and drugs, the intensity of their fears and anxieties about addiction and harmful consequences, their concern with loss of control, their traditional cake-and-candles view of parties and entertainment, and their personal care and love focused view of social relations and friends—are some of the characteristic details making up their different world.

To make practical use of these conclusions requires more than documentation that users and nonusers have different images, different perspectives, and a different outlook on drugs, entertainment, values, and so forth. Applying this information regarding perceptual and attitudinal dispositions to prevention programs requires that the processes and mechanisms that underlie the dispositions be recognized at a depth essential for their use in educational prevention.

The Cumulative Power of Perceptual Dispositions

The details presented on both users and on nonusers show that single mosaic pieces of perceptions and attitudes do not act alone but rather in combination. The effects are created by an extensive array of mosaic pieces and dominant trends of perceptions and attitudes working in combination to form propensities for use and propensities for nonuse. As the detailed data in these last chapters demonstrated, there is an impressive consistency in the perceptual and attitudinal dispositions of users supporting use, just as there are forces working against use in the case of the nonusers. What matters here is that the behaviors of use or of no use have a broad foundation in a system of perceptual and attitudinal dispositions that support use in the case of users and that resist use in the case of nonusers. These contrasting systems of behavioral dispositions work in opposing directions, the combined effects pushing users toward use and nonusers toward resistance. Recognition of this dynamic can enhance the understanding of how their subjective worlds have a different psychological foundation, with contrasting behavioral implications.

It follows from the broad systemic foundation that the power of the underlying psychological dispositions is cumulative. The aggregate character is affected by several dimensions and characteristics of the system as a whole. One important consideration is the generality of perceptual and of attitudinal dispositions. For instance, the tendency to overlook consequences and harm has emerged as a broad general trend characteristic of users in the context of all substances examined. It was also registered as a more dominant characteristic of users in the context of themes related to entertainment, problems, fears, and so forth. In contrast, the nonusers showed general trends of fear and concern with harm and consequences, trends of obviously opposing direction and motion registered in the context of alcohol and drug themes, as well as most themes related to entertainment.

Dominant perceptions and attitudes identified through image analysis revealed not only two contrasting worlds characteristic of users and of nonusers but also their foundation on a host of partially contrasting behavioral dispositions. This helps to explain how the differences in worlds become the foundation for contrasting behaviors. Each group shows remarkable consistency regarding all of the harmful substances covered by these investigations. Beyond the substances examined, aggregate measures of behavioral dispositions can offer insights into the impact of these dispositions on other behaviors, ranging from educational performance to various lifestyles.

A Force below Awareness and beyond Introspection

The perceptions and attitudes that support the use of harmful substances reinforce each other and produce combined propensities for use. This explains the deep systemic nature of the drug problem. Because dispositions are based on dominant perceptions and motivations, the person experiences them as reflecting plain and simple reality. The Users are unaware that they are predisposed by their own system of psychological dispositions to overate the appeal of drugs and alcohol, to underrate their harm and adverse consequences, and to overrate fun and entertainment.

They are unaware that their world creates strong natural dispositions for them to make the choices they are making, to view them as normal and natural, and to fundamentally overlook how much their choices follow compellingly from their inner world, the only world they know and consider to be unadulterated reality. The nonusers are similarly predisposed by their own subjective world to make the choices they make and to behave the way they do based on their sense of reality. For each group, their own behaviors seem "normal," whereas the behaviors of the other group seem "odd."

Perhaps the least understood and most confusing feature of psychological dispositions, and a key to their influence, is their hidden nature—their existence in the individual's subconscious. Much of what is revealed by comparative imaging about the worlds of the users and of the nonusers reflects two separate systems of mental representations. These systems follow different rationales, each of which has its own logic controlled by different rules imposed by different perspectives. The consistency reflected by these different perspectives is impressive, suggesting that what they reveal is something real and powerful, even though it is below the individual's awareness. The individual respondents are unaware of what their responses reveal or what their group is communicating, a group in which each is only one of 400 members. When one understands the operations of conflicting systems of behavioral dispositions, the consistency in the world of users and the consistency in the world of nonusers becomes comprehensible but still amazing.

Even more impressive is the consistency of the differences observed between users and nonusers. These contrasting perceptual and motivational factors can tell the secret that is the basis of their differences in behavior. Our comparisons show that differences in psychological dispositions go along with different choices and behavior by users and nonusers. They reveal behavioral dispositions that are dominant forces leading people toward the use of harmful substances or protecting them from the slippery slope of experimentation.

3

The System
Mapping the World of Users and Nonusers

The analysis has shown highly consistent differences between the images of those who use harmful substances and those who do not use them. As revealed by mapping, the users and the nonusers differ not only in single isolated images but also in their subjective worlds— in their system of cognitive–semantic representations. Mapping shows how they differ along such parameters as what is important to them, what is attractive, and what is related to what. The findings of our imaging and mapping show strong agreement with the latest views of neurobiology on the working of the neural system as the foundation of the neural representation of the world, as the foundation of behavior.

SHIFTING THE ASSESSMENT FROM SINGLE IMAGES TO THE SYSTEM— THE SUBJECTIVE WORLD

The strategy of comparative imaging, analyzing the mental images of people with contrasting behavior, is useful in identifying the perceptual and attitudinal dispositions at the foundation of their differences in behavior. This leads to the following questions: Since images are many and their one-by-one assessment is tedious, is there a way to simplify the process? In other words, what happens when we shift the focus from single images to larger units of cognitive–semantic representations and broader domains of people's subjective worlds?

Comparing Systems of Cognitive–Semantic Representations

The next few chapters offer answers to these questions and others regarding the practical use of the results. Some answers come from shifting the focus from the comparative analysis of single images to the comparative analysis of the systems of cognitive–semantic representations, more simply called *the subjective world* of users or of nonusers.

When the broad system of cognitive–semantic representations is the target of assessment, we use a variety of analytic measures. Each involves the computer-assisted analysis of thousands of responses elicited in the systematically designed multiple-response tasks. A sophisticated package of software programs has been developed for these analyses. Compared to imaging, the task is of a different nature. The analysis is fast, mechanized, and does not require any human decisions. The results are numerical, succinct, and conclusive, but at the same time, their best use calls for support from the imaging results. Reconstruction of the system along the various parameters of cognitive–semantic representations is called *cognitive mapping*.

Tracing Trends across Images and Domains

Our approach builds on the dominant perceptual and motivational dispositions of particular student populations. Targeting prevention programs on the most influential dispositions makes it desirable to identify them as sharply and unequivocally as possible. This requires tracing how the students' choices about the use of alcohol and other drugs are actually shaped by their dominant psychological dispositions.

From comparative imaging we have found, for instance, that lack of sensitivity to harm, the appeal of alcohol and other substances, entertainment orientation, and hedonism are important psychological dispositions of users. What single images cannot tell us is their combined effects. Should they be considered one-by-one or in combination? What we have learned, however, is that the decisions to use or not use harmful substances have a broad foundation in several domains of life. Many images and multiple domains are involved in decisions affecting use. There were indications that the combined effects of all of the domains or images involved should be considered as the effects of the entire system of cognitive–semantic representations.

Based on our representational model of behavioral organization, the answers to these questions can be found by extending the analysis to the system of cognitive organization. This means, naturally, the subjective world of users and that of nonusers that provides the framework or organization for their different choices and behavior. In order to understand how the system works and how it shapes behavior, we have to consider, beyond specific images, the effects of the system as a whole.

RECONSTRUCTION OF THE SYSTEM BY ITS NATURAL PARAMETERS

Our behavior is organized and controlled by our inner worlds, our subjective representations, and our personal understanding of the environment. In the simplest terms, what we do depends on how we see and understand the world. We are guided by what we consider to be important. We make choices based on what is appealing to us. Knowing what is important or dominant, what has appeal, and what is related to what in our own worlds are valuable keys to understanding what we choose and what we actually do. To enhance our understanding the behavior of users and of nonusers, subjective images offer insights here as well, but not on the basis of comparing single images. In the context of the system, we analyze the images along some of the natural parameters, using the measures we have developed for their assessment.

DOMINANCE—WHAT IS IMPORTANT TO USERS AND TO NONUSERS

The importance of a particular image is inferred from the number of responses elicited. The Dominance measure, which is discussed in the appendix, shows the subjective importance of a particular image, theme, or subject for a person or a group. This measure is built on the recognition that these things have different psychological importance. This is a basic fact of life demonstrated and measured as one of the characteristics of specific images.

Remember that an important characteristic of the AGA technique is that respondents are not *asked* to judge what is important to them. They reveal what is

TABLE 3.1. Dominance Scores of Users and Nonusers

Domain/theme	Users	Nonusers	Domain/theme	Users	Nonusers
Self and family			Social values		
ME	5873	6047	AUTHORITY	6455	7099
I AM	6590	7053	DISCIPLINE	5968	6188
FAMILY	8074	8940	RELIGION	7224	8089
FATHER	6924	7112	RESPONSIBILITY	6664	6301
mean	6865	7288	mean	6578	6919
Social institutions			Alcohol and drugs		
SCHOOL	7875	8561	ALCOHOL	7700	7251
CAMPUS	7221	7625	DRUGS	7437	7621
SOCIETY	4801	5123	MARIJUANA	7829	7397
GOVERNMENT	6702	7155	DRUNK	7259	6858
mean	6650	7116	mean	7556	7282
Friends and entertainment			Problems		
FRIENDS	6935	7110	PROBLEMS	6650	6480
FUN	8190	7912	HOOKED	6005	5672
PARTY	8594	8537	SMOKING	7762	7927
GETTING HIGH	6165	5670	FEAR	5657	6061
mean	7471	7307	mean	6519	6535

	Users	Nonusers
Overall mean	6940	7075

important or dominant to them without being aware that they are doing so by giving many or few responses to a given stimulus word. Noble (1952) introduced a similar measure (meaningfulness). Through comparisons of Dominance scores of each theme, we can determine their ranking of priority within the system of a particular person or group, as well as the differences in priorities between two systems. In the present context, the comparisons show how users and nonusers differ in what is important or meaningful to them.

Table 3.1 compares the Dominance scores of users and of nonusers in the six domains of life included in our study. The average scores for the four alcohol and drug images, 7,556 for users compared to 7,282 for nonusers, show the greater importance of alcohol and drugs for the users than for the nonusers. Both ALCOHOL and DRUNK have more psychological importance to the users than to the nonusers. Yet it appears to be inconsistent and counterintuitive that nonusers showed higher dominance scores for DRUGS. An explanation can be found from closer examination of the image data on DRUGS, particularly two response categories on which the nonusers scored higher than the users. One involves negative consequences and negative evaluations of drugs. The other involves references to medicine and health that reflect the popularity of prescription and over-the-counter medications. The nonusers' attention to these components is what made their Dominance score outweigh the users' dominance score. This example illustrates the advantage of using several complementary analytic procedures. MARIJUANA, as expected, has a higher Dominance score for the users. As a closer look at the image data supports, the direct personal experiences of the users with this substance, with the related paraphernalia, and with a particularly rich stock of slang for marijuana, the plant and its effects result in a higher Dominance score.

Regarding the domain of Friends and Entertainment, the users scored higher than the nonusers on three of the four images—FUN, PARTY, and GETTING HIGH—suggesting that these images are richer in content or meaning for users. The exception is FRIENDS, on which the nonusers scored noticeably higher. It may be debatable whether GETTING HIGH is more a drug use word or an entertainment word. The answer may depend again on the population considered.

Dominance scores in the Social Values domain indicate that values are more important to nonusers than to users. Differences are particularly striking regarding the subjective importance of RELIGION, which appears to be more meaningful to nonusers than to users. AUTHORITY also holds more weight among the nonusers. The issue of RESPONSIBILITY, however, is a more important one for the users.

These measures offer quick insights into what the users consider important in their world, and what is relevant in making their choices. It is intriguing that these insights into dominant priorities come from the respondents mostly without their awareness. They are similarly unaware of these dispositions when they are making decisions regarding the use of harmful substances.

Evaluation—What Is Positive and Appealing and What Is Not

The Evaluation measure reflects respondents' attitudes. It is derived from the attitude scales administered anonymously to groups at the time they respond to the set of stimulus themes. When used on a group basis, the Evaluation score reflects the average attitude expressed by the group members toward each stimulus theme. The scores range from +3.0 (strongly positive) to –3.0 (strongly negative). We have developed other evaluation measures, as discussed in the appendix.

Table 3.2 compares the users' attitudes and those of the nonusers. In the six domains considered within the users' system, their most positive attitude is toward social relations (note their scores in the Friends/Entertainment and Self/Family domains). Within the nonusers' system, the most positive attitudes are toward Self/Family and Social Values.

As expected, the greatest contrast between the two groups is in the Alcohol/Drugs domain where the nonusers were extremely negative (–2.6) and the users were neutral or slightly positive (0.4). More specifically, users were slightly positive in their ALCOHOL, MARIJUANA, and DRUNK images, whereas the nonusers were firmly negative. The second domain characterized by the largest differences in attitudes involves Social Values. A third domain involves Entertainment. These

TABLE 3.2. Evaluation Scores of Users and Nonusers

Domain/theme	Users	Nousers	Domain/theme	Users	Nousers
Self and family			Social values		
ME	1.8	2.0	AUTHORITY	.0	1.2
I AM	1.8	2.0	DISCIPLINE	.7	1.5
FAMILY	2.4	2.7	RESPONSIBILITY	1.6	2.0
FATHER	2.0	2.2	RELIGION	1.0	2.0
mean	2.0	2.2	mean	.8	1.7
Social institutions			Alcohol and drugs		
SCHOOL	1.3	1.8	ALCOHOL	.9	–2.4
CAMPUS	.9	1.2	DRUGS	–.3	–2.5
GOVERNMENT	–.5	.4	MARIJUANA	.6	–2.7
SOCIETY	.0	.3	DRUNK	.3	–2.6
mean	.4	.9	mean	.4	–2.6
Friends and entertainment			Problems		
FRIENDS	2.6	2.6	PROBLEMS	–1.2	–.8
FUN	2.8	2.6	HOOKED	–1.1	–1.3
PARTY	2.2	.9	SMOKING	–1.0	–2.4
GETTING HIGH	.6	–2.3	FEAR	–.9	–.8
mean	2.1	.9	mean	–.7	–.9

	Users	Nonusers
Overall mean	.8	.3

differences offer a quick summary view showing what attitudinal differences are behind the observed differences in behavior in the case of users and nonusers.

Attitudes are recognized as a particularly important category of psychological dispositions that influence behavior. The diverse AGA attitude measures offer insights of varying depth. The direct measures, like the scaling reported here, offer simplicity and comparability. The inferential measures, like the Evaluative Dominance Index (see appendix), reflect more on implicit cognitions and are totally nontransparent. The various attitude measures rely on different methods of assessment, but they have in common the intent to identify the attitudes shaping each group's behavior toward alcohol and other drugs.

Affinity–What Is Intrinsically Related to What

With the AGA method we have developed several measures of affinity to reconstruct how images are related for one group compared to another. They provide a means for assessing how particular groups organize and interrelate elements of their subjective worlds. The affinity measures indicate which images and themes are related by a group to which other themes and to what extent. The degree of relationship among these elements of a group's subjective world is an important parameter in their system of cognitive–semantic representations.

Using a formula described in the appendix, we calculate affinity scores to assess how each image is related to every other image. The higher the score, the more closely related the images. The resulting matrices of interrelatedness reveal the cognitive–semantic organization characterizing each group under study. For example, in analyzing affinities in the domains of Alcohol and Entertainment for users and for nonusers (see Table 3.3), we found that these domains were very closely related for users but not for nonusers. Nonusers see very little relationship between friends

TABLE 3.3. Affinity Scores of Users and Nonusers

Domain/Theme	Alcohol		Drunk		Drugs		Mariju.		Friends		Fun		Party		Getting high	
	user	non	user	non	user	non	user	non	user	non	user	non	user	non	user	non
Alcohol/drugs																
Alcohol			48	44	18	33	20	32	19	5	24	8	35	17	26	31
Drunk					20	29	16	22	21	5	24	10	38	17	26	35
Drugs							35	41	11	3	8	3	16	9	39	42
Marijuana									12	1	11	2	18	6	50	44
Entertainment																
Friends											24	21	26	22	24	5
Fun													40	32	21	7
Party															34	13
Getting high																

and alcohol or other drugs, and getting high is strictly a drug concept and does not overlap with their views of friends or entertainment as it does for the users. Comparisons of these matrices of relatedness reveal similarities as well as differences in the cognitive organization of users and of nonusers. The independently obtained results are in line with the basic conclusions of our comparative imaging analysis. They reflect differences in the respondents' subjective worlds, built on their different images and differences in organization. The findings support the idea that there is a hidden underlying organizational structure that can be identified by independent methods of assessment. They support the model of cognitive–semantic representations. How much this cognitive–semantic organization effectively controls the respondents' behavior is demonstrated in the following chapters.

Psychological Distance—How Far Apart Are Users and Nonusers?

Psychological distance is expressed by a single numerical value that indicates how far apart individuals or groups are in the images reconstructed by the imaging process. We are especially interested in differences in images that are related to differences in behavior between users and nonusers.

Within the AGA technology there are several measures of distance (see appendix). In this comparative study of users and nonusers, we use the Distance score found by calculating the degree of overlap of the response sets from the two groups (i.e., their similarity) and subtracting that number from 100% (perfect)

TABLE 3.4. Distance Score of Users and Nonusers

Domain/Theme	User-nonuser distance	Domain/Theme	User-nonuser distance
Self and family		Social values	
ME	32	AUTHORITY	24
I AM	31	DISCIPLINE	30
FAMILY	20	RESPONSIBILITY	30
FATHER	25	RELIGION	24
mean	27	mean	27
Social institutions		Drugs and alcohol	
SCHOOL	26	ALCOHOL	41
CAMPUS	25	DRUGS	38
SOCIETY	34	MARIJUANA	48
GOVERNMENT	28	DRUNK	44
mean	28	mean	43
Friends and entertainment		Problems	
FRIENDS	27	PROBLEMS	28
FUN	32	HOOKED	23
PARTY	31	SMOKING	31
GETTING HIGH	66	FEAR	28
mean	39	mean	28
Overall mean	32		

overlap. The larger the Distance score, the more the two groups are different with respect to their dominant perceptions and attitudes revealed by their reactions to the select stimulus themes. The Distance measure is inversely related to the degree of similarity of the user and of the nonuser responses to the same stimulus concept: the more alike the two groups are, the smaller the distance between them.

The Distance scores offer another empirical measure to test the assumption that people who behave differently also think differently. Although the Distance measure does not tell what the dominant psychological dispositions are or what to do about them, it offers a clear indication of where to look for them. Distance scores calculated for 24 stimulus words ranged from 20 to 66, with a mean score of 32 (see Table 3.4). The users and nonusers agree the most on the theme of fAM-ILY with a relatively small distance score of 20. The greatest distance (least overlap) between the groups was 66, measured on the theme of GETTING HIGH.

The average user–nonuser Distance of 43 for the four alcohol/drug-related images was much greater than the average Distance of 30 for the other 20 images. This sizable difference in distance scores offers further support that the alcohol- and drug-related images are important and influential in shaping substance abuse behavior. The Distance is large for ALCOHOL and for DRUNK. This indicates that users and nonusers are further apart on these images than on any other images that we compared. Users and nonusers are less far apart in the Friends/Entertainment domain, except regarding their views of GETTING HIGH.

Whereas we have begun our presentation with the two domains that we found most informative for explaining the differences in behavior between users and nonusers, it is not surprising that the images in those domains have among the largest Distance scores. These findings are supported by literally hundreds of thousands of spontaneous responses elicited by the imaging technology and are in fundamental agreement with logical expectations. They offer a simple and direct measure that shows how the images of users and of nonusers compare in terms of their overall similarity or distance. In comparing users and nonusers, the Distance data show on what images and domains the users and nonusers are the closest and on which ones they are farthest apart. Considering our focus on psychological dispositions leading to substance abuse, the images and domains that show the largest distance are of particular interest. In accessing the hidden worlds of users and of nonusers, large distances are indicative of differential perceptual and attitudinal dispositions that accompany their differences in behavior.

Used in combination with comparative imaging, the Distance measure offers a simple diagnostic tool that can be used to identify the images and domains that deserve closer attention. Then, comparative imaging offers a means of identifying the particular perceptual and motivational dispositions that differentiate users and nonusers. In planning and targeting prevention programs, the identification of these differential dispositions is of considerable practical interest.

Compared to the Affinity measure, which reveals the cognitive organization of each group's world and the cognitive–semantic organization of their behavior, the Distance scores show how select images in two different worlds compare. To understand these invisible systems, it is helpful to reconstruct them along the main parameters informative on their functioning.

MODELS OF COGNITIVE–SEMANTIC REPRESENTATIONS

As we have said, the comparison of users and nonusers serves a dual purpose. First, it is informative to know how different they are in their images, and second, their differences in perceptions and attitudes reveal psychological dispositions that are at the foundation of their differences in behavior. We trace the system of cognitive–semantic representations along several parameters of organization. We look at the dominance scores to see which are the most important images and which are the least important ones shaping behavior regarding alcohol and other drug use. The evaluation scores tell us which attitudinal differences are the most influential in affecting substance use. The affinity scores reveal how the images cluster and are consistent with use. The Distance measures show which images have the largest differences and the most influence on substance abuse.

Recognizing that these parameters are interrelated, we aim to reconstruct the system of cognitive–semantic representations regarding its impact on the behavior of substance abuse. Figure 3.1 presents a schematic model of cognitive–semantic

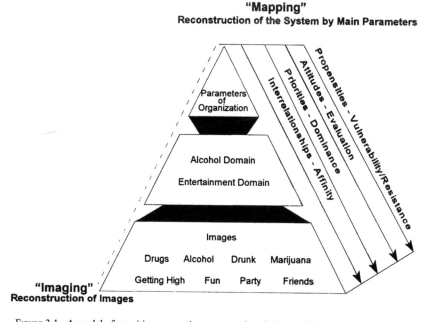

FIGURE 3.1. A model of cognitive–semantic representation: Sphere of "Alcohol, Entertainment".

representations to illustrate the relation between imaging and mapping as two complementary approaches in the task of multidimensional assessment.

In this model, mapping relies predominantly on analyses performed along the vertical dimensions of this system; comparative imaging is focused on the images, their relationship, and the dispositions they reveal across units of cognitive–semantic representations; they are characterized primarily by horizontal ties.

The findings presented in these chapters tell us a great deal about the system of cognitive–semantic representations characteristic of users and of nonusers. They show that groups with different behaviors differ in their overall systems as well as in their particular images. Before going further with this subject, we take a look at information available on the working of the system, as offered by other scientific disciplines.

An Independent View of Images and Systems from Neurobiology

Systems and their impact on behavior are not among the popular research topics of behavioral science. An important exception is neurobiology. With its interest in the neural system as the key to human behavior, neurobiology is a discipline of exceptional knowledge about the role of the neural system in organizing and directing behavior. In previous decades when stimulus–response behaviorism discouraged scientists from looking behind and beyond observable behavior, the neurobiologists kept acquiring a unique treasure chest of information far ahead of most other behavioral science disciplines.

In a recent book, *Descartes' error: Emotion, reason and the human brain*, neurologist Antonio Damasio (1994) offers a state-of-the-art account of the working of the body/mind as a single integrated system of neural representations and organization. This system, built on trillions of synapses, billions of neurons, and miles of neural connections provides guidance and organization that assures a continuous adaptation of the person to a constantly changing world.

The discipline of neurobiology offers fascinating new insights into the functioning of the neural system and its central role in organizing and shaping behavior. Parallel to the principles identified by Damasio (1994), our findings offer specifics on how images work reflecting on dispositions and on propensities to use or not to use harmful substances. As the reader is aware, our findings are based on large samples of student populations.

The System of Neural Representations Is Built on Images

How does the neural system, the body/mind system, guide the organism in ways essential to its survival? How does the neural system receive and retain information on the changing environment? How does it use the information to adapt behavior to thrive in a world filled with changes and challenges? According to Damasio and other neurobiologists and brain researchers, the center of this enigma is a system of neural representations built on "topographically organized neural images" (A. R. Damasio & Damasio, 1993; Kosslyn *et al.*, 1993; Shepard & Cooper, 1982).

In contrast to the popular tendency to view images as simple, static visual representations of persons, events, and so forth, Damasio (1994), Dennett (1991), and others describe neural images as different in several important ways. They are composite products of changing composition. They are pieced together from elements of past and of present experiences. They involve highly selective reproductions of elements of the external realities.

Our findings on mental images support Damasio (1994) and other neuroscientists who discuss neural images, their nature, composition, and functioning. We may consider, for instance, the image of ALCOHOL, one of the many images we discussed in some detail in the first few chapters. Figure 3.2 presents the mental image as a "semantograph"; the main components of the users' image are depicted by the black bars, and those of the nonusers' image by white bars in a circular arrangement. On three main components—Bad , Stupid . . . , Party, Bar . . . , Fun, Good . . .—the mosaic pieces of the users' and nonusers' images revealed by their actual responses and their score values are presented in detail. The images of ALCOHOL and all of the other images presented in previous chapters show wide variations by image and by group. The wide range in score values shows how the salience of the specific mosaic elements varies. The images show how different experiences influence the composition of a particular image. They show how images are subjective representations that omit certain details of the external world and include others that exist only in the mind of the observer. They show how the neural images are shaped and how they vary by parameters in the system of neural representations of particular populations (e.g., users and nonusers). Whereas the conclusions of neurobiology are based on the working of the neural system, ours are based on the reconstruction of mental images in the system of cognitive–semantic representations. Figure 3.2 presents a semantograph of the mental image of ALCOHOL and highlights some clusters in the image that may be helpful in the following discussion to convey the similarities between our work with mental images and Damasio's (1994) work with neural images.

Neural Images Are Built from Sensory and Emotional Elements

Damasio's (1994) explanation of the foundation of neural images on the system of the neural representations is based on the observations of neurobiologists about the working of the neural system. Neural representations are aggregates of past experiences which retain sensory as well as emotional elements. They accumulate over the history of the person and retain elements of past experiences. Compared to the sensory elements of experiences registered in the neurocortex, Damasio identifies a second category with emotional content registered by limbic centers

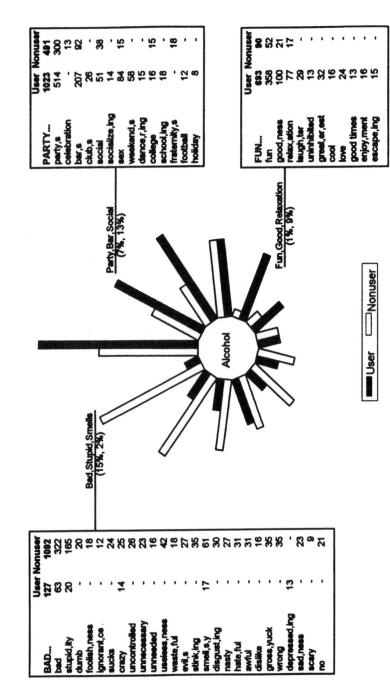

BAD...	User	Nonuser
bad	127	1092
stupid,ity	63	322
dumb	20	165
foolish,ness	-	20
ignorant,ce	-	18
sucks	-	12
crazy	14	24
uncontrolled	-	25
unnecessary	-	26
unneeded	-	23
useless,ness	-	16
waste,ful	-	42
evil,s	-	18
stink,ing	-	27
smell,s,y	17	35
disgust,ing	-	61
nasty	-	30
hate,ful	-	27
awful	-	31
dislike	-	31
gross,yuck	-	16
wrong	-	35
depressed,ing	13	35
sad,ness	-	23
scary	-	9
no	-	21

Bad, Stupid, Smells
(15%, 2%)

PARTY...	User	Nonuser
party,s	1023	491
celebration	514	300
bar,s	-	13
club,s	207	92
social	26	-
socialize,ing	51	38
sex	14	-
weekend,s	84	15
dance,r,ing	58	-
college	15	-
school,ing	16	15
fraternity,s	18	-
football	-	18
holiday	12	-
	8	-

Party, Bar, Social
(7%, 13%)

FUN...	User	Nonuser
fun	693	90
good,ness	358	52
relax,ation	100	21
laugh,ter	77	17
uninhibited	29	-
great,er,est	13	-
cool	32	-
love	16	-
good times	24	-
enjoy,ment	13	-
escape,ing	16	-
	15	-

Fun, Good, Relaxation
(1%, 9%)

Alcohol

■ User □ Nonuser

FIGURE 3.2 The image of ALCOHOL by users and nonusers reflecting different mosaics in their perceptions and evaluations.

outside of awareness. As the example of ALCOHOL illustrates, in some cases it is easy to differentiate elements that come from the sensory centers (e.g., smell) from emotion-laden elements (e.g., disgusting); however, the majority of image mosaics suggest a mixture that has sensory content with emotions attached (e.g., laughter, relaxation). Some of these mosaic pieces of images have a directly observable physical foundation, whereas others exist only in the person's mind or in their system of cognitive–semantic representations.

The image of ALCOHOL, for example, includes elements from friends, entertainment, harm and risks, family, children, love and sex, and other domains of life. How far-branching are its connections across other domains varies according to the experiences of the particular group, such as users and nonusers.

As the ALCOHOL example illustrates, these connections involve contrasting perceptions and attitudes that, in turn, serve as the foundation of two contrasting behaviors. The relation between contrasting choices in behavior and contrasting trends of perceptions and attitudes is explicit and consistent. The scores for the mosaics of perceptions and attitudes in a component of negative evaluations (*bad, stupid, useless*) are consistently more salient for nonusers than are the responses from users in this same category (Figure 3.2), indicating that these elements are shaped not simply by single experiences working in isolation, but by systemic influences.

Neural Images Are Integrated Units of a System of Multidimensional Representation

As part of a broad systemic foundation, neural images work as integrated units of representation. As demonstrated decades ago by Jones and Powell (1970), various centers of the cortex do not connect directly with each other or with the motor controls. According to Damasio (1994), at the level of the cerebral cortex, for instance, each sensory area must talk first to a variety of interposed regions which talk to regions further away, and so forth. Thus, the communication among input sectors and between input and output sectors is not direct but rather intermediate. There is a complex architecture of complex neuron assemblies that provide flexibility and integration. Similarly, investigators focusing on particular cortical representations of different sense modalities—visual (Tononi, Sporns, & Edelman, 1992; Zeki, 1992) and auditory (Adolphs, 1993; Konishi, Takahashi, Wagner, Sullivan, & Carr, 1988)—show that sensory data from diverse cortical centers do not activate behavior directly; only after they have been integrated with each other do they activate behavior.

Our Affinity scores (Table 3.3) further illustrate differences in the foundation of the mental images. They reflect that the relationship among the domains of life do differ for users and nonusers. As we have seen, the image of ALCOHOL had more in common with their image of FRIENDS for users than for nonusers. The results in

Table 3.3 show that this relation has a broad foundation that goes beyond a single image. In the case of the users, the domain of Alcohol and Drugs has across the board a stronger affinity to the domain of Friends and Entertainment.

Neural Images Have a Dispositional Foundation

Neural images are characterized as *dispositional representations,* conveying that they not only represent external and internal realities but also dispositions toward certain choices and behaviors regarding the world that they represent. The mental images identified through comparative imaging reveal in a similar vein dominant perceptual and motivational dispositions to behave as directed by the very nature of these mental representations.

The specific response mosaics in the three highlighted components of the image of ALCOHOL (Figure 3.2) reveal some strong foundations in emotions and in positive or negative attitudes. The contrasting perceptions and attitudes of users and of nonusers clearly convey that members of these groups have internal dispositions to make contrasting choices regarding alcohol. The perceptions and attitudes shown by the users predispose them to vulnerabilities and the propensity to use alcohol. The perceptions and attitudes of the nonusers show the contrasting dispositions, that is, a propensity to resist alcohol use. Such contrasting dispositions are revealed by comparative imaging. Another way to assess behavioral propensities from the imaging data is by obtaining prevalence scores calculated across one or more domains. Profiles of prevalence scores are constructed based on the categories of responses whose scores were consistently higher for one group (e.g., users) contrasted with the response categories whose scores were higher for the other group. The prevalence profiles of users and of nonusers in Figure 3.3 are the result of analyses based on the comparison of 400 users and 400 nonusers on six response categories on which users scored higher contrasted with the prevalence scores of nonusers on six contrasting response categories. The prevalence profiles offer a brief summary.

The difference between the users' and the nonusers' total score for a cluster is the Prevalence score (e.g., if the score was higher for users than for nonusers, it indicates a prevalent user trend). Figure 3.3 shows the following distinctions: Users are clearly preoccupied with social entertainment—fun, parties—to a far greater extent than Nonusers; their social interest is also evident in their greater attention to friends and other people. Users obviously emphasize alcohol, drugs, getting drunk and high, and smoking. Nonusers, on the other hand, are very critical of alcohol and other drugs, describing them as bad and stupid; they are especially concerned with the dangers, harm, and the possibility of death. Health has a high priority. Nonusers show greater concern with abuse and addiction. There is also more emphasis among nonusers on loving, caring, and helping others.

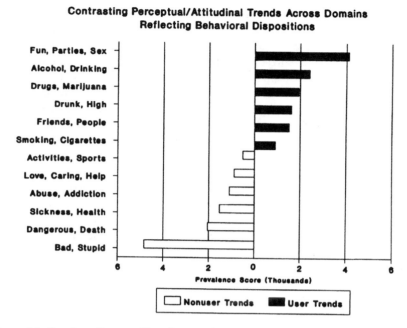

FIGURE 3.3. Prevalence Score profiles of users and nonusers based on the domains of Alcohol and Drugs, Problems, and Friends and Entertainment.

The images, which serve as the foundation of prevalence trends, their positive/negative affect loading, and the consistency differentiating users and nonusers of harmful substances convey clearly a sense of how certain attitudes and perceptions promote the propensity to use harmful substances and how others promote resistance to use them. The push and pull of these contrasting propensities offer a sense of the dynamism of contrasting behavioral dispositions promoted by neural images.

The following chapters show how dominant perceptual and attitudinal dispositions serve as the foundation for the identification of users and of nonusers. Our research has shown that a person's choice about using harmful substances is consistent with his or her propensities of vulnerability or resistance, as inferred from the mental images.

Images: Neural Representations—"On Line"

A particularly important implication of the dispositional character of neural images bears on their role in shaping behavior. As Damasio (1994) characterizes the process, the neural representations aggregated from different cortical and subcortical limbic centers form neural images, and these neural images are continuously modified and updated by new experiences. Most important, they remain continuously "on line," as Damasio puts it, ready to make their input to behavior as aggregate representations of integrated knowledge and experience.

In the imaging and mapping approach, the perceptual and attitudinal mosaics serve a similar purpose. The relation between mental images and behavior is demonstrated by our measure of aggregate propensities of vulnerability and of resistance, a measure of dispositions to use or not to use harmful substances. In the following chapters we explain the process by which vulnerability and resistance is measured and how behavioral influences are validated.

In the final chapter we return to the discussion of the close parallels between our work and neurobiology and how our approach relates to some of the latest developments in other fields. In the context of our immediate interest in explaining how images influence behavior, our findings are consistent with findings in neurobiology that show that images are more than simple visual facsimiles of objects and people in the environment; they are immensely more complex products of neural representations that include not only the sense modalities but also symbolic/semantic representations and the invisible influences of past positive and negative experiences. These composite images become influential in shaping choices and behavior without the person's awareness. We show how these mosaic elements of representation vary by comparing the images of users and of nonusers. How mental images influence personal choices and decisions is shown and validated by the results in the following chapters.

When we return at the end to neurobiology and its three main conclusions, which are of special relevance to our results, we will be in a better position to place the system of neural representations in proper perspective regarding its fascinating role in shaping people's worlds in many ways beyond their conscious awareness. Though neurobiology has no specific interest in substance abuse or in its prevention, we hope that the capability we are developing to identify categories of behavioral dispositions as they affect behavior may have some relevance to neurobiology as well.

THE WORLD OF USERS AND OF NONUSERS AS SHOWN
BY THE PARAMETERS

The imaging and mapping findings we have presented on users and on nonusers offer new insights from a number of different perspectives—what is important, what is related, and so forth. How these different perspectives affect the worlds and the dominant perceptions and attitudes of users and of nonusers has been assessed by several independent measures. The findings obtained by these independent measures showed the following trends.

The differences between users and nonusers appeared with a high degree of consistency across the six domains compared. The findings were consistent in showing how the domains examined had different effects, following a clearly identifiable order of magnitude regarding their relative impact on drug-related decisions and behaviors. The domain of Alcohol and Drugs has shown the most difference, followed by the domain of Fun and Entertainment.

An essential agreement emerged, despite the clear differences revealed by the independent measures. The parameters traced by different measures of assessment are indeed part of a large system of cognitive–semantic representations. This is the foundation for different systems of behavioral organization, one for users and one for nonusers, one leading to use and the other to nonuse. Further examples in the appendix show differences in the system of cognitive–semantic representations of other student samples of different ages.

The differences demonstrated along the parameters of this analysis show how the differences in behavior have a broad foundation in the inner worlds of these two groups. Although we already demonstrated this in the context of selected images, the present chapter goes a step further to show that the differences in images are part of a broad system of cognitive–semantic representation. The system can be analyzed and described along selected parameters of organization in the mind of the group.

Practically all of the findings have their foundation in the users' and the nonusers' images that, in our theoretical model, are the building blocks of the inner world—the system of cognitive–semantic representations. This system serves as the organizing force of choices and behavior (e.g., to use drugs or not use them). The practical value of a system-based analysis will become increasingly apparent from the comparison of the image-based analysis and the systemic analysis performed along select parameters.

Complementary Insights from Imaging and Mapping

In contrast to the detailed findings from comparative imaging, the analyses performed along the select parameters of the system produce general information on the world of users and of nonusers in a concise form. Whereas comparative imaging focuses on the specific images of users and of nonusers, the analyses we have discussed in this chapter focus on the reconstruction of larger and larger areas of the groups' subjective world along selected parameters. This second, more inclusive systemic analysis is what we refer to as cognitive mapping. Each of these two main assessment strategies has its own distinct advantages, and the novelty and value of the information they produce are the result of their combined use. Since we have already discussed results produced by comparative imaging, we can now turn our attention to cognitive mapping and how it helps to expand and to use what we have learned from comparative imaging.

As a simple analogy we like the example of the blindfolded scientists trying to describe the elephant, each tapping a different part of it. The cognitive map offers a proportionate reproduction of the elephant that shows where the specific parts that each one is tapping fit into the whole image. The map, produced along the various parameters, helps to place the various parts in proper relation to each other. The Dominance data show what is dominant in the eyes of the users and what is dominant in the eyes of the nonusers. The Attitude data show what the users like in contrast to the nonusers. The Affinity data show that the elephant has a somewhat different structure (e.g., African vs. Asian elephants) in the sense that its parts stand in somewhat different relation to each other in the two systems as they do in the worlds of users and of nonusers. The Distance data offer another useful perspective for identifying pieces that require attention.

The findings produced by imaging are in no way contradictory to the results of the mapping. They are in fact complementary. With this awareness, any initial impressions of being overwhelmed by detailed image data is likely to disappear. Just as for the blindfolded scientist who did not know what part of the elephant he was touching, uncertainty disappears once there is access to a map that shows where each part is in relation to the whole. Also, if he realizes that this is not the part in which he is interested, the map tells him what to look for and where to go.

The cognitive map provides orientation in the private world of cognitive–semantic representations. In this new world the cognitive maps have two main functions. They show where to look for what we are interested in and they show what is important and related in the world of users and in the world of nonusers and where to find it. Once the relevant area of interest is located, the detailed image data are rich in information that suggests its best use.

Finally, the new data on the cognitive maps and their main parameters offer compelling empirical evidence that human behavior has a solid foundation in a cognitive-behavioral organization:

- Behind the images there is a powerful system of cognitive–semantic representations which is different for Users and for Nonusers.
- What we identify as the world of Users and the world of Nonusers appears to be the source of their differences in behavior.
- The system provides a natural framework for the images we have analyzed: it determines their place, their role, and their functioning as well.
- Information on the system provides an overview and reduces the need to know all of the details about the many differences between Users and Nonusers. The generic maps reconstructed on the system along its main parameters make it possible to use the image data more selectively as required by particular applications.

As we discuss in the later chapters on applications, a combined use of the image data and the results of cognitive mapping offers two categories of new information on the dominant psychological dispositions and environmental conditions that lead to substance abuse. This new information and technology can be used in the development of prevention programs systematically targeting the key factors that can make a difference.

The System's Relevance to Substance Abuse

We have discussed the reconstruction of the system of cognitive–semantic representations along such parameters as what is of importance, what has appeal, and what is related to what in the subjective worlds of users and of nonusers. Using analytic measures developed to assess these parameters, we mapped two systems of cognitive-behavioral organization, one characteristic of users and the other characteristic of nonusers. Cognitive mapping of these two systems provides the guidance and orientation for using the extensive information produced through comparative imaging. Understanding the system of cognitive–behavioral organization as a whole is important to the use of the new information in planning and development of effective prevention programs.

Up to this point we have been laying the essential groundwork for the introduction of another parameter of the system: Vulnerability/Resistance. Since the late 1980s we have focused on an assessment of the aggregates of psychological dispositions, those promoting substance abuse as well as those resisting it. Compared to other parameters that bear on other behavior besides substance abuse, the Vulnerability/Resistance measure has been designed to reflect the overall aggregate of positive versus negative propensity for substance abuse.

In this chapter we have discussed, beyond the specific images and their differences, the organization that holds the images together. We have attempted to explain how an organized system of images directs behavior. This lineage of connection and behavioral organization is generally not understood because it is not directly observable, but it is central in the identification of dominant psychological dispositions that differentiate users from nonusers. It is also central in the development of systematic strategies and programs targeting variables that can make a difference.

The system, as introduced and measured along several dimensions in this chapter, plays a critical role in determining a person's general propensity to use or not use harmful substances. Much of our research has dealt with the systematic development of a measure built on the aggregates of dispositions that either promote or work against decisions to use these substances. To distinguish this multidimensional assessment from comparative imaging, we discuss it under the more generic label of cognitive mapping. Cognitive mapping is the topic of the following chapters in which we introduce this specialized measure for assessing aggregate propensities along two complementary directions: those promoting substance abuse and those working against it in the world of the student, considered individually as well as collectively.

Part II

The Assessment of Vulnerability/Resistance
through Cognitive Mapping

The Measurement of Vulnerability/Resistance
The Propensity for Substance Abuse

Dominant trends of perceptions and attitudes provide the foundation for contrasting sets of psychological dispositions. In turn, they provide information about powerful influences affecting drug use. This chapter introduces the tool for tracing and mapping these hidden influences by the measure of Vulnerability/Resistance. Based on computer-assisted mapping of the users' and of the nonusers' worlds, this diagnostic tool gauges the respondent's propensity to use or not to use harmful substances. We describe the computation and scoring system developed to identify dominant perceptual and motivational dispositions and measure their combined effects resulting in the contrasting propensities for use and for resistance to use.

THE COMMON EXPERIENCE OF VULNERABILITY OR SUSCEPTIBILITY

It is a common experience that some people are more prone than others to accidents or sickness. Elderly people are vulnerable to falling and fracturing their bones. By diagnosing the vulnerabilities and identifying the fact that frequent fractures are related to osteoporosis, a deficiency of calcium in the bones, we can begin to explain their frequent accidents. By identifying the cause of the vulnerability it is possible to develop methods, such as diet and medication, to function as effective preventive measures. Vulnerability to bone fractures is different in many important ways from vulnerability to substance abuse. Whereas many of the differences are important and consequential, what they have in common is that by identifying the sources of vulnerability, it is possible to trace the relevant causes. Identification of causes is the most important prerequisite of scientific prevention.

Vulnerability to Substance Abuse

It is becoming increasingly common to speak of vulnerability to substance abuse based on the growing recognition that people vary in their predispositions to become involved in drug use. Leading drug researchers, such as Glantz and Pickens (1992), Sher (1994), and Tarter and Vanyukov (1994) speak in a general sense of vulnerability to substance abuse. They recognize that certain dispositions and conditions make some people prone to use or abuse alcohol and other drugs and other people more likely to avoid such abuse. We think that vulnerability is a key to the enigma of substance abuse as a broad psychosocial problem. We define *vulnerability* as a composite of psychological dispositions toward experimentation and habitual use of alcohol and other drugs. The propensity to use harmful substances contrasts with a propensity to avoid experimentation and to remain drug free.

In line with our interest in diagnostic applications, we use vulnerability as a scientific construct that can be empirically linked to the use of alcohol and other drugs. The construct of vulnerability is strongly founded in the etiology of substance abuse and on psychological factors operative in the phase preceding chemical dependence or addiction.

In every aspect of life scientific prevention depends on systematic control of the key contributing factors to the problem. In substance abuse prevention, *psychological vulnerability* refers to dispositions that promote substance abuse and that need to be redirected through effective prevention strategies. That is why we focus on the empirical identification and measurement of dominant dispositions that are contributing to experimentation and to use.

Our interest has taken us beyond talking about vulnerability in general terms and on to the challenge of measuring it. As in the case of measuring intelligence or achievement motivation as scientific constructs, measuring vulnerability to substance abuse requires the specification of a procedure to operationalize it. Our Vulnerability measure is based on the dispositions differentiating users and nonusers, which we found through the comparative imaging process discussed earlier. In introducing vulnerability, we are aiming to say more than that users are vulnerable to substance abuse or that elderly people are vulnerable to osteoporosis. Our objective is to provide a quantitative diagnostic measure of practical value to effective prevention. To achieve that objective we must have criteria by which to test and to validate the results.

What We Have Learned from Comparative Imaging

In the first chapters we traced specific perceptual and attitudinal trends through comparative imaging. We found that the contrasting behavioral choices to use or not use alcohol and other drugs correlate closely with trends of perceptions and attitudes that emerge from our imaging method. The images of ALCOHOL, DRUGS,

MARIJUANA, and GETTING HIGH, as well as others have shown with considerable consistency that habitual users tend to perceive drug-related themes in a way that supports use. The nonusers tend to perceive these same themes in contrasting ways revealing perceptions and evaluations that support abstinence.

The contrasting trends of perceptions and evaluations for users and for nonusers suggested hidden dispositions that in the case of users revealed vulnerability and in the case of nonusers revealed sources of resistance. The mosaics of the perceptual and motivational trends emerging from the imaging process offer strong support for the measurement of vulnerability and resistance to substance abuse. They support the rationale of contrasting behavioral dispositions and offer a rich source of information on propensities leading to one behavior or to the other. In an indirect way the results of imaging also suggest that a systematic strategy for measuring the aggregate effect of vulnerabilities and resistance may offer a key to substance abuse prevention. Just as the identification of calcium deficiency was a key to finding effective prevention and treatment for osteoporosis, the identification of contributing factors in substance abuse is also a critical prerequisite to effective prevention.

There are some important distinctions to consider. In the case of osteoporosis, there is a single main cause and simple tests to measure bone density and calcium deficiency. Once identified, preventive measures can readily follow. In the case of substance abuse, there is no single cause but rather a variety of contributing factors. Their systematic and inclusive assessment presents a complex and demanding requirement.

What Have We Learned from Mapping

The perceptual and motivational trends in the domains of Drugs, Entertainment, Family, and Values provide ample indications of the users' dispositions to use harmful substances. Although these trends certainly suggest vulnerabilities, they do not in themselves fit the requirements for an effective diagnostic instrument.

In Chapter 3 we discussed our Dominance measures, Evaluation (attitude) measures, and Distance measures that further show that the world of users differs from the world of nonusers, not only in their images of ALCOHOL, DRUGS, and ENTERTAINMENT but also in some fundamental dimensions such as what they consider to be important, desirable, relevant, and so forth. In other words, users differ from nonusers in their internal world along select parameters that are fundamental to the organization of their behavior.

The findings suggest that a parameter of special interest to us in our research in substance abuse prevention may be assessed just as in mapping cognitive–behavioral organization along other parameters. The strategy described in the following was developed as a cognitive mapping task to measure vulnerability/resistance by identifying contrasting propensities for use or nonuse.

MEASURING VULNERABILITY TO SUBSTANCE ABUSE

The assessment of overall vulnerability/resistance approaches psychological dispositions from the opposite end of the spectrum. Instead of focusing on specific images, the aim is to reconstruct the system of cognitive–semantic representations along select parameters, which provides the foundation for behavioral organization. This mapping process relies on the computer-assisted analysis of thousands of spontaneous responses. By focusing on the differences between users and nonusers we arrive at the construct of vulnerability/resistance. The accumulation and aggregation is performed by computer, following the algorithm of specially developed software that operationalizes the key theoretical assumptions. Although the process of calculation is too extensive and technical to describe here, this step-by-step mapping analysis has the advantage of providing concise and conclusive results.

The Central Assumption

The assessment of vulnerability/resistance is based on the central assumption that people's choices regarding the use of alcohol and other drugs (as well as other behavior) is shaped by their internal world and by their dominant perceptions and motivations. Seeing the world as does a habitual alcohol/drug user produces natural propensities to engage in experimentation and to get progressively involved with drugs. In other words, the more a person perceives and evaluates the world as does a user, the stronger is his or her vulnerability to engage in drug use. In contrast, the more a person perceives and evaluates the world does as a nonuser, the stronger is his or her resistance to use drugs.

The imaging and mapping strategy offers a practical method to assess dominant perceptual dispositions, to map systems of mental representations, and to measure similarity to the world of users or to that of nonusers. These analytic capabilities make a systematic assessment of vulnerability/resistance possible. Habitual users and nonusers represent the groups at the opposite ends of a broad continuum. The vulnerability/resistance measure is based on the assumption that the more a person reveals aggregate propensities for use, the more vulnerable he or she is. We infer a person's position on a continuum of vulnerability/resistance by measuring the similarity of the respondent's world with the users' and with the nonusers' to get a measure of his or her vulnerability or resistance to substance abuse.

The imaging and mapping technology offers a solid foundation for testing these complementary assumptions. The results of such tests give conclusive feedback on the utility of the aforementioned principles to provide an empirically based measure of vulnerability/resistance.

Contrasting Propensities of Users and of Nonusers

Figure 4.1 is a schematic presentation of the contrasting trends observed between users and nonusers in some of their dominant perceptions and attitudes. The boxes on the left and on the right in Figure 4.1 show the contrasting perceptions of users and nonusers in the context of the domains identified in each circle. Each person or group reveals, by the nature and spontaneous distribution of its responses, dispositions to perceive these selected stimulus themes in the same way

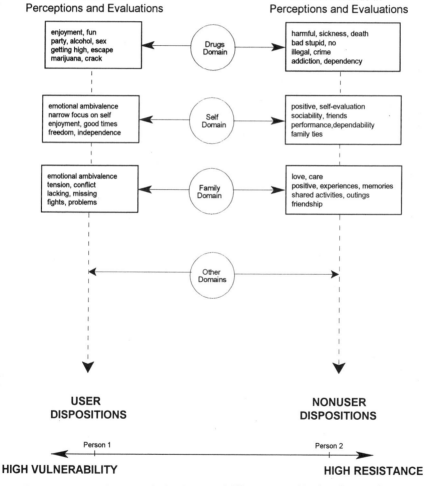

FIGURE 4.1. Perceptions and attitudes: Sources of different propensities for substance abuse.

as do users or nonusers. Based on such spontaneous response distributions, it is possible then to localize people along the continuum of high versus low vulnerability at the bottom of the diagram. Toward the left we show a score indicating high vulnerability, and to the right is a score at the low vulnerability (high resistance) end of the scale.

The response trends we have tracked in numerous groups over the many years of our research support the conclusion that there is a direct relation between substance abuse behavior and the users' system of dominant perceptions and attitudes. The stability of this relation and the sensitivity of our technology to map it made it possible to offer new empirical measures of vulnerability and resistance with a high degree of accuracy.

How We Measure Vulnerability/Resistance—Overall Propensity for Substance Abuse

Step 1. Identification of Responses that Differentiate Users from Nonusers (Reference Norms). First we selected a sample of frequent users of alcohol and drugs and a sample of nonusers from a pool of several thousand college students who provided data regarding use. Users are heavy alcohol users (daily or almost daily) or frequent alcohol users (1–3 times/week) who have used any illicit substance. Nonusers are students who have never used drugs or alcohol. We then identified the specific responses to each theme (ALCOHOL, FRIENDS, etc.) that had the largest difference in frequency for the two groups. We defined *discriminators* as any response that had a score difference of at least 30 and built a list of prevalent user responses and a list of nonuser responses. Figure 4.2 shows the responses to DRUNK that best differentiate users from nonusers.

USER RESPONSES		NONUSER RESPONSES	
(Score +1 for each match)		(Score -1 for each match)	
alcohol	party,s	accident,s	harm,ful
bar,s	problem,s	alcoholic,s	hate,ful
beer	puke,ing	bad	idiot,ic
drink,ing	sex	bum,s	irresponsible
fall,ing	shot,s	car,s	jail
forget,ing	sick,ness	crazy	kill,ing
friend,s	sleep,ing	danger,ous	m.a.d.d.
fun	sloppy	dead,ly	man,men
girl,s	stumble,ing	death	never
hangover,s	tipsy	disgust,ing	sad,ness
happy,ness	tonight	drive,ing	stupid,ity
keg,s	too much	driver,s	why
laugh,ter	wasted	dumb	wrong
me	weekend,s		
often			

FIGURE 4.2. Responses differentiating users and nonusers on the image of DRUNK.

Step 2. Comparison of the Individual's Responses to User and Nonuser Reference Norms. The Vulnerability/Resistance score for an individual is obtained by comparing his or her responses to all the stimulus themes to those on the user and nonuser response lists. A score of +1 is assigned for every response that is the same as one on the user list and a score of –1 is assigned for every response that matches one on the nonuser list (responses not on either list are not scored). Figure 4.3 displays the test slip responses of three different people to the stimulus word DRUNK and shows the Vulnerability scoring that would be made. Many of Person A's responses are like the responses of users, Person B's responses are more often like the responses of nonusers than users, and Person C has responses that are not consistent with either users or with nonusers.

Step 3. Calculation of the Cumulative Vulnerability/Resistance Score. As with the above example for DRUNK, there is a computerized Vulnerability scoring process that can be performed for each of the 24 stimulus themes, from FAMILY to GOVERNMENT and from FRIENDS to RESPONSIBILITY. The total Vulnerability/Resistance score for a person is compiled from the scoring for all of the stimulus terms. Typically, a person's total Vulnerability/Resistance score will be the net scoring from 150 to 200 individual responses. The individual's overall Vulnerability/Resistance score indicates the degree to which the person's perceptual disposition is more like a user or a nonuser. The higher the score, the greater the vulnerability. Students whose Vulnerability/Resistance scores fall in the negative range (below zero) are classified as Resistant. Their psychological dispositions are more like those of nonusers. We considered a student correctly identified if he or she was classified by the Vulnerability/Resistance score as Vulnerable and self-reported using alcohol or other drugs, or was classified as Resistant and self-reported abstinence.

Person A DRUNK			Person B DRUNK			Person C DRUNK		
DRUNK	*alcohol*	+1	DRUNK	*party,s*	+1	DRUNK	*driving*	-1
DRUNK	buzz,ed		DRUNK	*drive,ing*	-1	DRUNK	*alcohol*	+1
DRUNK	*fun*	+1	DRUNK	*kill,ing*	-1	DRUNK	*bar,s*	+1
DRUNK	fuzz,y		DRUNK	*stupid,ity*	-1	DRUNK	*party,s*	+1
DRUNK	*beer*	+1	DRUNK	funny		DRUNK	foolish,ness	
DRUNK	*stumble,ing*	+1	DRUNK	*happy,ness*	+1	DRUNK	fight,ing	
DRUNK	slur,s		DRUNK	*alcoholic,s*	-1	DRUNK	*stupid,ity*	-1
DRUNK	*friend,s*	+1	DRUNK	smoke,ing		DRUNK	*crazy*	-1
DRUNK	*party,s*	+1	DRUNK			DRUNK	not thinking	
DRUNK	college		DRUNK			DRUNK		
DRUNK	fraternity,s		DRUNK			DRUNK		
DRUNK			DRUNK			DRUNK		
Score for Drunk:		+6	Score for Drunk:		-2	Score for Drunk:		0

FIGURE 4.3. Sample test slips: How vulnerability/resistance is scored.

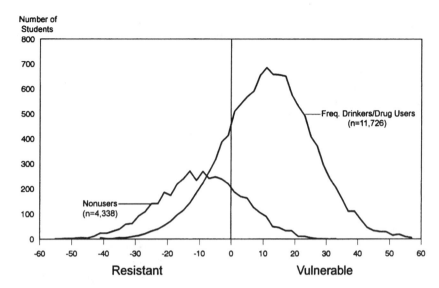

FIGURE 4.4. The distribution of Vulnerability/Resistance scores for nonusers and frequent drinkers/drug users in the college population.

We close this chapter by presenting in Figure 4.4, the distribution of Vulnerability/Resistance scores of 16,064 college students whose self-reports indicated they were nonusers or frequent drinkers/drug users. About 80% of the nonusers/abstainers, the smallest group of students, had Vulnerability/Resistance scores below zero, indicating resistance to substance abuse. The group of binge drinkers and drug users are located mostly on the other side of the scale (again, about 80% of these students) at varying degrees of vulnerability to substance abuse. Students who, based on their self-reports, were categorized as "occasional drinkers" ($N =$ 13,327) fall mostly in between. We use this visual presentation to convey the proportions correctly identified as frequent users and nonusers in the total population of the students tested.

Extending beyond the reference groups of Users and Nonusers, the findings support in general the following:

• Positive Vulnerability/Resistance scores can be used to identify habitual users with a high degree of accuracy.
• Negative Vulnerability/Resistance scores are useful to identify nonusers with a similar degree of accuracy.

These findings obtained on large samples offer strong support to our central assumption. They show that the cognitive mapping measures offer valid results by gauging the similarity of the respondents' world with that of reference groups of habitual users and nonusers. The general validation of this fundamental principle shown in Figure 4.4 opens the opportunity to test a series of hypotheses that will be helpful to examine the validity of the findings in further detail. The next chapter offers findings on vulnerabilities related to the use of various substances as shown by the Vulnerability/Resistance measure.

5

Vulnerability and Resistance
The Effects of Using Various Harmful Substances

To test the information value of the Vulnerability/Resistance measure, our large college student population offers a broad foundation. We computed Vulnerability/Resistance scores for each of the tens of thousands of students on whom we also had independent data regarding their self-reported use of alcohol and other drugs. The results showed a direct relationship between the propensity measured through mapping and the level of use reported. This relationship is very close on all substances examined, from tobacco to crack cocaine. Naturally, there are some characteristic variations in how the vulnerabilities measured are distributed across the various substances and populations.

Is the Measurement of Vulnerability a Pipe Dream or Reality?

Not only is our interest in vulnerability uncommon and nontraditional but our approach is as well. The question of vulnerability requires special attention. Is what we are measuring inherently linked to substance use? In other words, does vulnerability increase with greater frequency of use? Does the use of one substance affect vulnerability more than the use of another substance? How does the vulnerability measured in relation to alcohol use compare with vulnerability measured in relation to marijuana use? What is the nature and scope of similarity or difference? In general, how do survey data on the level of reported use of alcohol and other drugs compare with the vulnerability/resistance data obtained through mapping the vulnerability/resistance dimension?

Beyond the finding that the Vulnerability/Resistance measure could be used to identify users and nonusers at an 80% success rate, there are other ways to examine the validity of this new measure. Since we did ask the students about their use of particular substances, we could explore how the students' reported use compared to their Vulnerability/Resistance scores. In our research on college student drug and alcohol involvement, we calculated the Vulnerability scores for each student tested at all of the campus sites. The levels of measured vulnerability/resistance closely correspond with the levels of self-reported use of alcohol, tobacco, and other drugs.

How the Students' Vulnerability Compares to Their Self-Reported Use

Of our sample of nearly 30,000 college students, 15% were identified as nonusers (abstainers), and 40% were identified as frequent drinkers and/or illicit drug users based on self-reported use. This user classification includes students who reported

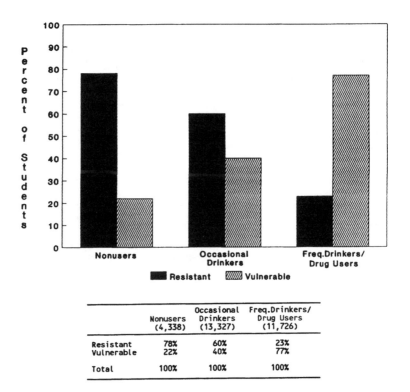

	Nonusers (4,338)	Occasional Drinkers (13,327)	Freq.Drinkers/ Drug Users (11,726)
Resistant	78%	60%	23%
Vulnerable	22%	40%	77%
Total	100%	100%	100%

FIGURE 5.1. Proportion of students vulnerable or resistant to substance abuse at three levels of reported use.

binge drinking at least once a week (i.e., 2 or more times in the past two weeks), consuming an average of 10 or more drinks per week, daily alcohol use, or any use of illicit drugs. The remaining 45% percent were classified as "occasional drinkers." Naturally, the pie might be cut in many other ways, depending on varying definitions of who is a user and who is an abuser, but for the purposes of exploring psychological vulnerability, we chose these three simple categories.

In Figure 5.1 we show the proportion of students in these three usage categories who were vulnerable or resistant to substance abuse. Students whose Vulnerability/Resistance score was above zero were classified as vulnerable to substance use because they were thinking and perceiving in ways more similar to users. About 80% of the nonusers appeared to be Resistant whereas only 23% of students who are frequent drinkers or drug users exhibited resistance. About 40% of the occasional drinkers showed vulnerability to substance abuse.

VULNERABILITY ASSOCIATED WITH USE OF SPECIFIC SUBSTANCES

Student Drinking and Vulnerability

If psychological dispositions, as measured by our Vulnerability/Resistance score, really do impact substance use, then we would expect to see Vulnerability/Resistance scores increase as self-reported frequency of alcohol use increases. The simplest way to test this prediction was to check the extent to which high Vulnerability corresponds with frequent use. We asked students on campus to estimate the average number of drinks they consumed in a week. We found that a third reported having less than 5 drinks a week and another third (37%) did not have any drinks on a weekly basis. The average consumption, based on this large college student population, was 5.5 drinks per week. Still, more than 10% reported having 15 or more drinks per week. Without asking the students directly, we were able to determine from their free responses to the imaging task whether their vulnerability increased along with their frequency of drinking. Figure 5.2 shows that, indeed, the students' level of psychological vulnerability rose with each increasing number of drinks.

Vulnerability is related not only to alcohol use but also to the use of many other substances. We used a number of questions to determine the extent of involvement with various substances and its impact on vulnerability to substance abuse. As a general indicator we simply asked, "How often do you drink alcohol?"; "How often do you smoke cigarettes?"; and "How often do you use marijuana?" When we examined the students' level of vulnerability along with their self-reported use of these substances, we found that vulnerability is directly tied to the level of use, regardless of the substance.

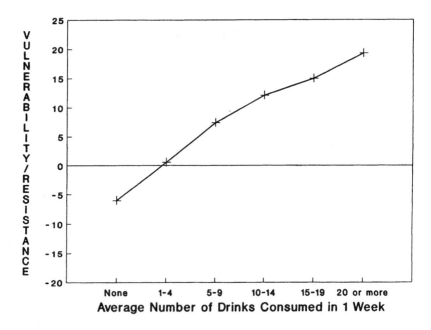

FIGURE 5.2. Reported weekly alcohol consumption and vulnerability.

Cigarette Smoking and Vulnerability

Unlike drinking behavior, where we found a fairly even distribution of students across the middle, but fewer at the extremes, we found most people at the extremes as nonsmokers or daily smokers. From the anonymous self-reports, the majority of college students (58%) do not smoke at all. In addition, there were 15% who only smoked on rare occasions (1–6 times a year). However, for those who do choose to smoke cigarettes, less than half do so in moderation. In our total student sample, 16% were daily smokers. Figure 5.3 shows vulnerability as a function of smoking frequency for the entire sample and demonstrates the following:

- As smoking frequency increases, Vulnerability to substance abuse also increases.
- There is a sharp increase in Vulnerability even among the rare smokers (1–6 times per year).
- Only 3% of the students who smoke abstain from alcohol and other drugs.

Marijuana Use and Vulnerability

Marijuana is the most widely used illicit drug among college students. In our research at over 50 colleges across the nation, prevalence of use (based on self-reports) ranged from 4% to 63%. In the total student sample, 29% reported us-

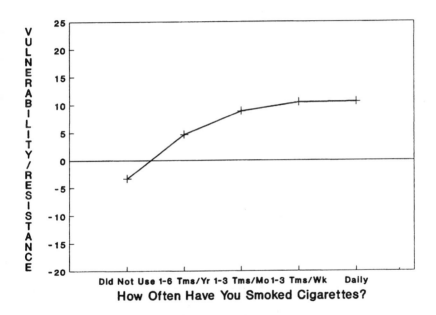

How Often Have You Smoked Cigarettes?	All Students (28,833)
Did Not Use	58%
1-6 Times/Year	15%
1-3 Times/Month	6%
1-3 Times/Week	5%
Daily/Almost Daily	16%
Total	100%

FIGURE 5.3. Reported frequency of cigarette smoking and vulnerability.

ing marijuana. About half of those are rare users (1–6 times/year). The relation between level of reported use of marijuana and psychological vulnerability to substance abuse is shown in Figure 5.4 and is summarized as follows:

- The 71% who do not use marijuana show resistance whereas those who do use marijuana show increasing vulnerability to substance abuse.
- The greatest increase in vulnerability is just at the point of experimentation: from no use to 1 to 6 times a year. Highest vulnerability is found among the daily users (less than 3% of the total student population).
- The levels of vulnerability among marijuana users are of a much greater magnitude than those found among alcohol drinkers: the vulnerability of weekly drinkers is roughly equivalent to that of students who use marijuana 1 to 6 times a year.

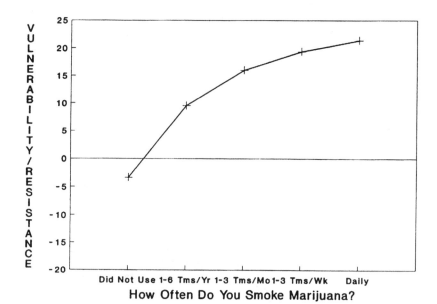

How Often Have You Smoked Marijuana?	All Students (28,239)
Did Not Use	71%
1-6 Times/Year	16%
1-3 Times/Month	7%
1-3 Times/Week	4%
Daily/Almost Daily	2%
Total	100%

FIGURE 5.4. Reported marijuana use and vulnerability to substance abuse.

Use of Other Drugs (Hallucinogens, Cocaine) and Vulnerability

About 7% of the students reported using hallucinogens in the past year. Very few reported more than rare use (1–6 times/year), and those who did tended to be male students (70%). Of the 2,000 hallucinogen users, 82% reported yearly use, 13% reported monthly use, and 5% reported weekly/daily use. Cocaine use was reported by less than 5% of the total student population tested. Less than 1% used more than 1 to 6 time/year. For hallucinogen and cocaine use, Figure 5.5 shows a similarly drastic increase in vulnerability among students who decided to experiment:

- Students who reported no use of hallucinogens (93%) or no use of cocaine (96%) showed little or no Vulnerability to substance abuse.

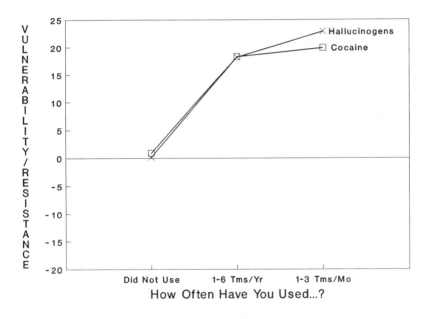

How Often Have You Used...?	Cocaine (28,865)	Hallucinogens (28,834)
Did Not Use	96%	93%
1-6 Times/Year	3%	6%
1-3 Times/Month	1%	1%
Total	100%	100%

FIGURE 5.5. Reported frequency of hallucinogen and cocaine use and vulnerability to substance abuse

- The rare hallucinogen and cocaine users who tried it 1 to 6 times in the past year showed an immediate and serious increase in Vulnerability.
- Increased use of hallucinogens is accompanied by a gradual increase in Vulnerability, slightly more than for cocaine users.

RELATIVE VULNERABILITY WITH ALCOHOL, TOBACCO, AND MARIJUANA USE

Regarding the generality or specificity of the Vulnerability measure, the findings showed that it is in a certain way generic. For practically all of the substances considered, we found that vulnerability did rise with each increase in the reported use of the particular substance. The more a person is thinking and perceiving in the same ways as frequent drinkers and drug users do, the more "vulnerable" he or she is to use harmful substances.

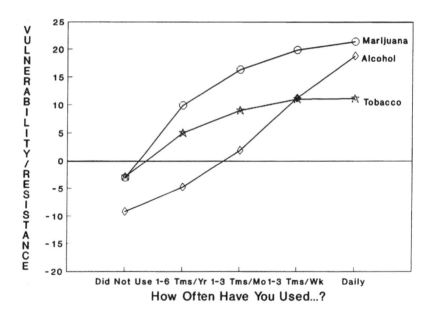

How Often Have You Used...?	Marijuana (28,945)	Alcohol (28,803)	Tobacco (28,833)
Did Not Use	71%	17%	58%
1-6 Times/Year	16%	24%	15%
1-3 Times/Month	6%	27%	6%
1-3 Times/Week	4%	29%	5%
Daily/Almost Daily	3%	3%	16%
Total	100%	100%	100%

FIGURE 5.6. Vulnerability by reported use of alcohol, cigarettes, and marijuana.

One important consideration is the different distribution of students, depending on the substance. Whereas drinkers/nondrinkers are fairly evenly distributed, for example, fewer students smoke, but if they do many tend to smoke on a regular daily basis; in the case of marijuana, most students either do not use it (71%) or use it only on rare occasions. Nevertheless, the impact on vulnerability is the same: increased substance use increases vulnerability.

At this point we want to consider how vulnerable are nonusers, moderate users and heavy users of each substance. Do nonusers of marijuana have higher vulnerability levels than nondrinkers? Are heavy pot users more Vulnerable than heavy drinkers? Figure 5.6 provides a summary view of how Vulnerability increases with the use of the three most popular substances: cigarettes, alcohol, and marijuana:

- Smokers showed higher vulnerability than most drinkers, partially because of the combined use: Smokers tend to be drinkers but drinkers are not necessarily smokers.
- Nondrinkers showed lower vulnerability than nonsmokers (who may be drinkers) or marijuana nonusers (who may drink and smoke).
- Drinkers do not rise to the range of vulnerability until they are drinking monthly, but smokers and marijuana users immediately show vulnerability.
- It appears that drinkers and marijuana users are becoming more and more similar as their usage increases (daily users are closest).
- Vulnerability does not appear to increase as drastically among smokers as it does among drinkers and marijuana users.

VULNERABILITY OF STUDENTS WITH DIFFERENT GENDER AND BACKGROUND

We are using a new technology and we are breaking new ground in measuring variables on which no empirical data are available. This makes it desirable to offer findings on parallel samples that differ only in certain ways but are otherwise comparable. Because the effects of high use environments versus low use environments promise particularly relevant insights, we include comparisons of students in different groups (male–female) and settings (high-use and low-use environments). The findings are based on the total college population of 30,000 students and subsamples of male and female students and students from three of the highest use colleges ($n = 1,000$) and three of the lowest use colleges ($n = 1,000$) in our studies.

Gender Differences in Alcohol Consumption and Vulnerability

Gender is another important issue regarding drinking on college campuses. As Figure 5.7 shows, there are consistent gender differences: 31% of the male students compared to 41% of the female students report no drinking at all. Conversely, 20%

of the men say they have more than 15 drinks a week, in contrast to only 5% of the women. Figure 5.7 illustrates these gender differences in vulnerability, which have been explored in greater depth regarding their specific perceptions and attitudes (Doherty & Szalay, 1996):

- Over three-fourths of the female students, the ones who have fewer than 5 drinks per week, exhibited resistance to substance abuse. For the male students, only those who reported no drinking showed resistance.
- Forty-two percent of the male students average 5 or more drinks per week and male Vulnerability is higher than their female counterparts at all consumption levels.
- The gender gap in Vulnerability narrows slightly as drinking levels rise.

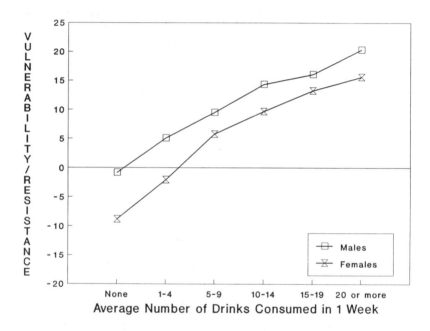

FIGURE 5.7. Reported alcohol consumption and vulnerability/resistance by males and females.

Average # of Drinks Consumed in 1 Week	Males (9,010)	Females (12,526)
None	31%	41%
1-4 Drinks	27%	35%
5-9 Drinks	12%	12%
10-14 Drinks	10%	7%
15-19 Drinks	4%	2%
20 or more Drinks	16%	3%
Total	100%	100%

Alcohol Consumption and Vulnerability
in Different Campus Environments

Sixteen percent of all students tested claimed to be nondrinkers, whereas only 3% said they were daily drinkers. To get a better idea about the frequency and amount of alcohol used by students in different campus environments, we compared their estimates of the average number of drinks consumed in a week. The Vulnerability to substance abuse rises sharply at both the low-use and high-use campuses with each higher category of consumption, as shown in Figure 5.8.

- Once beyond the majority of students who drink fewer than 5 drinks per week, vulnerability increased sharply, regardless of the college environment.

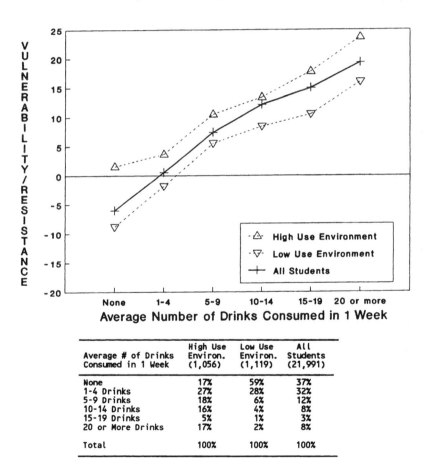

Average # of Drinks Consumed in 1 Week	High Use Environ. (1,056)	Low Use Environ. (1,119)	All Students (21,991)
None	17%	59%	37%
1-4 Drinks	27%	28%	32%
5-9 Drinks	18%	6%	12%
10-14 Drinks	16%	4%	8%
15-19 Drinks	5%	1%	3%
20 or More Drinks	17%	2%	8%
Total	100%	100%	100%

FIGURE 5.8. Reported alcohol consumption and vulnerability/resistance in different campus environments.

- At the low-use colleges, students who consume fewer than 5 drinks per week exhibited resistance; however, there was a bigger gap between these rare users and nonusers than there is on high-use campuses.
- At the high-use colleges even students who reported no use of alcohol showed some vulnerability compared to other nondrinkers.

COMMUNICATING FINDINGS AND THEIR VALIDITY WITH LINE GRAPHS

As we have just demonstrated, the worlds of users and nonusers involve different systems of cognitive–semantic representations. Our measurement of vulnerability is a product of cognitive mapping. Up to now no one has quantitatively measured vulnerability to substance abuse. Our Vulnerability measurements are the result of a computerized evaluation process based on the relation of response distributions involving thousands of spontaneous responses. The Vulnerability/Resistance measure offers insights into internal dispositions that were previously inaccessible. The line graphs reflect the effects of these dispositions and also inform on the validity of these new measurements.

To promote recognition of the influences of the hidden systems of cognitive–behavioral organization, we have included many visual presentations in the following chapters. We use line graphs to present trends, relationships, and the systemic effects of variables that were previously inaccessible. These can show how the hidden psychological factors interact and shape choices related to the use of harmful substances.

The first line graph in this chapter (Figure 5.2) shows in a simple way how vulnerability, as measured by our Vulnerability/Resistance scores, increases in proportionate increments in relation to increases in the frequency of alcohol use reported.

What Does the Slope of the Line Convey?

The slope of the line tells us several things about this previously unquantified relationship between alcohol consumption and vulnerability to substance abuse. First, it shows how the drinkers and nondrinkers compare in their relative vulnerability/resistance and how the vulnerability of nondrinkers compares to various groups of drinkers who report drinking with various frequencies. It shows how growth in vulnerability is linked to incremental increases in frequency of drinking. The percentage of the students in each response category gives a sense of proportion for how drinking at various levels and vulnerabilities are distributed across the total population of students. The steepness of the slope readily conveys the strength of the relationship between alcohol use and vulnerability: the steeper the slope, the stronger the relationship. To see a contrast in the strength of the rela-

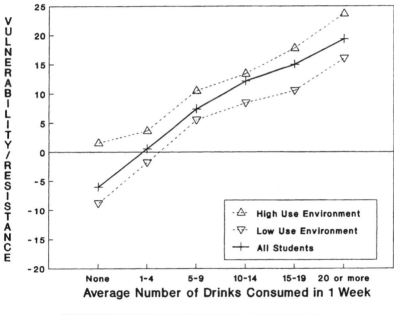

tionship, compare the slope of the line for vulnerability and weekly alcohol consumption (Figure 5.8) with that for vulnerability and class year (Figure 14.3).

Comparing the Lines

The visual presentation is used to convey a sense of proportion: first how the use of specific substances affects the aggregate propensity for substance abuse measured by the Vulnerability/Resistance scores and later how other variables affect this propensity. The graphs show how the consumption pattern varies by substance and how these variations affect the distribution of vulnerability among the students tested. We think this simple visual form helps to convey a sense of proportion for the effects of psychological dispositions that were previously unquantifiable.

Feedback on Validity of the Vulnerability/Resistance Measure

The lines provide a quick visual feedback on validity. The consistency of results conveyed by the line graphs offers a simple indication of validity of the Vulnerability measure. Although the Vulnerability/Resistance scores are the products of thousands of measurements, they could not be so clear if the underlying trends they measure were not also consistent and real. Considering the large number of respondents and their responses, interpretable results cannot be accidental. Whether the results are meaningful or to what extent they convey internally consistent trends can be readily seen from the line graphs.

The effects of gender and environment on vulnerability may be used as an example. The parallel lines reflect how females are consistently lower in vulnerability compared to males across the board in all reported use categories. This example shows, with a remarkable degree of consistency, differences in vulnerability in the expected direction. Male students at all levels of participation are more vulnerable than females, and students in high-use environments show greater vulnerability than do students in low-use environments. Comparison of the male–female and high–low use colleges reflect the same direction of difference. Again, the results communicated by the line graphs could not be accidental; they are based on tens of thousands of independent data points. The order and consistency of the data points represented in these line graphs offer clear evidence that the assumptions on which they were produced are valid. The line graphs depict relationships visually and can be used to show the relationship among several variables simultaneously, such as gender and environment. As we discuss later (Chapter 6), the slope of the lines, the relationships of the lines, the consistency of the trends, and the comparison of trends provide a great deal of feedback about the intrinsic characteristics of the results.

THE CENTRAL ASSUMPTION CONFIRMED

Our central assumption that the worlds of users and of nonusers offer solid insights into the foundation of their different behaviors was put to the test. In view of the lack of empirical information on the overall propensity to use or not use harmful substances, whether such an aggregate propensity exists, and what it does, and what it affects, the most natural point of departure was to explore how vulnerability relates to the use of specific harmful substances.

The results provided strong evidence that overall propensities do exist and that they can be identified through cognitive mapping procedures designed to measure vulnerability:

- Vulnerability was linked to the use of all the substances examined. In the context of all substances there was a linear relationship: more reported use results in more vulnerability.
- Substance-specific consequences were noted: the frequency of the use of substances varied in the population, and various substances have shown different effects on vulnerability.
- The expectation of increase or decrease in vulnerability based on present knowledge was affirmed: males were found to be more vulnerable than females, and students in high-use environments were consistently more vulnerable than students in low-use environments.

The findings support the hypothetical consequences that logically follow from our central assumption about vulnerability and that are testable at this point in combination with other commonsense trends considered fundamental to this field.

FOCUS ON ETIOLOGY: GRADUAL CHANGES IN DISPOSITIONS AND IN BEHAVIOR

Our work differs from the epidemiological fact-finding tasks of most surveys in the field of substance abuse. Our primary interest was not to assess the level of substance abuse at a particular campus, or for that matter at all the campuses tested across the country. Our interest is in learning more about the causes and key contributing factors that lead students to use harmful substances. In the pursuit of this interest the results on reported levels of use were provided as familiar reference points but our primary focus is on the relationship of key psychological and environmental factors affecting the level of substance abuse. What matters is not just who is using what substance with what frequency. It is essential to understand how internal systems promoting or resisting substance abuse differ in ways that shape decisions affecting use. We look for factors producing the most difference, those that deserve close attention in developing successful prevention programs.

Substance abuse, beyond chemical dependence, is a pathogenic behavior resulting from a combination of dominant behavioral dispositions promoted by environmental influences. The line graphs are helpful in illustrating how use is related to a combination of relevant behavioral dispositions and environmental conditions.

What is of special relevance to prevention is the extent to which this vulnerability exists before a person actually begins to use a particular substance. Although this question cannot be answered with the same conclusiveness as the others, all figures in this chapter that report findings from rare use to daily use show that the transition is gradual and involves changes in the psychological dispositions we have identified and analyzed in the earlier parts of this volume. The gradual change in the underlying psychological dispositions suggests that the lower stage prepares people for higher levels of involvement with the substance, frequently traceable to the influence of the environment. More use produces increased vulnerability. So vulnerability and use grow hand-in-hand: vulnerability increases the likelihood of involvement, and use increases vulnerability.

Beyond a generic vulnerability that is measurable in the context of each substance, there is a great deal of specificity in the vulnerability. The vulnerability observed with cigarettes is not distributed in the same way as with alcohol or with marijuana (see Figure 5.6). Although in all instances there is a demonstrable vulnerability, how it progresses, how sharply it increases, and how the previous stage prepares the people slowly or quickly for higher levels of use varies from substance to substance. In general, the results described in this chapter show conclusively that increasing vulnerability is linked to greater use, although the impact of progressive use on vulnerability depends on the substance under consideration.

These results support the general conclusion that vulnerability/resistance is an effective and sensitive measure of the aggregate propensities that characterize involvement with particular substances. The results suggest a high degree of validity of the measure, showing changes in Vulnerability as a direct function of changes in reported use. A more detailed discussion of the validation of these results and their implications is taken up in the next chapter.

Criterion and Construct Validation of the Vulnerability/Resistance Measure

The close agreement between the students' Vulnerability scores and their reported use of all substances, from tobacco to crack cocaine, offers evidence of the validity of the Vulnerability/Resistance measure. The results bear on additional aspects of the Vulnerability measure focusing on the accuracy of predictions. The first comparison tests the accuracy of identifying users of specific substances based on the students' Vulnerability scores. The second shows how the accuracy of identification based on the vulnerability alone can be increased (well over 80%) by using multiple predictors (gender, environment, etc.).

TESTING THE ACCURACY OF THE VULNERABILITY/RESISTANCE MEASURE TO PREDICT USE

As we said in the Introduction, we generated reference norms of perceptions and attitudes that differentiate users and nonusers based on the response distributions of a sample of 400 in each group. The users were people who self-identified as either using alcohol daily/almost daily or using alcohol 1 to 3 times/week, and using any illicit substances. The nonusers were a demographically matched group who self-identified as never using alcohol and never using drugs. The two groups responded to many stimulus themes in strikingly different ways, and these differences served as the basis for calculating the Vulnerability/Resistance scores.

Vulnerability/Resistance measures are calculated by assessing the similarity of a single person's responses to those typical of users and to those typical of nonusers. Using the rationale and procedures discussed in Chapter 4, we calculated Vulnerability/Resistance scores to measure the propensity of individual students and that of groups to use or not use alcohol and other drugs. We did this by mapping the similarity of their worlds with the contrasting worlds of users and of nonusers. In Chapter 5 we examined the relation of the Vulnerability/Resistance scores to the reported use of various substances as well as to gender and environment, variables known to affect substance use in predictable ways. The close agreement of the Vulnerability scores with reported usage of all substances, from cigarettes to hard drugs, demonstrates the viability and stability of the construct of Vulnerability/Resistance and of the way in which we measure its strength.

The question we address next is the accuracy or validity of the Vulnerability/Resistance scores—how well they predict substance use. To do this we looked at the percentage of students we could correctly identify as users or as nonusers on the basis of their Vulnerability scores as predictors and their self-reported use of alcohol and other drugs as the criterion behavior.

When we deal with concepts such as "intelligence" or "vulnerability to substance abuse," it is important to assess the extent to which they help to measure and explain behavior, even though the referents of these constructs are not directly observable themselves. For example, though intelligence makes itself apparent in many ways, it is not a tangible thing that can be seen or counted. If we can agree on a practical definition, or operational definition, of what activity or behavior demonstrates intelligence, then we can measure the behavior (things like problem-solving speed or how completely written material can be learned in a set time period) for different people and compare their performance scores. If we believe there are several kinds of behavior related to the construct of intelligence and people who get a high (or low) score on one behavior are observed to get a similarly high (or low) score on the other behaviors, we can say the construct has generality and utility.

With intelligence the next step might be to assemble brief samples of intelligence-related behavior and call the set of tasks an intelligence test. We could then

TABLE 6.1. Percentage of Users of Specific Substances Identified as Vulnerable Based on Their Vulnerability/Resistance Scores

Substance used	Number of users	Percent correctly identified
Cigarettes[a]	6,096	74%
Alcohol[a]	9,370	78%
Marijuana	8,371	82%
Speed	954	86%
Cocaine	1,024	88%
Inhalants	835	89%
Ecstasy	629	90%
Hallucinogens	2,054	93%

[a]Note: Results are based on weekly/daily users of cigarettes and alcohol and on any use of all other drugs listed.

use the test scores as an indicator of how much intelligence we would expect people to display in a variety of real-life circumstances. We would not always be correct but we would be correct most of the time. The degree to which we are correct is a measure of the validity of the test.

So it is with our concept of vulnerability/resistance to substance abuse. We want to confirm that the construct has real meaning, and we want to know that what we are measuring indeed bears on substance abuse behavior. Table 6.1 presents the results of identification of users of a variety of substances from their Vulnerability/Resistance scores. Students whose Vulnerability/Resistance score was above zero were classified as vulnerable; that is, as having psychological dispositions similar to users of alcohol and other drugs. If the student's Vulnerability/Resistance score was below zero, he or she was classified as resistant; that is, hav-

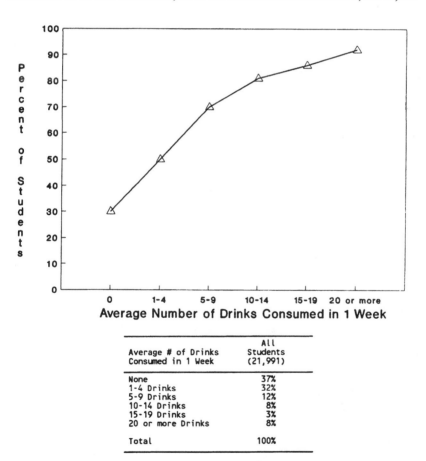

Average # of Drinks Consumed in 1 Week	All Students (21,991)
None	37%
1-4 Drinks	32%
5-9 Drinks	12%
10-14 Drinks	8%
15-19 Drinks	3%
20 or more Drinks	8%
Total	100%

FIGURE 6.1. Percent of students scored as vulnerable at different levels of drinking.

ing psychological dispositions more similar to nonusers. We considered a student correctly identified if he or she was classified by the Vulnerability/Resistance score as a vulnerable and self-reported using alcohol or other drugs or as resistant and self-reported abstinence. The rate of correct identification ranged from 74% of the smokers to 93% of hallucinogen users.

When we took a look at usage in general in Chapter 5, we identified 78% of the nonusers (abstainers from alcohol and other drugs) as resistant and 77% of the frequent drinkers and/or drug users as vulnerable, based on the student's Vulnerability/Resistance score. When we take a closer look at the relation between the Vulnerability/Resistance score and the degree of alcohol use, our identification of users as vulnerable to substance abuse increased as their frequency of use increased. An individual Vulnerability/Resistance score indicating vulnerability (scores above zero) was associated with 34% of the yearly drinkers, 54% of the monthly drinkers, 77% of the weekly drinkers, and 89% of the daily drinkers. We obtained similar results when we used the amount of alcohol consumed as the basis of comparison. Figure 6.1 shows the percentage of students who were classified as Vulnerable to substance abuse according to their average number of drinks per week.

CONSTRUCT VALIDATION

We have conceptualized vulnerability as a predisposition that makes some people prone to use harmful substances. Vulnerability is construed as a contrasting force to resistance, a similarly powerful set of dispositions that protects people from getting involved in experimentation. This construct of vulnerability/resistance is built on the following fundamental assumptions: The more people are predisposed to see the world as users see it, the more vulnerable they are to using alcohol or other drugs. Similarity in perceptions, or mental representations, among people indicates similarity in their dispositions leading to behavior. The similarity can be inferred from the distributions of free elicitations: the more similar the elicitations are, the more similar are their psychological dispositions. It is important to determine to what extent we can predict behavior based on our measure of vulnerability/resistance to gain confidence that the construct is valid and the outcome is neither accidental nor artificial.

The results presented in the line graphs show a surprising degree of regularity, as evidenced by the consistency of the slopes and the distance of the lines from each other. This is possible if the strategy of cognitive imaging and mapping works and both fundamental assumptions of the vulnerability construct hold; namely, that similarity with users' perceptions and attitudes indicates vulnerability and similarity with nonusers' perceptions and attitudes indicates resistance and that the Vulnerability/Resistance measure reflects an overall propensity to use harmful substances or to avoid them. This same reasoning holds for all the findings presented in Part III of this volume. Each figure depicts relations that are consistent with logical expectations that follow from the vulnerability/resistance construct. The advantage of having self-reported substance use as the criterion measure is that the "use" or "no use" alternatives and frequency of involvement are fairly simple and straightforward pieces of information. In circumstances such as with student populations, treatment centers, hospitals, and trauma centers, that information is readily available.

Although we do not directly validate piece by piece the specific perceptual and attitudinal trends found by comparative imaging, their contribution to shaping drug behavior is certainly represented in the process in which the Vulnerability/Resistance scores are validated against observed behavior. The Vulnerability/Resistance scores are aggregate measures that accumulate dominant perceptual and motivational trends along the principles specified by our theoretical assumptions. The remarkably close agreement of the Vulnerability/Resistance scores with reported or observed behavior offers solid validation for the working of the underlying psychological dispositions as stated and specified.

USE OF MULTIPLE INDICATORS TO ASSESS PROPENSITY FOR SUBSTANCE ABUSE

Along a different line of inquiry we examined ways to improve the power of the Vulnerability/Resistance measure to identify Users and Nonusers. This ambition does not stem from dissatisfaction with the established validity and performance of this new measure. Our general results of 80% correct identification based on 4,438 Nonusers (abstainers) and 11,726 frequent Users of alcohol and drugs are conclusive enough to tell us that we are on the right track. Nevertheless, we want to place the variables affecting substance abuse into broader perspectives. Interest in assessing the influence of psychological dispositions is not new, but we have been fortunate enough to gain access to these variables in a new and effective way. Now we are in the position to examine the effects of a diversity of variables through these new capabilities that help to reduce well-known methodological and diagnostic problems associated with the assessment of psychological factors shaping behavior.

We explored the possibility of improving the predictive value of the Vulnerability/Resistance score by combining it with data from other variables. What makes such an exercise interesting both from a practical and from a theoretical angle is that the Vulnerability/Resistance measure focuses on psychological dispositions, compared to social, biomedical, and other important factors in substance abuse.

Using a statistical technique called discriminant function analysis (DFA), we explored combinations of the Vulnerability/Resistance measure and various background and lifestyle variables to see what would give us the best prediction of usage. With DFA, the objective is to find the minimum number of predictors that will yield the best overall prediction. For this analysis we selected from the total database of 30,000 students a group of 4,338 nonusers (abstainers from all alcohol and drug use) and an equal-sized group of users (students who binge drink and/or who drink alcohol weekly/daily and use illicit drugs).

We then selected a few background and lifestyle variables that, based on our own research and others, could be expected to affect the students' use of alcohol and other drugs. More detailed findings on these factors are presented in part III. Peer influences were represented by the frequency of going out with friends. We also included a measure of the student's campus drug climate. On the basis of the percentage of frequent users at each college, we created a campus environment variable in which 49 colleges were categorized as high use (top 12 sites), low use (lowest 12 sites), or moderate use (middle 25 sites). Our research has also shown that religious involvement correlates with drug use. Level of academic achievement may also be informative in that heavy alcohol and drug use can be expected to adversely affect the student's grades.

Results of the DFA, in which we tested many combinations of variables, are selectively presented in Table 6.2. The percentage of nonusers who were correctly identified was consistently higher in all cases than the percentage of users who were correctly identified. The highest percentage who were correctly classified with the fewest variables was 88% for nonusers and 84% for users. We already know that we can identify 78% of the nonusers and 77% of the users just on the basis of their Vulnerability/Resistance score, which reflects the intensity that the student is similar in his or her psychological dispositions to users or to nonusers. Table 6.2 shows that adding information about frequency of contact with friends increases the accuracy of identification slightly, as does adding information about the environment. As would be expected, if we know the students' attitude toward

TABLE 6.2. Percentage of Users and Nonusers Correctly Identified Based on Their Vulnerability/Resistance and Other Background and Lifestyle Factors

	Percentage Correctly Identified			
Canonical correlation	Nonusers (4,338)	Freq. Users (4,338)	Total (8676)	Variables used in discriminant function analysis
.64	81%	78%	89%	Vulnerability/Resistance (V/R)+going out with friends
.66	83%	78%	81%	V/R+going out with friends+environment
.72	88%	83%	85%	V/R+going out with friends+environment+attitude toward alcohol
.73	87%	84%	86%	V/R+going out with friends+environment+attitude toward alcohol+religious attendance
.74	88%	84%	86%	V/R+going out with friends+environment+attitude toward alcohol+religious attendance+GPA

alcohol we can more easily predict their classification. Two other variables, religious attendance and grade point average, only slightly improved the accuracy of prediction. By taking into account these four variables along with the students' Vulnerability/Resistance score, the strength of the canonical correlation increased from .64 to .74, and we improved the percentage of students correctly classified on the basis of vulnerability/resistance alone from 81% to 88% for nonusers and from 78% to 84% for users.

The DFA results indicate that successful identification of people with propensities for substance abuse can be enhanced by including variables related to social influences (friends, environment), values (religion, attitudes toward alcohol), and behavior (academic achievement).

The results support the validity of the Vulnerability/Resistance measure with respect to substance abuse behavior. Moreover, validation of the general measure is an indirect validation of the specific results obtained on the differential perspectives of users and of nonusers. In Part V, we discuss the practical use of the generic vulnerability/resistance indicator and the specific information on dominant perceptions and attitudes.

Part III

Tracing the Effects of Background and
Lifestyle on the Use of Harmful Substances

7

Background and Group Membership
Factors Affecting Substance Abuse

The Vulnerability/Resistance measure makes the propensity for substance abuse identifiable and quantifiable based on the aggregate effects of psychological dispositions. In the previous chapter we examined the validity of the Vulnerability measure with respect to a range of substances, from tobacco to the various hard drugs. Now, we explore how that propensity is affected by a host of variables such as age, gender, ethnic–cultural background, and membership in certain groups (fraternities and sports teams). Though some of these are "fixed" variables in the sense that they are not amenable to change, they can affect the risk level for involvement with harmful substances.

In the previous chapters we introduced vulnerability/resistance and showed that it does exist and is measurable. Vulnerability goes hand in hand with the use of harmful substances and actually precedes substance abuse in a gradual transition from total abstinence to various degrees of involvement with them. Now that its existence has been firmly established and an analytic procedure for measuring it has been validated, we can apply the measure in contexts that may or may not involve substance abuse. We are speaking of such factors as the student's background, membership in various groups, and the social environment in general.

In real life these various factors do not work alone but in various combinations to shape decisions and behavior. A student who wants to remain drug free in order to maintain control over his or her life in a high-alcohol-use college environment and who is also interested in being popular is likely to be exposed to conflicting influences. The Vulnerability measure has been used to assess such contrasting influences in their interaction.

Over the next several chapters, we examine the role of background and lifestyle factors that affect substance use through shaping the students' perceptions and attitudes into the contrasting psychological forces measured by vulnerability/resistance. The results show that some of these variables promote vulnerability while others promote resistance to substance abuse.

Another category of variables that we know is important but about which less is known is the social environment. We assume that environmental factors are powerful in shaping perceptions and attitudes and drug-related decisions and thus deserve careful consideration. For this reason we have taken into consideration the student's campus environment (high-use vs. low-use colleges). With the exception of Figure 7.1, which includes all students classified into environments, the reference groups selected to represent high-use and low-use environments come from the extremes—the three highest use and the three lowest use colleges. We show its effects in combination with other variables in the line graphs presented in the following chapters.

THE IMPACT OF HIGH-USE AND LOW-USE ENVIRONMENTS
ON VULNERABILITY

Figure 7.1 shows the relationship between frequency of reported alcohol use and Vulnerability as measured in three different campus environments characterized by high, moderate, and low substance use. These results show consistent differences in vulnerability with large samples of 7,000 to 10,000 students. The effects of alcohol consumption in the high-use, moderate-use, and low-use campus environments show the same trend: more use resulted in proportionately more psychological vulnerability. The only difference observed under the three environmental conditions is in the general level of vulnerability, rising with use:

- Students who reported the least usage of alcohol have the lowest Vulnerability scores.
- Every increment in reported use shows a corresponding increase in Vulnerability. Students who reported the most frequent alcohol use (daily, almost daily) have the highest Vulnerability scores.
- Students in a High-use environment have consistently higher Vulnerability at all levels of reported use than do students in a Low-use environment. In all instances, environmental influences show the same consistent, quantifiable relation to use.

As we discussed in Chapter 5, the results could not be so orderly if the underlying thousands of data points that serve as their foundation were not also based on an essentially accurate assessment. They support the validity of the assumption that the more people drink, the more they are vulnerable, having perceptions and attitudes similar to those of known users. Under these conditions, it is compelling to accept the main point of these findings, namely that high-, moderate-, and low-use environments produce different, empirically quantifiable vulnerabilities.

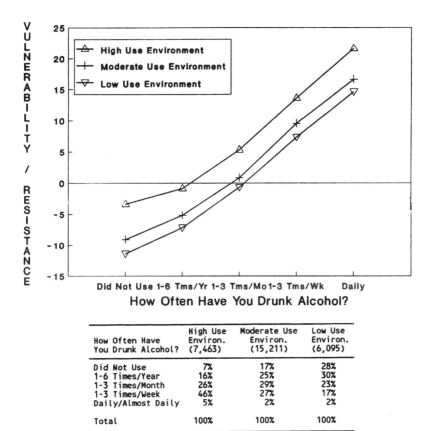

FIGURE 7.1. Frequency of alcohol use and vulnerability in high-use, moderate-use and low-use campus environments.

Next, we look at the students' frequency of going out with friends and its impact on vulnerability (Figure 7.2). Whereas we discuss this important social factor in more detail in chapter 8, here we want to consider how campus environment affects this relationship. A comparison of Figures 7.1 and 7.2 shows some important differences. Compared to the direct relationship between alcohol consumption and Vulnerability, going out with friends does not affect vulnerability in the same way.

General Effects of the Environment

Compared to alcohol consumption, where the level of use was the prime determinant of vulnerability, in the case of going out with friends, the environment is a critical factor shaping vulnerability. In the high-use environment (except for the 1% who reported never going out with friends), the students' vulnerability was shown to depend on the frequency of their social contacts. The more frequently they went out, the higher their vulnerability.

In contrast, in the Low-use environment only the students who reported going out "a lot" (19%) showed increased vulnerability. For all others, going out with friends did not promote their propensity for using alcohol or other harmful substances.

Frequency of Social Contacts in the Environment Makes a Difference

As we said in Chapter 5, the strength of the influence of a particular variable, such as drinking or going out, is indicated by the slope of the line. The steeper the slope, the stronger the influence. In the high-use environment, going out often or a lot in-

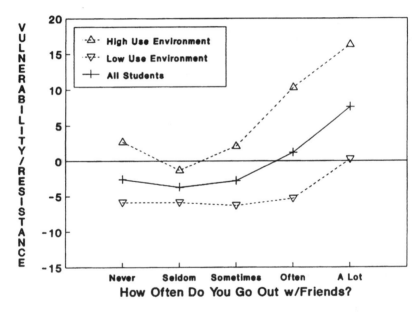

How Often Do You Go Out With Friends?	High Use Environ. (1,073)	Low Use Environ. (1,125)	All Students (28,787)
Never	1%	3%	1%
Seldom	6%	19%	10%
Sometimes	19%	32%	26%
Often	35%	27%	33%
A Lot	39%	19%	30%
Total	100%	100%	100%

FIGURE 7.2. Going out with friends and vulnerability in high-use and low-use campus environments.

creased the students' vulnerability intensively (see Figure 7.2). In fact, starting from those who reported going out seldom, the high-use environment has an amplifying impact on shaping vulnerability as a consequence of more frequent contacts. As this example illustrates, the slope of the line is informative both as a whole and in its individual segments. The resulting curves tell the story of a frequently complex interaction between the variable under consideration and the environment.

Interaction of Multiple Factors Affects Vulnerability/Resistance

The line graphs help convey the relation and interaction effects among several variables, as we just illustrated in considering environmental conditions, frequency of contacts, and vulnerability. In the following chapters we consider gender, age, grade point average, and other factors to gain insights into their relation and the effects of their interactions.

Because new insights about the interactive relation of several variables with the environment is a major interest, we use line graphs extensively in presenting our findings. In examining environmental effects, we take into consideration the relation of the lines depicting the relation between vulnerability and selected factors. Divergent lines indicate that the environmental conditions amplify vulnerability as a function of social contacts (e.g., see Figure 7.2).

What Proportion of the Student Population Is Affected?

We use line graphs in conjunction with tables that show the percentage of the student population represented in each response category on the graph. In Figure 7.2, for instance, 39% of the students in the high-use campus environment reported going out a lot, whereas in the low-use environment only 19% of the students reported going out that much (half the number in the high-use environment). This explains the increasingly close relation between vulnerability and the proportion of students in frequent contact in the high-use environment. To form a clear picture of what happens as a result of the interaction of these hidden psychological and environmental variables, it is important to take into account these percentage distributions of the student population under consideration.

Systemic Influences and Etiology

We are now in a good position to document the impact of various factors promoting or resisting the use of harmful substances as we trace them in their relation rather than in isolation. The results reveal the interrelationships that shape the decisions and behavior of students in high-use and low-use campus environments.

THE EFFECTS OF BACKGROUND ON PROPENSITIES FOR USING
OR NOT USING HARMFUL SUBSTANCES

Membership in certain sociodemographic groups cannot be altered (we are born males or females), whereas membership in other groups, such as social clubs, is largely a matter of choice. Both of these categories are relevant to prevention but in somewhat different ways.

Age, gender, and cultural background are generally well recognized as potential risk factors in the use of harmful substances. Although these are fixed variables that we cannot change, identifying the underlying psychological foundation of these risks is important for effective prevention of substance abuse.

Membership in other groups is mostly an individual choice, and these choices can also affect a person's propensity to use or not to use harmful substances. For instance, there is a considerable body of literature which shows that membership in college fraternal organizations is conducive to increased substance abuse. It is important to be aware of this second category of membership by choice because in some circumstances it can become a tool of social influence to decrease vulnerability.

Males Are More Vulnerable

Perhaps the most widely studied area among group risk factors is that of gender differences. Recent research has begun to identify some of the possible causal mechanisms underlying men's greater vulnerability to substance use. According to Kaplan and Johnson (1992), socialization plays an important role in creating differences in men and women that lead to different levels of substance abuse. Socialization leads men and women to value different outcomes and to follow different norms regarding appropriate behavior. For example, men are more concerned with physical effectiveness, whereas women are more concerned with physical attractiveness. Thus, men may be more likely to view substance use as a demonstration of their power and control.

Even with cigarettes, male smokers usually are portrayed as tough and macho. On the other hand, advertisers must work hard to portray attractive images of female smokers. Likewise, social norms regarding drunkenness admonish women that it is not ladylike, while suggesting to men that it is just part of boys being boys.

Men define risk taking and delinquency in positive terms more so than women. R. Jessor and Jessor (1979) found that marijuana use was correlated with alienation for females and social criticism was correlated with marijuana use for males. These social norms regarding sex-appropriate behavior and valued outcomes may be important factors in both men's and women's decisions to use or not use harmful substances.

Whereas some studies have shown that men engage in greater use of alcohol and other drugs than do women (Berkowitz & Perkins, 1987; Maney, 1990), others show no such differences, at least among college samples (Engs & Hanson, 1985). Our research has consistently shown that college men are more vulnerable and college women more resistant to substance use based on differences in attitudes, values, and beliefs that affect vulnerability to substance abuse (and also self-report).

Of all the background variables we studied, gender was the strongest factor affecting Vulnerability. Females were consistently less vulnerable to substance abuse than males, even when we included other variables such as age, environment, and so forth. The line charts on the following pages show characteristic trends across large populations tested. Although we have discussed gender differences in more specific terms elsewhere (Doherty & Szalay, 1996), Figure 7.3 shows gender differences in vulnerability; it also shows that campus climate does not noticeably alter the gender gap between males and females.

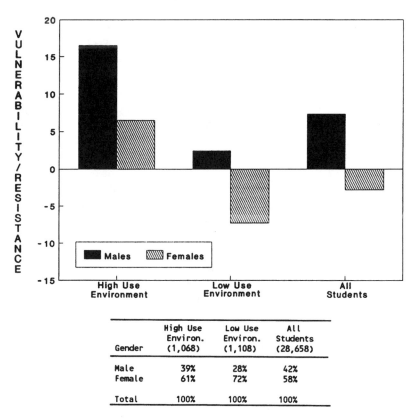

Gender	High Use Environ. (1,068)	Low Use Environ. (1,108)	All Students (28,658)
Male	39%	28%	42%
Female	61%	72%	58%
Total	100%	100%	100%

FIGURE 7.3. Gender and environmental influences on vulnerability.

There are sizable differences in the Vulnerability levels of male and female students in the high-use and low-use campus environments suggesting the important influence of social environment:

- Women in high-use colleges, although not as vulnerable as men, are at much greater risk than women at all colleges in general and women in low-use colleges. The same is true of men at high-use colleges.
- In the low-use colleges, women demonstrated resistance to substance abuse and men showed Vulnerability levels much lower than men in high-use colleges.

Rising Vulnerability Has Age Limits

Adolescence is a time of great emotional turmoil, caused by both hormonal changes and the challenge of facing new decisions and dilemmas with less adult supervision. As adolescents move towards establishing themselves as independent beings with their own identities, their peers take on a more influential role in their lives. Coombs, Paulson, and Richardson (1991) found that young people's behavior regarding the use of alcohol and other drugs was greatly influenced by their peers. Furthermore, those teens who had positive relationships with their parents were less likely to be involved in substance use. Those young people who experience the greatest emotional distress during adolescence may become vulnerable to using substances as a coping mechanism. It should not be surprising, then, that in the general population substance use increases with age throughout the teen years (S. Duncan & Duncan, 1994; Maggs, Almeida, & Galambos, 1995; Warheit, Biafora, Zimmerman, Gil et al., 1995; Williams & Smith, 1993). Previous research using the AGA method has shown that vulnerability to use illicit substances increases with age for elementary, middle, and high school students as social ties and peer group pressure become increasingly more important (Szalay, Inn, Strohl, & Wilson, 1993).

This increase in substance use with age through adolescence does not continue endlessly. Typically, use levels decrease as users progress into adulthood. As young adults begin to become involved with employment, marriage, and parenthood, patterns of use that developed in their late teens and early 20s become incompatible with daily reality. Research by Kandel, Simch-Fagan, and Davies (1986) has supported the role-conflict hypothesis, which explains the drop in use and abuse by the mid-20s.

Our data enabled us to explore this issue up to about age 45, at which vulnerabilities still exist but are substantially reduced. The data are probably atypical because they come from a college student population with an above-average education; we might get different results if we were dealing with the general population. There is some variation based on age as a biological factor as well as on age influenced by environment. The fact that a person moves from no substance use in

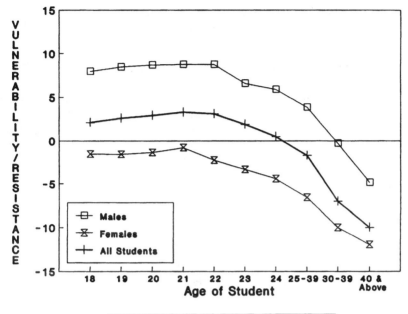

FIGURE 7.4. Age and vulnerability/resistance of males and females.

Age	All Males (12,072)	All Females (16,646)	All Students (27,957)
18	18%	21%	20%
19	18%	19%	18%
20	17%	16%	16%
21	15%	15%	15%
22	10%	8%	9%
23	6%	4%	5%
24	3%	2%	3%
25-29	7%	5%	6%
30-39	4%	6%	5%
40 & Above	2%	4%	3%
Total	100%	100%	100%

early childhood to the use of particular substances as he or she grows toward adulthood underscores the importance of developmental changes in general. The results presented in Figure 7.4 show the relationship between age and vulnerability:

- Vulnerability levels off during the college years and then, at about age 22, it begins to decrease with age.
- Over age 23, the vulnerability of males shows a gradual decrease, and the Resistance of females becomes stronger.
- Older, nontraditional-aged college students tend to have stronger, nonuser type psychological dispositions than those of traditional-aged college students.

Influences of the campus environment on the vulnerability of students of different ages are shown in Figure 7.5. They appear to be strongest among the younger
students:

- In the high-use college environment there was a decrease in vulnerability
  around age 21 and then some increases until after age 25.
- In the low-use college environment all students demonstrated resistance to
  substance abuse, but it was strongest between ages 19 and 21.
- Environmental influences appear to decrease as the students age and mature,
  as evidenced by the decreasing gap in the vulnerability of students over time.

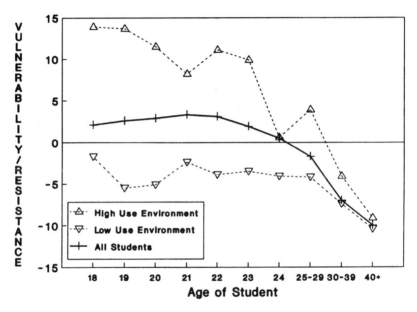

Age	High Use Environ. (1,056)	Low Use Environ. (1,080)	All Students (27,957)
18	19%	17%	20%
19	15%	15%	18%
20	18%	12%	16%
21	23%	10%	15%
22	12%	8%	9%
23	4%	4%	5%
24	2%	3%	3%
25-29	4%	9%	6%
30-39	2%	15%	5%
40 & Above	1%	7%	3%
Total	100%	100%	100%

FIGURE 7.5. Age and environmental influences on vulnerability/resistance.

Family History of Substance Abuse Increases Vulnerability

We asked the students in our samples whether their parents or grandparents had substance abuse problems. About one-fourth of the students said yes. A higher percentage of the female students believed there had been family problems of substance abuse. Figure 7.6 shows the vulnerability of students according to their family history of use:

- Vulnerability scores for students who reported a family history of substance abuse were higher than for students who did not.
- The vulnerability of students with a family history of substance abuse was higher for both males and females, but a higher percentage of females reported the problem.
- From this and other comparisons, we can conclude that the perceptions and attitudes of the children reflect the social influence of the family.

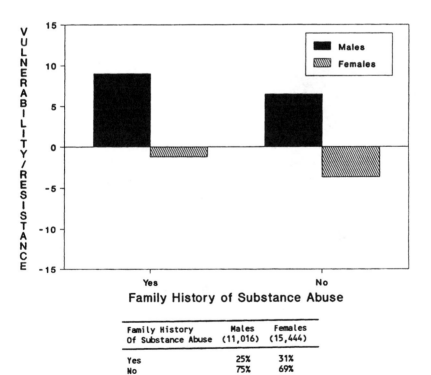

Family History Of Substance Abuse	Males (11,016)	Females (15,444)
Yes	25%	31%
No	75%	69%
Total	100%	100%

FIGURE 7.6. Family history and vulnerability/resistance for males and females.

Marriage Lowers Susceptibility to Substance Abuse

Bachman, O'Malley, and Johnston (1984) reported that marriage is associated with decreased drug use and our findings support this same conclusion. About 11% of the students tested were married. The reported alcohol and other drug use of married students was significantly lower than for single students. Among the single students, 43% reported binge drinking/drug use, whereas just 18% of the married students were in this category. The relationship between marital status and vulnerability is shown in Figure 7.7.

- Married students are at much lower psychological risk of substance abuse than are single students.
- The decrease in vulnerability related to marriage is about the same for males and for females.

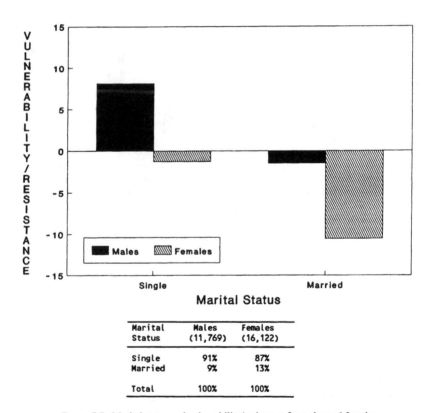

FIGURE 7.7. Marital status and vulnerability/resistance for males and females.

Minority Students Are at Lower Risk than the Caucasian Mainstream

Race and ethnicity have been examined extensively as factors in substance use. Although many racial differences in behavior have been described, little work has been done to try to specify some of the causal variables that underlie such differences (Yee, Fairchild, Weizmann, & Wyatt, 1993). The picture is made even more complex by consideration of other important variables, such as socioeconomic status.

Recently, several researchers within the field of substance abuse have begun to address this void. Group differences due to ethnic origin are, to a large extent, the result of shared experiences within a particular group that, in turn, affect their perceptions and attitudes. These perceptual differences can leave some groups more vulnerable to substance abuse and others more resistant to it.

In the present study we found distinct differences among the four main ethnic populations in our student samples: Caucasians, African-Americans, Hispanic-Americans, and Asian-Americans. Of the eight subgroups, African-American women had the lowest vulnerability score (highest resistance to substance abuse). The average vulnerabilities by Hispanic-Americans and Asian-Americans are similar to each other and fall midway between Caucasians and African-Americans. The results presented here do not show the deep differences that exist across ethnic groups. That information is available from our more narrowly focused studies, like our acculturation study of Puerto Ricans in the United States (Szalay, Canino, & Vilov, 1993).

According to Brunswick, Messeri, and Titus (1992), socioeconomic status is a vulnerability factor for inner-city African-Americans. As we have noted previously, there is typically a drop in substance use for Caucasians in their mid-20s that often is explained by the role-conflict hypothesis, which states that as one assumes adult roles (marriage, work, etc.), substance use becomes an incompatible behavior. Since a large number of African-Americans (especially males) experience delays in assuming these roles (unemployment rates are higher, marriage rates are lower), they are likely to stay involved with substance use to a more advanced age. That leaves them at higher risk than higher-economic-status others, Black or White. This explanation is supported by the work of Glantz and Pickens (1992), who reported that low involvement in organizations that support traditional norms and values, such as church, was an especially important risk factor among African-Americans.

However, whatever general observations others have made about ethnicity as a factor in drug and alcohol use, college students, particularly in the case of ethnic minorities, represent a highly select subpopulation. This apparent discrepancy with the research cited previously may be a reflection that the college goers are a select group different from the majority in their interests and motivation or it may be related to the effect of the new environment. Just by being in college, they have adopted a value central to mainstream society and in doing so they are preparing to assume conventional adult roles. Thus, we would not expect to see the same relationship between race and vulnerability in our college sample as Brunswick and his associates (1992) did in their inner-city sample.

Although over 90% of the students tested were Caucasian, there were significant numbers of African-Americans, Hispanic-Americans, and Asian-Americans for comparison, as shown in Figure 7.8.

- The Caucasian students had the highest vulnerability of the four ethnic groups and the African-American students reflected the least vulnerability.
- Gender emerged as a distinctly more powerful factor than ethnicity regarding vulnerability/resistance.
- For all four ethnic groups, the Vulnerability scores for males were much higher than for females. In fact, all the female groups had scores at the resistance end of the scoring spectrum.

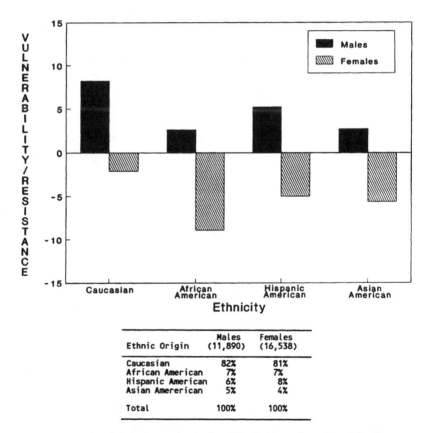

Ethnic Origin	Males (11,890)	Females (16,538)
Caucasian	82%	81%
African American	7%	7%
Hispanic American	6%	8%
Asian Amererican	5%	4%
Total	100%	100%

FIGURE 7.8. Ethnic background and vulnerability/resistance for males and females.

GROUP MEMBERSHIPS IMPACT MORE THAN SOCIAL LIFE

Sociodemographic background cannot be changed, but prevention practitioners must be aware of the associated propensities in order to be effective. Membership in most social groups and voluntary organizations is changeable. By knowing which group memberships promote resistance and which ones increase vulnerability, prevention practitioners can use the social influences of group membership as a tool of prevention.

Who Is More Vulnerable—Freshmen or Upperclassmen?

There are conflicting reports about the relationship between class year and substance abuse. Williams and Smith (1993) found that substance abuse increased with age until age 21, and on that basis we would expect juniors and seniors to show the highest vulnerability. However, Perlstadt, Hembroff, and Zonia (1991) found that freshmen reported are the greatest use of alcohol.

Our research across all the colleges tested shows that there is a sort of leveling off of vulnerability from the freshman year through the senior year. However, this across-the-board generalization does not hold when we look at specific colleges. Compared to the overall slight decrease across the board, there are some colleges that show a distinct increase in vulnerability by class year. This suggests the presence of a particular drug climate at those campuses and contradicts the assumptions of some other researchers. It is clear from our results that vulnerability must be considered the result of two major factors: one is the maturational biological process and the other is the net environmental effect at a particular college. Figure 7.9 shows that these effects can vary depending on the campus climate:

- Freshmen at high-use colleges are much more vulnerable to substance abuse than are freshmen at low-use colleges.
- At the high-use colleges, upperclassmen were less vulnerable than underclassmen whereas at low use colleges, class year made less difference.
- At College #73, vulnerability rose as students progressed through their college years, suggesting that this particular environment is in some way conducive to use.

The Benefits and Risks of Joining a Fraternity/Sorority

There is a continuing debate on the college campus regarding the benefits of fraternities and sororities as social organizations. Administrators are concerned that they are a source of substance abuse on campus, whereas members argue that their

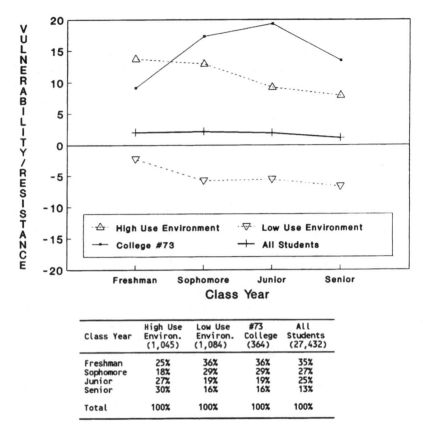

FIGURE 7.9. Class year and environmental influences on vulnerability/resistance.

organizations foster friendships and that their philanthropic interests promote healthy lifestyles. Recent studies (Goodwin, 1990; Klein, 1992; Montgomery, Benedicto, & Haemmerlie, 1993) have found that fraternity members are the heaviest consumers of alcohol on campus. Kuh and Arnold (1993) concluded that the values and beliefs of fraternities encourage alcohol consumption. Seventeen percent of the students we tested were members of fraternal organizations, and in most cases they did show higher than average vulnerability (see Figure 7.10). Varied results on a campus-by-campus basis as well as in high- versus low-use environments suggest the need to be cautious with generalizations and the need for further research:

- At the high-use campuses and among all campuses, membership in fraternal organizations was generally associated with higher Vulnerability scores.
- At the low-use campuses, fraternity membership was associated with lower Vulnerability scores (higher Resistance) than nonmembership. However,

only 4% of our low-use campus sample was involved with fraternities, so this result may be unstable.

- In the total student population sample, membership showed less, but still noticeable effects on vulnerability.

Does the Student's Choice of Major Suggest Greater Risk of Substance Abuse?

Any student's major field of study reflects his or her preferences, values, attitudes, and goals, which in turn may be related to behavioral propensities for substance abuse. This idea has not been broadly discussed in the literature; however, our data suggest that there may be subconscious selectivity or group influence affecting

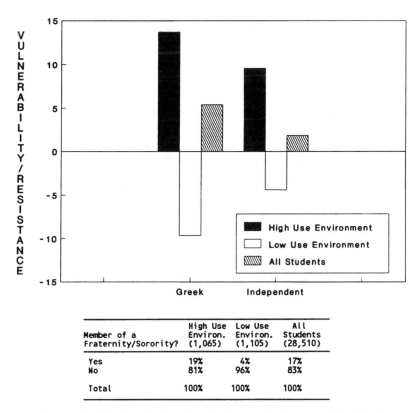

Member of a Fraternity/Sorority?	High Use Environ. (1,065)	Low Use Environ. (1,105)	All Students (28,510)
Yes	19%	4%	17%
No	81%	96%	83%
Total	100%	100%	100%

FIGURE 7.10. Membership in fraternity/sorority and environmental influences on vulnerability/resistance.

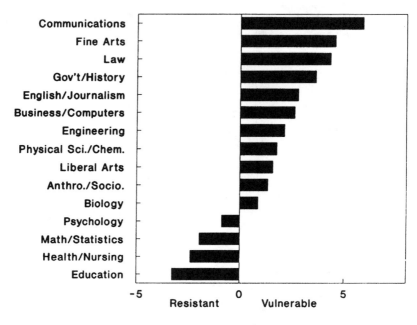

Major	# of students	Major	# of students
Communications	1147	Liberal Arts	463
Fine Arts	501	Anthro./Socio.	730
Law	727	Biology	1273
Gov't/History	1015	Psychology	2740
English/Journalism	953	Math/Statistics	320
Business/Computers	5038	Health/Nursing	2257
Engineering	1549	Education	3269
Physical Sci./Chem.	448		

FIGURE 7.11. Major field of study and vulnerability/resistance.

dispositions related to vulnerability/resistance. This issue obviously requires closer investigation, but our results are unlikely to be entirely accidental. Though our conclusions are based on 30,000 students, some of the specific fields had been selected by rather small subgroups, so we do not consider these conclusions to be generalizable. In Figure 7.11, we show the top 15 major fields pursued by the students in our sample, along with the average Vulnerability/Resistance score in each field's subset of students.

As shown in all of the figures presenting differences between students in high-use and in low-use environments, the environment has an impact on the student's propensities. In all of the variables we explored, there were significant differences in the vulnerability level of students living in high-use and in low-use environments. People who do not use drugs but who live in a high-use environment were found to have higher Vulnerability than comparable students in a low-use environment. We think these environmental influences deserve particular attention because we have found them to be strong and also because they work in combination with background variables that are already a part of contemporary risk assessments. Most important, our investigations of the impact of environment underscore the conclusion that vulnerability/resistance to substance abuse involves both psychological and environmental factors that need to be considered in combination. In Chapter 12 we return to this issue of environmental and cultural influences on substance abuse.

8

Lifestyles Affecting Vulnerability to Substance Abuse

The Vulnerability/Resistance measure was found to be a sensitive tool for assessing how various activities and lifestyles promote vulnerability or resistance to substance abuse. As the findings show, this question is best answered in the context of the environment. We found that many activities are neutral in themselves but can promote vulnerability in a high-use environment. This is characteristically true about certain sports and leisure activities. Certain lifestyles and activities increase a person's vulnerability in high-use environments where practicing a particular lifestyle involves frequent interactions with users.

CONFLICTING REPORTS OF LIFESTYLE INFLUENCES ON SUBSTANCE ABUSE

It is a much discussed topic in the literature that various behaviors and lifestyles do influence students' involvement with alcohol and other drugs. In the research literature on lifestyle, ambiguities related to practically every lifestyle factor have led to conflicting results. Most investigations have relied on self-reported behavior, which leaves open questions about cause and effect. Even strong correlations with reported substance abuse cannot be taken as proof of causation, unless the direction of the influence can be established conclusively. *Lifestyle* as we use it here refers to an enduring, routine behavior or activity that has a significant correlation with the use of harmful substances. Some lifestyle choices, such as joining a fraternity, are widely thought to promote substance abuse (Lo & Globetti, 1995), while others, like active attendance of religious services, seem to strengthen resistance to substance abuse (Cochran, 1993).

In our review of the literature, we observed that most social influences on drug and alcohol abuse are explained in terms of peer pressure. We think this has become popular largely because it is more readily researchable by direct methods than are more subtle, but frequently more powerful influences. In our view, students generally follow internal motives and needs of which they are unaware, and only in later reflection do they suggest that peer pressure was active. On the limitations of such tasks that assume the validity of introspections, the recent literature on implicit versus explicit cognitions and mental representations is rich and relevant (Greenwald & Banaji, 1995; Nelson, Schreiber, & McEvoy, 1992; Stacy, Ames, Sussman, & Dent, 1996). This is further discussed in Chapter 18.

Beyond peer pressures there are other mechanisms of social influence: culture change, social change, group influences, and various modalities of socialization and acculturation. These are recognized by sociologists and anthropologists, are widely discussed and speculated about, but mostly have not been empirically assessed. We address social influences in more depth in part IV. The following results bear on some of the most widely discussed lifestyle alternatives addressed in the literature on prevention. They provide information about other factors that have not been well recognized. In this chapter, we consider the following lifestyle elements: interaction with friends and peers of the same or opposite sex, participation in sports, and TV watching. We make several types of comparisons. First, we show how the reported frequency of an activity covaries with the reported frequency of alcohol and drug use. Then, for each activity, we show how the frequency covaries with the Vulnerability/Resistance measured and explore the differences based on gender, substance use involvement, and campus climate regarding substance use. Finally, we relate the results obtained through our comparative imaging and mapping techniques to the relevant literature. The Vulnerability/Resistance measure offers useful results on several fronts:

- Development of information about variables that appear to be relevant to prevention
- Resolution of conflicting research results on specific variables
- Identification of lifestyle alternatives that have the most promise of promoting resistance and reducing vulnerability as part of systematically planned and targeted prevention programs

SOCIAL CONTACTS: GOING OUT WITH FRIENDS AND DATING

Can Going Out with Friends Put Students at Greater Risk of Substance Abuse?

There has been a good deal of interest in how interaction with friends and peers affects the use of specific substances such as cigarettes (Feigelman & Lee, 1995), alcohol (Epstein, Botvin, Diaz, & Schinke, 1995; Johnson, Bachman & O'Malley, 1989; Weill & Le Bourhis, 1994), and various illicit drugs (Madianos, Gefou, Richardson, & Stefanis, 1995; Wallace & Bachman, 1991). There also has been interest in how ethnic-cultural background (Barnes, Farrell, & Banerjee, 1994; Madianos et al., 1995; Wallace & Bachman, 1991) and gender (Bahr, Marcos, & Maughan, 1995; Diem, McKay, & Jamieson, 1994; Weill & Le Bourhis, 1994) affect the interaction. In these and other contexts age is also considered a factor in shaping substance use (Diem et al., 1994; Keefe, 1994).

Parents often encourage their children to socialize and develop peer relationships. However, Bachman, Johnston, O'Malley, and Humphrey (1988) found that increased marijuana use was associated with greater frequency of going out at night. In our studies we found that frequent users are more likely to engage in extroverted activities, such as hanging out with friends and going to parties, and that this behavior is associated with increased vulnerability. Students who go out "a lot" with friends tend to drink more often and more excessively than students who go out less. Only 16% of the nonusers go out "a lot," whereas 43% of the heavy users do. High-frequency contact is clearly an important factor related to substance abuse.

The Vulnerability/Resistance measure has a broad multidimensional foundation in the respondents' dominant psychological dispositions relevant to decisions related to substance abuse. The reader may recall the results reported in part I. Frequent users were found to be very interested in social contacts, interaction with friends, the importance of going out with friends, and relating parties and bars to alcohol and drugs. Fun and entertainment were important features in their world. They were attracted to alcohol, drugs, and marijuana and paid little attention to potential harmful and negative consequences, such as addiction and other health hazards. Nonusers, on the other hand, had a much stronger interest in deeper, more meaningful personal relationships and tended to think about harmful and negative consequences of drugs and alcohol. As a result, they reject alcohol and drugs as stupid and socially unacceptable.

The practical application of these findings is related to the psychological dispositions underlying vulnerability/resistance. Therefore, a prevention effort might focus on finding a way to nurture serious friendships among students and to challenge the more casual socializing that may revolve around alcohol and drugs.

From our research, we have found that the effect of "going out with friends" on alcohol and drug use depends on the two primary variables of frequency of contact and social environment. Depending on how these interact, the effects of going out with friends can be positive or negative with respect to vulnerability. Under conditions of low contact with friends, the effects are slight, but as the frequency of contact increases, so does the likelihood for use. High social contact combined with high-use social environments increase vulnerability to substance

abuse in a major way. As shown in Figure 8.1, in the low-frequency contact categories the relation was generally flat; in other words, infrequent social contact did
not affect vulnerability. However, the number of students in the *never* and *seldom*
categories accounted for only about 10% of the population tested. Frequent contact was linked to an increase in vulnerability that was observed consistently for
90% of the students. The results show that friends, and the social environment in
general, are a powerful source of influences promoting vulnerability:

- Students who go out with friends "often" and "a lot" showed a sharp increase in vulnerability.
- The campus environment appears to have a greater impact on vulnerability
  as the student's frequency of social contact increases, as indicated by the
  growing gap between students in the high-use and low-use environments.

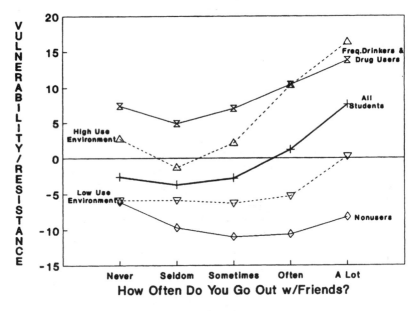

How Often Do You Go Out With Friends?	High Use Environ. (1,073)	Low Use Environ. (1,125)	Freq.Drink. Drug Users (11,648)	Nonusers (4,325)	All Students (28,787)
Never	1%	3%	1%	3%	1%
Seldom	6%	19%	6%	17%	10%
Sometimes	19%	32%	17%	34%	26%
Often	35%	27%	33%	30%	33%
A Lot	39%	19%	43%	16%	30%
Total	100%	100%	100%	100%	100%

FIGURE 8.1. Vulnerability/Resistance by frequency of going out with friends.

- At the low-use colleges only the students who went out "a lot" exhibited vulnerability; the general resistance of the majority of students was unaffected by contact with peers.
- The vulnerability of frequent alcohol/drug users rose the more they went out with friends, as it does for all students in high-use environments.
- Nonusers who never go out are less resistant than nonusers who have more frequent social contacts.

The vulnerability findings are singular in showing the multidimensional influences of the campus environment. The impact of the campus environment is clearly evident among students who are more actively involved with friends. Students in low-use campus environments have low vulnerability almost across the board. However, for students in high-use campus environments the use level and frequency of contact combine to produce additive effects, as suggested by the steep increase in vulnerability. The lines representing the vulnerability of students in high-use and in low-use environments are consistently far apart. Their distance shows how the differences between the high-use and the low-use environments entails differences in the students' propensity for substance use. As a measure of the effects of the campus environment, nonusers in a high-use environment show higher vulnerability than nonusers in a low-use campus environment. Results of analyses that systematically controlled for environmental effects have further demonstrated this conclusion (Szalay, Inn, & Doherty, 1996).

The impact of the environment with respect to drugs goes beyond direct, face-to-face peer influences of which students are aware. The effects of the social climate or of the social environment also include norms and standards of behavior and the prevailing views and attitudes about drugs and alcohol. Compared to the more readily researchable peer influences, there are many forms of subtle but powerful environmental effects of socialization, culture change, and *Zeitgeist* that operate below the students' conscious awareness (see part IV).

Figure 8.2 highlights gender differences and shows that, although males are more vulnerable than females (as we have seen in Chapter 7), the frequency of going out with friends has the same impact on vulnerability for both sexes. This is clearly demonstrated by the two closely parallel curves:

- Going out with friends frequently can significantly increase vulnerability to substance abuse, and male students tend to go out more often than the female students.
- Male students are much more vulnerable than female students, particularly when they go out "a lot."
- Female students exhibit resistance to substance abuse, except for those who go out with friends "a lot."

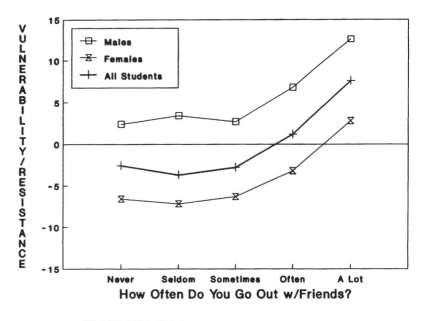

FIGURE 8.2. Frequency of going out with friends and vulnerability/resistance: Male–female differences.

Going Out on a Date Has a Different Impact
from Going Out with Friends

Although going out with friends had similar impact for both genders, we found somewhat different results regarding dating. For single males, dating is a source of slowly increasing vulnerability, rising with the frequency of dating. However, for single women, dating had no significant relationship with vulnerability (Figure 8.3):

- For females, going out on dates did not adversely affect their resistance.
- For males, vulnerability increased with dating.
- The biggest gender gap in vulnerability was among students who date "a lot."

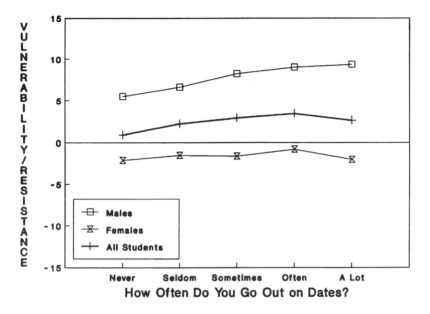

How Often Do You Go Out on Dates?

How Often Do You Go Out On Dates?	Males (11,775)	Females (16,444)	All Students (28,219)
Never	9%	14%	8%
Seldom	20%	18%	19%
Sometimes	29%	26%	28%
Often	23%	22%	24%
A Lot	19%	20%	21%
Total	100%	100%	100%

FIGURE 8.3. Dating and vulnerability/resistance for males and females.

The findings are consistent with the main conclusions of the literature, but they also introduce perspectives beyond what have commonly been discussed. The main difference in perspective between the traditional literature and our own research is that the traditional interest is in the role of behavior with respect to particular substances, whereas our work has focused on psychological dispositions that can be shown to be factors leading to substance abuse in general. From our perspective, differences in substances appear to be less consequential than the general propensities for substance abuse. As our results show, there is much more sharing of propensities among users of diverse substances than we, or any other researchers, anticipated.

Social influences resulting from interaction with friends appear to have a critical role in promoting propensities for substance abuse, and this role is broader and deeper than the narrow definition of peer pressure. Social activities vary in their impact on the propensity for substance abuse depending on several factors, such as the frequency of contact, environmental conditions, gender, and reported use. Based on large samples, we have identified particular social activities (e.g., going out with friends) that are associated with increased vulnerability and other activities that promote resistance. Depending on certain key factors, such as frequency of social contact and specific environmental conditions, some activities can have diverse, even opposing, effects.

The findings support several options for practical applications:

- Use the information offered by comparative imaging and mapping to reconcile conflicting results in the literature resulting from limited attention paid to psychological dispositions.
- Develop and use opportunities for social contact that optimize positive social influences while reducing the effect of influences promoting vulnerabilities.

What matters is not just the activity itself but also its role in promoting positive or negative influences shaped by the dominant psychological dispositions of the participants. Opportunities to assess the modalities of behavior and lifestyle in planning effective prevention programs are nearly unlimited.

PARTICIPATION IN SPORTS—THE HIDDEN HEALTH RISK

There is also conflicting research about whether participation in sports is a risk factor or a protective factor for substance abuse. In the mid-1980s the investigations of Rooney (1984) were published under the title of "Sports and clean living: A useful myth?" They are characteristic of several successive projects, both in their approach and in their conclusions. The research was based on questionnaire responses from close to 5,000 high school students from 6 states. As Rooney reported, the use of alcohol and various mind-altering substances did not decrease as a result of reported involvement in sports, although there was a slight reduction in smoking. He concluded that participation in all types of sports has very little effect on the use of mood-altering drugs.

During the next decade, numerous studies reached similar skeptical conclusions about the positive effects of sports on substance abuse. Most of these used questionnaires and reported mixed findings, depending on the focus of the research. Frintner and Rubinson (1993), with an interest in the effects of team membership, found a direct relationship between sports and alcohol use. In contrast, Vilhjalmsson and Thorlindsson (1992) concluded that sports have beneficial effects on the health status of the participants. Yet another study on the effects of extracurricular activities on alcohol and substance abuse, conducted with 16,000 students in Brazil, showed that sports participation did not have conclusive benefits, but religious involvement did (Carlini-Cotrim & Aparecida de Carvalho, 1993). Buckhalt, Halpin, Noel, and Meadows (1992), reporting on 130,000 students surveyed, found positive effects of academic and church involvements, but no significant effects of team athletics. However, based on an extensive review of the literature, Swisher and Hu (1983) concluded that certain activities like religious activities, sports, and academics detract from alcohol and drug use, whereas others, such as social entertainment and certain vocational activities, frequently act as facilitators.

As the literature indicates, it is customary to refer to the effects of sports in general and even to mix sports with other subjects, such as extracurricular activities or social entertainment. This diversity of referents is obviously one source of the varying conclusions reached by these investigations. Our view is that it makes

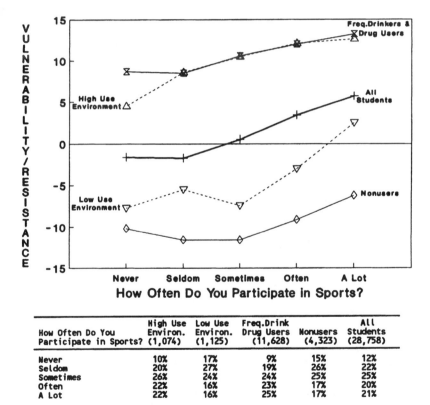

How Often Do You Participate in Sports?	High Use Environ. (1,074)	Low Use Environ. (1,125)	Freq.Drink Drug Users (11,628)	Nonusers (4,323)	All Students (28,758)
Never	10%	17%	9%	15%	12%
Seldom	20%	27%	19%	26%	22%
Sometimes	26%	24%	24%	25%	25%
Often	22%	16%	23%	17%	20%
A Lot	22%	16%	25%	17%	21%
Total	100%	100%	100%	100%	100%

FIGURE 8.4. Sports participation and vulnerability/resistance for frequent drinkers/drug users and for nonusers.

considerable difference regarding which sports are being considered. There are team sports and individual sports, spectator sports that lead to social entertainment, and sports activities that require intense personal physical exertion, concentration, and discipline, and they each can have a different impact.

For Some, Being Active in Sports Increases Vulnerability

When we administered the AGA task to our samples of college students, we posed the question about sports involvement in a general way: "How often do you actively participate in sports?" Almost half of the binge drinkers and drug users participated actively (often, a lot) in sports, in contrast to just a third of the nonusers.

Although our results varied from campus to campus, the overall picture drawn from the large student sample suggests that more active participation in sports is related to greater vulnerability to substance abuse. Figure 8.4 compares survey-based results with scores on the Vulnerability/Resistance measure:

- Across the board, the more frequently students participated in sports, the higher their vulnerability score.
- Frequency of participation in sports had the greatest impact on vulnerability among students in the low-use college environments.

What Sport Are We Talking About?

The literature on the relationship between sports and alcohol/drug use is conflicting and inconclusive, and our own findings provide only a partial explanation. Our data on frequent drinkers and on students in high-use environments supports the conclusion that sports participation is a contributor to vulnerability. However, nonusers have a different pattern. For these people, sports participation appears to have less effect on their vulnerability.

Beyond the social influences, another source of differences is the different meanings of sports. The situation is complicated by diverse interests and approaches of different investigations. Most research reported in the literature considers sports for its intervention value or remedial potential, whereas our interest in sports is in its value for shaping students' dispositions in ways that build resistance to substance abuse. In the American college scene, "sports" has diverse meanings, often with an emphasis on physical performance and often seen as entertainment. Our research in many college settings underscores the importance of making such a distinction. Our analysis of perceptions and attitudes has shown that nonusers tend to value individual and small-group sports activities, including skiing, running, mountain biking, exercising, and hiking. Frequent users are more interested in intramural, team and spectator sports, and large-group sporting events. Often such sporting events and competitions are seen as another chance to party with friends and are closely associated with alcohol use. Our very general question about sports participation hampered our ability to provide more differentiated results, but the results suggest the need to seek, beyond the entertainment-focused aspect of the term *sports,* more specific categories of sports with better-differentiated attributes. We now know that the role of sports cannot really be studied unless the general concept is broken down into more specific subparts or particular sports. What seems to make a difference is the level of physical involvement, discipline and endurance, and whether it is the sporting events that have more of the element of social entertainment that likely involves the use of alcohol, cigarettes, and sometimes drugs.

HOW TV VIEWING HABITS CAN AFFECT VULNERABILITY

A subset of our sample (2,058 college students tested at six different campuses in 1994) were asked about their television-viewing habits. One third of the students said they watched TV less than a hour a day. Another third spent 1–2 hours a day in front of the TV, and the rest watched for more than 2 hours. We found the level of watching and the level of alcohol consumption to have little relationship to each other. The level of watching did not show any significant relationship to vulnerability for females and only little relationship to it for males.

We also asked students whether they believed that there is too much violence on television. Over 70% agreed that there is too much. We noted strong gender differences: 80% of females agreed, in contrast to 55% of the males. On the other hand, 21% of the male students disagreed with the statement compared to 4% of the females. A larger portion of the frequent drinkers and drug users did not find television violence excessive.

We found a stronger effect regarding the issue of TV violence. Students who appeared to be less sensitive to violence on television also tended to drink more and to be generally more psychologically susceptible to substance abuse. Again, these results were stronger for males than for females. Figure 8.5 shows the Vulnerability/Resistance levels of nonusers and frequent alcohol drinkers in relation to their opinions of TV violence:

- Students who perceived less violence on TV showed increasing vulnerability to substance abuse.
- Even students who are neutral on this issue showed higher vulnerability than did students who took the position that the violence is excessive.
- The nonusers generally showed resistance, although it was significantly lower when they disagreed on this issue.

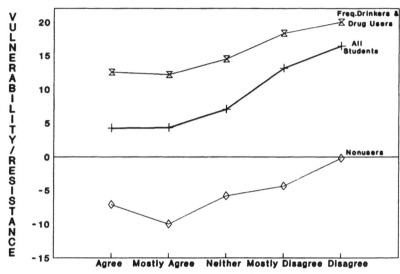

There Is Too Much Violence on TV

There Is Too Much Violence On TV.	Freq.Drink. Drug Users (1,170)	Nonusers (217)	All Students (2,005)
Agree	35%	47%	39%
Mostly Agree	32%	25%	32%
Neither	19%	21%	18%
Mostly Disagree	5%	2%	5%
Disagree	9%	5%	6%
Total	100%	100%	100%

FIGURE 8.5. Opinions of TV violence related to vulnerability/resistance of frequent drinkers/drug users and of nonusers.

We did find some gender differences. Females who agree that TV violence is excessive average 4.6 drinks per week, not much less than females who disagree (6.1 drinks per week). For males, however, perception of violence on TV is closely associated with their drinking: males who agree average 9.9 drinks per week but those who do not think there is too much violence on TV report an average of 15.6 drinks per week. The average number of drinks per week for this college population is 5.5.

Figure 8.6 presents the psychological vulnerability associated with these different positions toward violence on television for male and female students. Although students who exhibited the highest vulnerability regardless of gender were those who disagreed that there is too much violence, the female students' vulnerability was lower overall and did not rise as sharply as that of the male students.

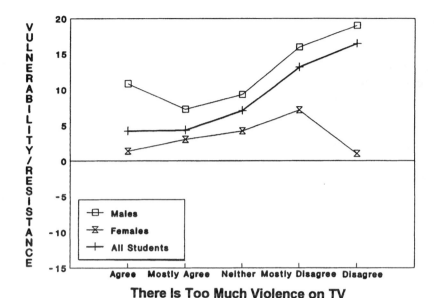

FIGURE 8.6. Opinions of TV violence related to vulnerability/resistance of males and of females.

Also, males who strongly agreed showed more vulnerability than do males who "mostly" agreed. This was not true of the female students:

- Regardless of gender, opinions on TV violence are clearly related to the students' vulnerability/resistance to substance abuse.
- Male students showed higher vulnerability than female students, even when they shared the same opinions about TV violence. The largest gender gap in vulnerability was observed at both extremes. A larger proportion of male students (21% in contrast to 5% of the females) disagreed.
- Of the female students, 80% agreed that there is too much violence on TV and these students showed lower vulnerability. However, so did the few female students at the other extreme.

The results suggest two types of conclusions. On the relationship between the amount of TV watching and vulnerability to substance abuse, there were distinct gender differences based on reported TV watching and reported substance use: there was a strong relationship between drinking and TV watching for males but not for females. The findings also suggest differences between frequent drinkers and drug users compared to nonusers. Whereas frequent users show a slow general increase in vulnerability that accompanies more time spent watching TV, in the case of generally resistant nonusers there is a slight increase in resistance with hours of TV watching.

Regarding perceived violence on TV, the data on reported substance use and reported perception of violence showed a much stronger relation than was found regarding hours of TV watching in general. The frequent drinkers and drug users were less likely to perceive violence, whereas almost three-quarters of the nonusers agreed that there is too much violence on TV. The vulnerability of the students was clearly linked to the degree to which they perceived violence of TV. Differences were found between males and females in that the vulnerability of males increased more dramatically as their perception of violence decreased.

9

Academic Performance and Lifestyles That Build Resistance

Behaviors and lifestyles found to promote resistance to substance abuse vary in their impact. Across the lifestyles examined, the effects of the social environment were more articulate in promoting vulnerability than resistance. The lifestyles found to promote resistance include academic performance, class attendance, religious attendance, and volunteering. The influences of the high-use vs. low-use campus environments were found to vary considerably.

ARE ACADEMIC MOTIVATION AND ACADEMIC PERFORMANCE SERIOUSLY COMPROMISED BY ALCOHOL AND DRUG USE?

In view of the debilitating consequences of substance abuse, there never has been much doubt that excessive alcohol and other drug use is incompatible with high academic performance. However, there are some popular assumptions that low-level alcohol use and recreational drug use have few negative consequences and could even be beneficially stimulating. Glantz and Pickens (1992) and other groups differentiate between drug use, drug abuse, and addiction, but considering our focus on prevention, such distinctions are of little interest to us. Our approach is to explore substance use along the entire spectrum, and where to draw the line between use and abuse is secondary in our discussion of academic motivation and performance.

The majority of research literature indicates that an inverse relationship exists between academic performance and substance use. Bahr, Marcos, and Maughan (1995) found that students in grades 7 to 12 with strong educational commitment tended to drink less frequently and in smaller quantities. Thomas and Hsiu (1993) found that GPA was among the four strongest predictors of substance abuse among 9th to 12th graders. Based on a survey of 130,000 7th, 9th, and 11th graders, Buckhalt, Halpin, Noel, and Meadows (1992) found that students who reported greater involvement in school also reported less involvement with drugs.

Academic Motivation—Students Who Skip Classes Are Thinking Like Users

As a simple indicator of academic motivation, we asked the students in our samples about their frequency of skipping classes. Though over 70% of the students said that they seldom or never skip classes, we found that class attendance and substance use are significantly related. Thirty-nine percent of the frequent drinkers and drug users say they skip class in contrast to 15% of the nonusers.

Figure 9.1 illustrates the relationship between class attendance and vulnerability among various categories of college students. The results parallel the relationship with self-reports of alcohol and drug use and show that the more frequently students skip classes, the more vulnerable they are to substance abuse. The results show that Vulnerability scores increase as class skipping increases and reach a peak with a high level of truancy in the high-use environment.

It is important to remember that "vulnerability" and "resistance" are not simply synonyms for "substance use" and "abstinence." Rather, they represent something much deeper: students who skip classes have attitudes, values, and beliefs that are similar to those of frequent users. More specifically, students who skip classes (and have higher Vulnerability scores) are more like users, who typically value their education less and have a more negative attitude toward school. Their more negative attitude toward school and learning and nonacademic self-concept leave them vulnerable to substance use, particularly when they are attending a college where alcohol and other drugs serve as a convenient distractor to education:

- The more regularly students followed their academic schedule, the stronger was their disposition not to be involved in the use of harmful substances. Skipping class, indicative of low academic interest, was associated with higher vulnerability: Students who often skip class are at greater risk because they are thinking and feeling in ways that are similar to heavy users.
- At the low-use colleges, most students indicated that they seldom or never skip class and these students showed greater resistance than their classmates who skip more often, despite the dip at the end where there are too few students to obtain reliable results.

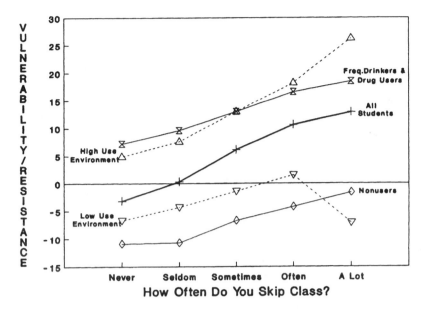

FIGURE 9.1. Class attendance and vulnerability/resistance by environment and use.

- Skipping classes had less impact on vulnerability in the low-use campus environments than in the high-use ones where more students skipped and there were much larger increases in vulnerability with greater frequency of absence.
- Frequent alcohol/drug users, like students in the high-use environment, showed higher than average vulnerability even when they do not skip class, but skipping class appeared to increase their Vulnerability to even higher levels.

We also found that male and female students differ with respect to skipping classes. Although the relationship between the frequency of skipping class and the increase in vulnerability is very similar for men and women, men have higher vulnerability at all levels of class attendance.

Academic Achievement Builds Resistance

Many studies have shown that high academic achievement is associated with lower levels of substance abuse. This relationship may seem obvious, because a student who abuses alcohol and other drugs will have less time and less cognitive capacity to devote to his or her studies. However, what survey research does not provide is an indication of the values, attitudes, goals, and beliefs that either increase motivation for academic success or increase vulnerability to substance abuse. What perspectives do the high achievers have that can be nurtured, encouraged, and rewarded to keep them from using alcohol or other drugs?

As a measure of academic achievement, we asked the college students to report their GPA. As might be expected, we found the largest proportion of abstainers and occasional drinkers among students reporting the highest grades: thirty percent of nonusers had a GPA of at least 3.5, whereas only 12% of the heavy alcohol/drug users reached that level of academic achievement. Conversely, the heaviest alcohol and drug use occurs among students who reported the poorest grades.

We examined the relationship between academic performance and Vulnerability/Resistance levels for various groups of students in low-use and in high-use college environments. Figure 9.2 illustrates the inverse relationship we found:

- Students with a GPA of 2.4 or less had greater vulnerability than students who reported better academic performance, regardless of the environment.
- In the high-use college environment, even students with good grades had more vulnerability than students in other college settings.
- Students with average grades were much more vulnerable on high-use campuses than on low-use campuses.
- In low-use campus environments, students generally showed resistance to substance abuse, but those with high GPAs showed the strongest resistance.
- Frequent drinkers and drug users who maintained a high GPA did show lower vulnerability than users with lower academic achievement.

We found similar, strong relationships between vulnerability/resistance and both academic motivation and academic performance. The frequency of skipping classes (our index of motivation) showed a direct relationship with vulnerability. Academic performance, measured by GPA, had a consistent relationship to vulnerability/resistance: students who performed well were more resistant, and poor or marginal students were increasingly vulnerable. For both academic factors, their relationship to vulnerability was particularly strong in the high-use environment and for frequent users. Males and females showed parallel trends, though males were found to be more vulnerable and females were found to be more resistant across the board.

As we described in part I, the mosaics underlying vulnerability and resistance suggest that nonusers take their role as students more seriously and define the

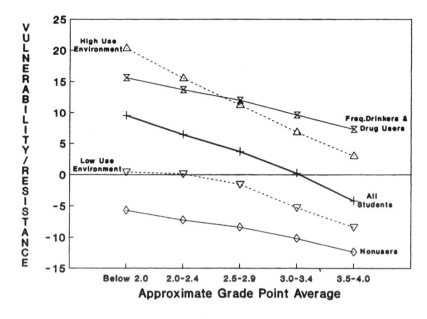

FIGURE 9.2. Academic performance and vulnerability/resistance by environment and use.

Approximate Grade Point Average	High Use Environ. (1,053)	Low Use Environ. (1,096)	Freq.Drink. Drug Users (11,359)	Nonusers (4,194)	All Students (28,787)
Below 2.0	3%	1%	3%	1%	2%
2.0-2.4	19%	9%	17%	8%	13%
2.5-2.9	42%	25%	35%	24%	31%
3.0-3.4	28%	39%	33%	37%	35%
3.5-4.0	8%	26%	12%	30%	19%
Total	100%	100%	100%	100%	100%

campus as a place of learning and study, whereas users are more focused on the social and nonacademic aspects of campus life. The consistency of our results demonstrates that high academic performance has a solid foundation in high abstinence and low vulnerability.

ANY VOLUNTEERS?

Volunteering has not been discussed much in the scientific literature as a lifestyle factor relevant to substance abuse prevention. Nevertheless, volunteering is a unique and important facet of the American culture. It ties in with fundamental characteristics identified by the foremost students of the American cultural scene (Hofstede, 1980; Hsu, 1981; Triandis, 1990) such as self-reliance, individualism,

and an action orientation. In our own comparative research conducted since the late
1960s with many samples from both American cultures and a number of others, we
have seen how American individualism and ideocentrism provide the foundation
for many of the behavioral dispositions that nurture volunteering. We found a sharp
contrast between Caucasian Americans and Hispanic Americans, Caucasian Americans and Arabs, and Caucasian Americans and Chinese.

Students Who Volunteer Show More Resistance to Substance Abuse

In our research on college campuses we included volunteering as a variable
in order to explore its potential for supporting prevention. We examined the general level of volunteering as well as the student's interest in four specific types of

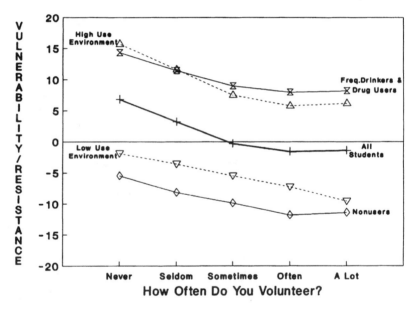

How Often Do You Volunteer?	High Use Environ. (1,069)	Low Use Environ. (1,124)	Freq.Drink. Drug Users (9,931)	Nonusers (3,245)	All Students (22,449)
Never	20%	20%	24%	15%	19%
Seldom	35%	30%	35%	28%	33%
Sometimes	29%	31%	26%	34%	30%
Often	11%	12%	10%	16%	12%
A Lot	5%	7%	5%	7%	6%
Total	100%	100%	100%	100%	100%

FIGURE 9.3. Volunteering and vulnerability/resistance by environment and use.

volunteering: peer counseling, community service, academic tutoring, and promoting a drug-free environment. Our analysis, based on 22,000 students, shows that volunteering is clearly associated with greater resistance to substance abuse.

Nearly 80% of the students reported participating in some level of volunteer services. Generally, a higher proportion of the nonusers than the frequent users were active volunteers (*often* or *a lot*), whereas a higher proportion of the frequent users seldom or never volunteered. Although the relationship between usage and volunteering is not striking, the students' vulnerability/resistance clearly is related to their decisions regarding volunteering (Figure 9.3).

- At high-use colleges, students who actively volunteered were at much lower risk than fellow students who were less involved.
- At the low-use colleges, all students showed resistance, which increased with degree of involvement in volunteering.
- Frequent alcohol/drug users who volunteered showed lower vulnerability than those who did not.

Even an Expressed Interest in Volunteering Is Linked to Lower Vulnerability

We asked students about their interest in volunteering for peer counseling, for community service, for academic tutoring, and for a drug-free environment. Table 9.1 shows their responses by the levels of reported use. Most interest was expressed in

TABLE 9.1. Vulnerability/Resistance of College Students Interested in Volunteering

Interest in volunteering	Nonusers (*n* = 4,338)		Freq. drinkers & drug users (*n* = 11,726)		All students (*n* = 23,191)	
	%	V/R score	%	V/R score	%	V/R score
as peer counselor?						
No	56%	−8.1	52%	12.2	53%	3.0
Yes	44%	−10.5	48%	9.9	47%	1.0
for community service?						
No	50%	−7.6	54%	12.5	52%	3.8
Yes	50%	−10.8	45%	9.1	48%	.2
for academic tutoring						
No	69%	8.3	78%	11.5	74%	3.0
Yes	31%	−11.1	22%	9.1	26%	−.7
for drug-free environment?						
No	59%	−8.1	84%	12.0	73%	4.1
Yes	41%	−10.8	16%	5.8	27%	−3.5

community service. The Vulnerability/Resistance results indicate that students who may not presently be active in volunteerism but who are interested in volunteering show greater resistance to substance abuse than do students who have expressed no desire to serve.

Strengthening Resistance to Substance Abuse through Volunteering

Previous research has suggested that volunteering produces personal experiences that deepen motivation and involvement. Volunteers working for a homeless shelter, for instance, were observed to enhance their related experience as well as their dedication. Peer volunteers offer important advantages in reaching members of their own age group. Using their own language and their own style of thinking and reasoning, peer volunteers can overcome communication barriers and other obstacles that stem from generational differences in views and perspectives. In the field of substance abuse prevention the importance of such differences in perspectives cannot be exaggerated.

In Part I, users of alcohol and other harmful substances are characterized as students leaning toward social alienation and expressing skepticism toward authority, society and government. They also show a strong tendency to overlook negative consequences of their behavior and to ignore harm in general and the possibility of addiction in particular. Because of these dispositions, young students in their most vulnerable periods of life are particularly hard to reach by people who are older and who represent the "establishment," authority figures, and whose discussion of consequences tend to be dismissed as scare tactics.

The University of Michigan surveys could not be more clear and convincing about the importance of perceived harm as the single most powerful factor shaping the ups and downs of substance abuse among students in the United States since the late 1970s. Whenever the students tend to ignore harm, the level of substance abuse rises, and when the students tend to recognize harm, the level of drug use decreases. Teachers, experts, and older people in general are at a grave disadvantage in delivering an effective message. Overcoming the students' tendency to ignore harm as well as allaying their suspicions of being manipulated are particularly difficult tasks for educational prevention. Relying on volunteers of the students' own age appears to be a promising approach.

Along this line volunteering offers two important opportunities:

- *Volunteering can be an effective tool of communication* to bridge differences in frames of reference and to communicate potential dangers to students who obviously lack the experience.
- *Volunteering as a lifestyle alternative* can effectively promote experiences that reduce vulnerability and build resistance to substance abuse.

AN ACTIVE RELIGIOUS/SPIRITUAL LIFE BUILDS RESISTANCE
TO SUBSTANCE ABUSE

Many references in the literature have shown that religious involvement, participation in religious services, and various other manifestations of religious convic-
tion correlate negatively with substance abuse. That is, the more involved an
individual is with religious practice, the less likely it is that he or she will be involved with substance abuse. This conclusion is supported by a host of investigations since 1992 which have used large samples of adolescents (Hardert & Dowd,
1994), high school students (such as McGee & Newcomb, 1992) and college students (Free, 1994). Conflicting evidence is rare and focuses primarily on the use
of hallucinogenic drugs to promote "religious," or "mystical" experiences.

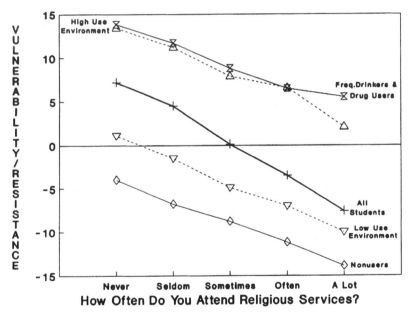

How Often Do You Attend Religious Services?	High Use Environ. (1,070)	Low Use Environ. (1,124)	Freq.Drink. Drug Users (11,614)	Nonusers (4,317)	All Students (28,716)
Never	35%	15%	32%	15%	24%
Seldom	34%	26%	35%	16%	29%
Sometimes	14%	18%	17%	15%	18%
Often	9%	17%	9%	19%	14%
A Lot	8%	24%	7%	35%	15%
Total	100%	100%	100%	100%	100%

FIGURE 9.4. Religious attendance and vulnerability/resistance by environment and use.

We used the imaging and mapping procedure to test the assumption that the values associated with most organized religions deter members from using harmful substances. The process allowed us to identify the particular values or beliefs that promote resistance to substance abuse as well as those that promote religious attendance. We found that nonusers embrace social values and institutions as good and necessary features in their lives. For them, religion provides support, love, comfort, morality, structure, and salvation. Users tend to be much more cynical about social institutions and values and question the authority and restrictions imposed. We have also found that male students are critical of religion, seeing it as stupid, while female students have doubts as to the benefits religion has to offer.

In our investigations, we asked students about the frequency of their attendance at religious services as a reflection of their religious orientation and as an indicator of behavior and lifestyle. The majority of students (53%) reported seldom or never attending religious services. One third of the nonusers attended services a lot, whereas only 7% of the frequent drinkers and drug users did. In general, the students who indicated more frequent attendance also reported less alcohol and drug use.

The results based on the total student population suggest that religious attendance is one of the strongest indicators of resistance to substance abuse. Those who attend religious services regularly reveal much lower vulnerability than students who seldom or never attend. Figure 9.4 presents findings on various categories of students in high-use and low-use environments as follows:

- Students who actively participated in religious services had lower vulnerability than students who participated less often or not at all.
- Students who attended religious services often or a lot had the strongest resistance at the low-use colleges and lowest vulnerability at the high-use colleges.
- Students who never attended religious services were the most vulnerable.
- Among the frequent drinkers and drug users, those who were more actively involved in their religion showed lower vulnerability to substance abuse than those who were less actively involved.

The linear relationship presented in Figure 9.4 is particularly steep, reflecting the strength of the relationship. Also, the distance between the vulnerability/resistance measured in high-use environments and in low-use environments was the largest on religious participation. Similarly, the distance between the lines representing nonusers and frequent users is also unusually large. Students who attend religious services least frequently are the most vulnerable to substance abuse and those who attend the most frequently are the most resistant to it.

In the research reported in part I we showed the perceptual and attitudinal foundation of this lifestyle of religious involvement. Some of the characteristics of users, their pleasure-centered world, their stronger materialism, hedonism, their stronger focusing on self rather than others, and their dismissiveness of harm, addiction, and consequences reveal the perceptual and attitudinal dispositions that are behind their vulnerability to substance abuse. The users consistently show preoccupation with pleasure and instant gratification, entertainment, sex, and so forth. In contrast, certain key attributes we identified as characteristic of the nonusers serve as the main psychological dispositions behind their resistance to substance abuse. The nonusers tend to be less centered on self and pay more attention to positive interpersonal relationships and the needs and interests of others. They place more emphasis on responsibility, future consequences, and personal and social harm.

As we know from the literature, denomination and formal affiliation make little difference except in their degree of tolerance toward alcohol. What appears to be truly consequential is the existence of an organized system of perceptions and attitudes that provides a coherent interpretation of the world with a focus on norms regulating interpersonal relationships. Another factor recognized in the literature is that *religiosity*, the lifestyle of religious attendance and practice, commonly has a strong foundation in family background and education. It is a propensity that can have deep roots and can promote resistance both in the short and in the long range.

CONVERGENT FINDINGS INDICATE PROPENSITIES WITH DEEP ROOTS AND STRONG IMPLICATIONS FOR PREVENTION

An important element of the lifestyle data is the high level of agreement between the Vulnerability measure and self-report data. Academic performance and lifestyles are areas where self-report data are available and can generally be trusted. Thus, we have even stronger support for the validity of the Vulnerability measure—its ability to measure propensities independent of biases usually associated with self-report measures of substance use. The results available on variables on which this direct comparison is possible lend confidence to the behavioral implications of factors on which the comparative data necessary for validation have not been available. For example, the findings of the imaging and mapping process support the idea that involvement in sports can promote both resistance and vulnerability to substance abuse. Apparently, a critical factor is the type of sport being considered (individual, intramural) and the nature of "involvement" (spectator, participant). Sports can offer a practical way to promote prevention, once it has been clarified what type of involvement promotes resistance to substance abuse.

Our results regarding academic motivation and performance suggest that active involvement promotes resistance. The students' higher performance emerges clearly as a result of a combination of psychological dispositions that support achievement. It is of special relevance to the task of prevention that fighting vulnerability goes beyond reducing propensities for substance abuse; it also involves promoting psychological dispositions that not only increase the students' resistance to substance abuse but also appear to be beneficial to their academic achievement.

The findings on volunteering indicate that it can be a useful activity for promoting resistance. The more volunteering students reported, the higher their Resistance score. Even students in high-use campus environments and frequent users of alcohol and other drugs show lower vulnerability when they volunteer. Volunteer work provides a simple and effective way to approach students through their peers. Efforts could be made to recruit students who do recognize the harm and are sensitive to the negative consequences of substance abuse. Their experience of helping others may lead to changes in their own attitudes, priorities, and values that make them more resistant to substance abuse. Volunteers who serve as academic tutors, peer counselors, or in other roles of student leadership may be successful in reaching students who are vulnerable. The impact can be twofold. For example, an academic tutor can help to boost the recipient's GPA, academic self-concept, and values concerning class attendance. The indirect influence can simply be the increased social contact between the recipient, who may be vulnerable to substance abuse, and the more resistant tutor (or peer counselor). Whether by example or additional social contacts outside of the volunteer/recipient relationship, the tutor can be a positive social influence for those he or she tutors.

In the research literature, religious participation has a universally positive effect on reducing the use of harmful substances. Our findings also show that religious involvement reduces vulnerability and enhances resistance.

Certain lifestyles may at first appear unrelated to substance abuse. Our results offer some new insights and evidence of how lifestyles promote various propensities, some promoting substance abuse and some protecting against it. Students with a commitment to academic achievement, those who attend classes regularly and obtain high grades, and those who attend religious services possess psychological dispositions that help them be more resistant to substance abuse than those who do not. Conversely, students who place priority on hedonistic values and entertainment, go out frequently, and are involved in social activities or entertainment-oriented sports have dispositions that leave them more vulnerable to engagement in substance abuse. Our findings across a variety of different lifestyles support the following conclusions:

- Although lifestyle choices may be the single most important measurable variable, the choices reflect the underlying dispositions that make an important difference.
- The intensity with which students practice a particular lifestyle or activity is a direct factor.

- The environment in which the activity is carried out can make a difference: for any given lifestyle choice, high-use and low-use environments can produce different effects on vulnerability or resistance to substance abuse.

In the various validation experiments, the consistency of results showing that vulnerability rises with the increasing use of any specific substance gave us confidence to explore how this measure may help in clarifying the effects of other variables that have been linked to substance abuse. In the last three chapters we have examined how the students' background, environment, academic performance, and lifestyles affect their propensities for substance abuse, as measured by their Vulnerability/Resistance scores.

In the context of background variables, we identified some with vulnerability and others with resistance. These findings are important from the angle of risk assessment even though such background factors as gender and ethnicity are fixed and unalterable. Nevertheless, these are not the most important factors to consider in prevention program development that is actively oriented to increase resistance and reduce vulnerability by targeting the students' psychological dispositions. We found that the students' lifestyle choices do vary in their consequences to promote vulnerability or resistance. We could clearly identify some lifestyles or activities which are associated with vulnerability, such as skipping classes and a high frequency of going out with friends. We also identified other lifestyle choices, such as academic achievement and religious attendance, associated with lower vulnerability and higher resistance.

A particularly important conclusion we can draw from examining the interrelationship of these many variables is that in many instances it is not the lifestyle alone that makes the difference but the lifestyle choices in combination with the environment. Going out with friends, for instance, can be very much a source of increasing vulnerability in a high-use campus environment. On the other hand, frequent going out with friends had little negative effects in environments characterized by low use. These findings underline the importance of considering the important variables in combination in order to draw meaningful conclusions about their effects.

Part IV

Tracing Environmental Influences,
Cultural and Social

Cultural Factors in Substance Abuse

From the angle of behavior, cultural factors create psychological dispositions rooted in people's histories and shared experiences that shape their world and actions, mostly without their awareness. These dispositions are of natural interest to professionals whose success in providing effective help and services depends on their ability to take the dispositions of their clients into consideration. This is a particularly demanding requirement in servicing minority populations with backgrounds different from the American mainstream. The main instruments used in the field of substance abuse and prevention are acculturation questionnaires. Our measure of cultural distance is a comparable tool based on imaging and mapping.

THE CASE OF HISPANIC-AMERICANS

In the following discussion we rely on the example of Hispanic-Americans. Our choice of population is based on several considerations. Hispanic-Americans represent the fastest growing minority population characterized by a language other than English in the United States. Despite sharing Spanish as their traditional language, Hispanic-Americans, as we will see, are highly diverse. According to the 1990 U.S. Bureau of the Census, there are more than 20 million Hispanics in the United States. Approximately 63% are people of Mexican origin residing in the Southwest and in the West, 12% are mainland Puerto Ricans located in the Northeast, and about 5% are Cubans residing in the Southeast. Current projections indicate that Hispanic-Americans will be the biggest minority group in the United States between the years of 2000 and 2010.

For several decades now statistics on a variety of individual and social problems, including substance abuse, have shown disproportionately high incidence rates among Hispanic-American populations. The New York City Board of Education's Annual Drop-out Report (1987–1988) stated that among New York City high school students, 39% of the dropouts were Hispanic-American, compared to 5% Asian-American, 39% African-American, and 17% Caucasian-American (New York City's high school population for that same time period was 30% Hispanic-American, 8% Asian-American, 40% African-American, and 23% Caucasian-American). Brenner and Meagher reported in 1970 that nearly three out of every four addicts were non-Caucasian (Hispanic-Americans, African-Americans), and there is evidence that Hispanic-Americans have a higher rate of substance abuse than African-American and Caucasian-Americans. In 1977, Martinez noted that there was a disproportionate number of Puerto Ricans reported in New York as narcotic addicts and drug abusers. Ten years later, according to the 1986 New York Statewide Household Survey of Substance Abuse (Frank, Schmeidler, Marel, & Maranda, 1988), Hispanic-Americans had a higher rate of use of the most frequently used illegal drugs—marijuana, cocaine, and heroin—than non-Hispanics. There is also evidence that Hispanic-American drug users engage in riskier and more dangerous habits involving substance abuse: among Hispanic-American drug users 21% regularly inject drugs compared to 10% of African-Americans and 2% of Caucasian-Americans.

Culture: The Hidden Dimension

It is generally agreed that the sources of contemporary inequities do not involve innate differences in intelligence or academic aptitude. Rather, these differences result from differences in background or culture. The literature on the importance and role of culture is rich and voluminous, yet since culture is characteristically evasive to objective empirical assessment, the scientific value of much of what is offered is frequently debated. Nevertheless, culture is one of the most powerful and ubiquitous realities of human existence. During the 1900s, hundreds of dedicated anthropologists have studied cultures across the globe and produced valuable knowledge supporting its hidden nature and its universal influence. Of special relevance here are the works of cultural and psychological anthropologists like Ruth Benedict (1935), Margaret Mead (1928), Francis Hsu (1961), Bronislav Malinowski (1944), Clyde Kluckhohn (1959), and Florence Kluckhohn and Fred Strodtbeck (1961). The most favored anthropological method of participant observation has offered useful insights for those practicing it in the field.

The resulting monographs provide rich illustrations of how behavior varies across cultures based on different experiences and resulting in different worlds. They illustrate how culture predisposes people to see the world and its problems in different ways, and these different ways of seeing result in fascinating differences in behavior. Their observations help us to appreciate culture as a ubiquitous force shaping our world as well as the world of others. Based on these insights Margaret Mead (1953) reached the following conclusion:

> A primary task of mid-twentieth century is the increasing of understanding, understanding of our own culture and of that of other countries. On our capacity to develop new forms of such understanding may well depend the survival of our civilization, which has placed its faith in science and reason but has not yet succeeded in developing a science of human behavior which gives men a decent measure of control over their own fate.

As the leading anthropologist Edward T. Hall, author of *The silent language* and *The hidden dimension*, put it : "People from different cultures not only speak different languages, they inhabit different sensory worlds" (1966, p. 2). Culture influences what we think and do, controlling human behavior in deep and persisting ways without our awareness. "Like an iceberg, culture hides more than it reveals, and strangely enough, what it hides, it hides most effectively from its own participants" (Hall, 1959). Cultural factors are frustratingly evasive to empirical assessment, and consequently, there is a natural inclination to ignore them in contemporary research. As Hall (1966) cogently observed:

> . . . we have consistently failed to accept the reality of different cultures within our national boundaries. Negroes, Indians, Spanish Americans, Puerto Ricans are treated as though they were recalcitrant, undereducated middle class Americans of northern European heritage instead of what they really are: members of culturally differentiated enclaves with their own communication systems, institutions, and values. (p. 183)

Within our own country Oscar Lewis and his associates (1966) analyzed forms of abject poverty which shape perceptions, attitudes, and outlook on the world in a way analogous to culture. Lewis even coined the phrase "culture of poverty" to describe how different economic conditions create vastly different world views, even within the same national borders. This culture of poverty, once established, can maintain itself by weakening people's natural coping potential to improve their situation.

Although these outstanding scholars of cultural anthropology placed the fascinating subject of culture in its proper perspectives, they were less successful in addressing the problem of the individual. They showed that culture can be at the source of many human problems, from poverty to mental illness, but could offer little practical help on how to alleviate these problems.

There is a lot of agreement between cultural anthropologists and some of the leading representatives of cross-cultural psychology (Berry Strimble, & Olmedo, 1986; Hofstede, 1980), an interdisciplinary field with a stronger focus on individual behavior. This agreement is particularly relevant to our interest in Hispanic-Americans and their problems with substance abuse. Cultural anthropologists and cross-cultural psychologists have both identified some of the differential characteristics of Hispanic-Americans and Anglo-Americans. For example, in the world of Hispanic-Americans, attachment to and identification with the family-is central and influences personal choices and relationships. The influence of family-based inter-personal relationships is not limited to childhood but shapes the Hispanic-American throughout life. The family structure is based on somewhat contrasting but complementary male–female roles and relationships. Personalism, dignity, and respect are central values. The world of the Latinos or Hispanic-Americans is dominated by an intensive sense of interdependence. This world differs characteristically from the world of the more materialistic, pragmatically oriented, self-reliant and individualistic Anglo-Americans.

The problem is, however, that the rich literature and characterizations available on Hispanic–Anglo-American differences have been of limited practical use to those providing educational, mental health, and substance abuse treatment and prevention services to individual Hispanic-Americans or their institutions and communities. Such knowledge has not furthered the ability of predominantly Anglo-American social services to reach the Hispanic-American communities in this country.

Cultural Diversity Is Often a Source of Confusion and Complexity

Part of our inability to meet the needs of Hispanic-Americans may be due to several factors. First, non-Hispanic mental health workers may underestimate the influence of culture and fail to recognize the disparity between one's native culture and the new, American culture, and the problems that arise when trying to reconcile the two cultures in one generation. Attempts to help may take on different meanings and significance when interpreted through the culture gap. Once we recognize the importance of culture, however, we may be further hampered by our tendency to view Hispanic-Americans as all members of one and the same culture. Health and mental health professionals of Hispanic-American background trained in various fields of behavioral and medical sciences do recognize the importance of culture and the dominant perceptual and attitudinal dispositions of their clients. They are aware that the dispositions characteristic of their Hispanic-American clients frequently differ from those of their non-Hispanic-American clients. Furthermore, based on their professional training and personal experiences, they become increasingly aware that their Hispanic clients are by no means homogeneous; they come from large, variously segmented Hispanic populations of Mexican-Americans, Puerto Ricans, Cubans, and Central and Latin American immigrants. Some are descendants of early settlers living for centuries in the United States, whereas others are more recent immigrants or fall into the category of "illegal alien." Some are thoroughly acculturated, that is, practically indistinguishable in their psychological dispositions from Anglo-Americans, and others still represent very much the culture of their native land and origin. These differences are critical to addressing the needs of each individual.

Considering the many problems Hispanic-Americans living in the United States face, from high rates of substance abuse to the low use of mental health services, it is of critical importance that those who provide the relevant human services know their clients in a larger context than their immediate need. The more it is understood that Hispanic-Americans can differ in many important ways from each other as well as from Anglo-Americans, the more it is pressing to know how to approach a particular client, how to identify his or her problem, how to establish rapport and generate confidence, how to develop a valid and useful diagnosis, how to generate trust, how to overcome social and cultural barriers, and how to proceed with counseling or therapy or the pursuit of a particular educational objective. It depends largely on the level of education and sophistication of the service provider how much attention the Hispanic background of the client is likely to receive. Familiarity with Hispanic culture can help to recognize the diversity of this large population.

If a service provider is not specially trained or has little experience with Hispanic-Americans, he or she may use simple indicators, like Spanish surname or accent to identify Hispanic-American clients. However, as our findings show, some Hispanic-Americans with Spanish surnames will think and see the world as most Anglo-Americans do, yet others will differ in significant ways. Identifying who is an Hispanic-American in legal or demographic terms versus identifying the psychological dispositions that shape personal choices and behavior are very different considerations. The language differences are obvious and readily recognizable, and yet the choice of English or Spanish is only remotely relevant to the meaningful cultural identification of Anglo-Americans and Hispanic-Americans. Indicators such as Hispanic surname, accent, or darker complexion have little bearing on the deep human dispositions that the word "culture" represents, or should represent to be a useful concept for professionals, treatment specialists, educators, and others who are serving Hispanic-Americans. Klor de Alva (1988) has characterized the situation in the following way:

> The mass media, advertising firms, government agencies, and the non-Hispanic population attempt to simplify their response to the burgeoning Spanish-speaking population by obscuring their substantial differences through collective labels (like their "Hispanic") and stereotypical assumptions concerning their supposed common cultures and socioeconomic conditions. Different Hispanic groups, generally concentrated in different regions of the country, have little knowledge of each other and are often as surprised as non-Hispanics to discover the cultural gulfs that separate them. (p. 107)

Despite the general agreement about the psychocultural attributes of Hispanic-Americans, Hispanic-American scholars emphasize the differences particular Hispanic populations have among each other. There are literally dozens of ethnic labels that continuously change over time, some that overlap, and others that refer to groups that sound distinctly different. The extent to which the different labels refer to identifiable differences in people's thinking and behavior remains mostly an open question. As the following findings demonstrate, differences between Hispanic-American and Anglo-Americans vary.

Measuring Acculturation by Questionnaire and Scaling Techniques

Leading Hispanic American professionals such as Amado Padilla (1980) and Jose Szapocznic (1978) have developed their own tools to measure acculturation by asking questions and presenting scales. What these measures of acculturation share in common is that they present the respondents with choices regarding preferred language, food, and style of dressing from Anglo-American versus Hispanic-American alternatives. The more a particular respondent prefers the Anglo-American alternative, the higher is his or her acculturation score. Some of the most widely used acculturation scales include:

- The Acculturation Rating Scale for Mexican Americans (ARSMA) developed by Cuellar, Harris, and Jasso (1980) to provide a measure of acculturation for both normal and clinical Mexican-American populations.
- The Feminine Interest Questionnaire (FIQ) developed by Miller (1977) to measure attitudes toward modern and traditional sex roles. It has been validated for use with Hispanic women by Ortiz and Casas (1990).
- The Hispanic Stress Inventory developed by Cervantes, Padilla, and Salgado de Snyder (1990) to assess psychological stress. It comes in two forms: one for immigrants from Latin America and one for later-generation Mexican-Americans.
- TEMAS (Tel-Me-a-Story) developed by Constantino, Malgady, and Rogler (1988) as a thematic apperception test developed specifically for African-American and Hispanic children but useful with all children.
- The Value Orientation Scale (VOS) developed by Szapocznik, Scopetta, Kurtines, and Aranalde (1978) as part of a process to establish a therapeutic model appropriate to the cultural characteristics of Cuban-Americans.

By using the various acculturation measures researchers seek up-to-date information on the relevant psychological makeup of their clients. Negy and Woods (1992), discussing the problems associated with the use of acculturation scales, observed that the primary deficiency is in the lack of agreement as to the definition of the construct of acculturation, along with the problems of effectiveness in assessing acculturation and the overall reliance on self-report. Some of the relevant issues cutting across these diverse approaches to acculturation have also been addressed by Berry, Trimble, and Olmedo (1986).

Measuring Acculturation by Cultural Distance

Our investigations in the fields of education and mental health, including substance abuse treatment and prevention, have indicated this general tendency to apply the Spanish–English language contrast to approach cultural differences between Anglo-American and Hispanic-Americans. We could not say how fallacious this tendency to focus on language is until we had solid research findings showing that Hispanic-Americans, including Mexican Americans, Puerto Ricans, and Cubans as well as recent immigrants from Latin America, differ from each other in their dominant psychological dispositions that shape their behavior.

Since the late 1970s, we have accumulated a broad, international database on Hispanic-American groups, using the AGA to measure their perceptions, subjective meanings, and mental representations. Cross-cultural studies sponsored by NIMH, NIDA, the Department of Education, the Office of Naval Research, and others have been pursued along a variety of objectives in the fields of mental health, education, multicultural training, and language training. The studies empirically measured Hispanic and Anglo-American psychocultural similarities and differences. The results on psychocultural distances underscored the need to pay attention to the level of acculturation of Hispanic groups. In our research on Hispanic-Americans we defined the level of acculturation as the extent to which the group was similar to a comparable Anglo-American group. We found striking and systematic differences in the level of acculturation reached by Mexican-American, Puerto Rican, Cuban, and other Latin-American immigrant samples.

Four in-depth comparative analyses of Hispanic and Anglo-American cultural samples were done. Each included samples of 100 respondents of matching sociodemographic composition. One study sponsored by NIMH compared five Hispanic-American samples (Puerto Ricans in San Juan and in New York, Mexican-Americans in El Paso and in Los Angeles, and Cubans in Miami) with Anglo-Americans (in New York and in Los Angeles). Each of these seven samples involved users of mental health service programs (25%) and their family members (75%) and equal numbers of males/females, young/old, and lower/higher income people (Szalay, Diaz-Royo, Miranda, Yudin, & Brena, 1983; Szalay, Ruiz, Lopez, Turbyville, & Strohl, 1978).

A second study, sponsored by the Office of Naval Research, involved Hispanic-American student samples from four regions of the United States (Puerto Ricans in New York, Mexican-Americans from El Paso and Tempe, and Cubans from Miami) and an Anglo-American student sample from New York and Washington, DC. The student sample consisted of juniors and seniors from high schools in these different locations (Szalay, Diaz-Royo, Brena, & Vilov, 1984).

A third study involved 100 students from universities in the Washington, D.C. metropolitan area and 100 university students from Bogota, Colombia (Szalay, Vasco, & Brena, 1982). The fourth comparative study involved the same Washington, D.C.

based samples and a matching sample of Mexican university students from Mexico City (Szalay & Diaz-Guerrero, 1985). The third and fourth studies were sponsored by the Division of International Education of the U.S. Department of Education. The samples included an equal number of male and female undergraduates chosen to represent a broad variety of major fields of study.

The results of all four studies showed that the psychocultural distance measured between U.S. mainstream and certain accultured population samples (e.g., Mexican-American) can be minimal. Simultaneously, the distance between Hispanic-American regional samples (e.g., highly accultured Mexican-Americans from San Antonio) and the more traditional Puerto Ricans from San Juan can be rather dramatic (Szalay & Diaz-Guerrero, 1985). The perceptions, subjective meanings, and mental representations of the many Hispanic groups provide a rich resource of psychocultural information for use in education, mental health services, program management, training, and communication as well as in substance abuse treatment and prevention.

THE MULTIPOLARITY OF HISPANIC-AMERICAN POPULATIONS

The most striking conclusion from the cultural distance results is the rich multipolarity among the Hispanic-Americans studied. As we said earlier, we tend to assume a simple bipolarity in American–Hispanic cultural relations (Figure 10.1), with Anglo-Americans at one end and Hispanic-Americans at the other. We tend also to view acculturation as a linear progression from one pole to the other.

However, our findings suggest that acculturation is not necessarily a linear process. What emerged from our studies is a clear and consistent picture of multipolarity (see Figure 10.2). The cultural distance data support this pluralistic model with extensive details discussed in publications of each of these investigations. The studies produced several main findings on the relationship of Hispanic-American regional populations to each other as well as to East Coast Anglo-Americans and to West Coast Anglo-Americans. One major finding is the diversity among Hispanic peoples in the United States. The millions of Puerto Ricans, Mexican-Americans, Cubans, and other Hispanic-Americans and Latin-Americans show an unexpected diversity among themselves and in their relationship to the American mainstream.

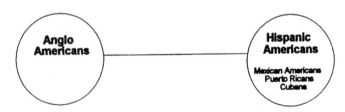

Figure 10.1. The bipolar model of Anglo-American and Hispanic-American interethnic relations.

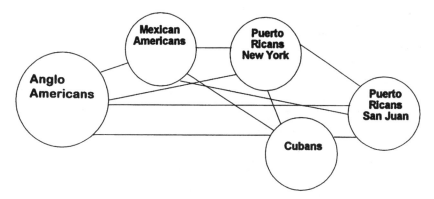

Figure 10.2. Psychocultural distance measured between Anglo-American and Hispanic-Americans.

Figure 10.2 illustrates the point that Hispanic-Americans are not merely different from Anglo-Americans; rather, subgroups of Hispanic-Americans are different from each other and in some cases more so than they are from Anglo-Americans.

A second major finding is the similarity of the Anglo-American samples selected in the representation of the "American mainstream" in Los Angeles and in New York. The high degree of cultural similarity among Anglo-Americans in these two physically distant locations is eventually an even more striking finding for Anglo-Americans, who can be individually widely different. Experiences of individual differences create a sense of diversity that works against the recognition of how much individual Americans have in common in their subjective worlds and perspectives. We will return later to the question of how the subjective worlds of Americans are affected by other factors such as economic status (see Figure 10.4 later).

DEPTH AND SPECIFICITY OF THE NEW KNOWLEDGE
ON CULTURAL INFLUENCES AND BARRIERS

The mapping of various cultural worlds, such as Anglo-American, Puerto Rican, and Mexican American, and of the psychological dispositions shaping their behavior offers a way to trace not only the commonalities that facilitate understanding and communication but also the barriers that were previously hidden and incomprehensible. To recognize the practical value of this new knowledge it is important to consider it in the context of coping with cultural factors affecting substance abuse. Much depends here on the depth and specificity of the knowledge and on the opportunities it offers for effective prevention and intervention.

The cultural distance data reflect the hidden realities of group relations as they are based on shared psychological dispositions that shape the behavior of the various culture groups in question. The Distance scores indicate the overall distance: the higher the score, the greater the distance. Take, for example, the relationship of Americans and Puerto Ricans. Table 10.1 shows the consistency of the Distance scores as well as the differences calculated between Anglo-Americans and Puerto Ricans in San Juan and between Anglo-Americans and Puerto Ricans in New York. Across domains, there is a high consistency in the findings. For example, the distances measured between San Juan Puerto Ricans and Anglo-Americans were, in every domain, larger than the differences between New York Puerto Ricans and Anglo-Americans.

Looking at the specific Distance scores calculated in ten domains of life, we find a great deal of agreement with the literature. For instance, the large distance measured between Anglo-Americans and Puerto Ricans in San Juan reflects broadly recognized cultural differences. The Distance scores provide practical indicators of where there is likely to be contrasting views that affect communication and behavior. For example, the results in Table 10.1 show that there is little distance between Anglo-Americans and Puerto Ricans in the career domain. Regarding work, job, or profession, people of different cultures show much more similarities than they do regarding ethnic images, their own as well as those of others. Where there is greater distance, there are frequently contrasting perspectives that are particularly relevant. In the case of ethnic images, they can reveal sources of ethnocentrism that require attention in order to overcome ethnic differences through communication and education. What the differences involve in terms of specific perceptions and attitudes can be determined by carefully looking at the

Table 10.1   Distances Between Anglo American and Hispanic American Groups
Measured in Selected Domains

Domain	P.R., San Juan and Anglo-Amer.	P.R., N.Y. and Anglo-Amer.	Mex,-Amer., L.A. and Anglo-Amer., El Paso
Ethnic images	.81	.44	.20
Social images	.44	.23	.20
Career orientiation	.27	.13	.08
Military service	.43	.15	.12
Achievement motivation	.60	.42	.16
Social values	.29	.22	.12
Leadership values	.44	.33	.16
Goals	.61	.27	.03
Leisure time	.46	.28	.19
Government	.51	.28	.16
Overal mean coefficients[a]	.47	.26	.13

[a]The mean coefficients were calculated by the formula $d = 1 - r$. The mean r values (Pearson's coefficient) are based on response distributions obtained for 12 themes per domain including about 3,000 pairs of observations. Z-transformation was used to calculate the means.

domains of greatest differences. The results are consistent with the extensive literature describing the importance of family and social relations for Hispanic-Americans (Gfroerer & de la Rosa, 1993; Padilla & Lindholm, 1983; J. Smart & Smart, 1993; Szalay et al., 1978; Triandis, 1994).

The monographs of our Puerto Rican (Szalay *et al.*, 1993) and Mexican (Szalay, Canino *et al.*, 1983) studies present extensive details on cultural similarities and differences based on imaging and mapping. They offer timely information on the cultural groups compared. They did not focus on substance abuse, but they offer relevant information on that subject as well as many others involving cultural differences. The data on specific images is the foundation of the distance between Anglo-Americans and Puerto Ricans in the domain of interpersonal relationships, which is again a mean calculated on the specific themes representing the domain. Our focus on substance abuse does not allow for much elaboration here; however, to illustrate the nature of the specific information, we use the image of marijuana for Anglo-American students and for Puerto Rican students in Puerto Rico (Figure 10.3). The students selected for these comparisons were 100 college students from the University of Maryland and from the University of Puerto Rico at Mayaguez.

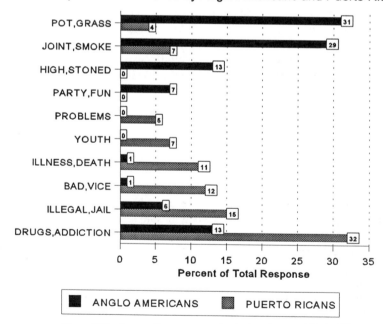

Figure 10.3. Image of MARIJUANA BY Anglo Americans and Puerto Ricans.

The attention Anglo-American students and Puerto Rican students paid to different perceptual and attitudinal dimensions indicates two different sets of perspectives. In this study we did not ask the students about their use of marijuana or other drugs. Still, the results show definite cultural differences, such as the Puerto Ricans' stronger preoccupation with illegality and the Anglo-Americans' tendency to view marijuana as fun and entertainment. The results also suggest the Anglo-Americans have had more direct experience with marijuana than the Puerto Ricans, who tended to reject and condemn marijuana outright.

CULTURAL DISTANCE IS A FUNCTION OF MANY BACKGROUND FACTORS

As a last point about the Distance data, we may briefly mention that it is not only culture that produces differences between people but also gender, age, economic conditions, and other factors as well. Economic conditions are sources of particularly conspicuous differences in people's existence. The differences in the living conditions of the rich and of the poor are among our most prominent national concerns. We have used the Distance measure to explore the extent to which income level is a source of differences in people's subjective worlds. Figure 10.4 shows distances based on two income levels (high, low) for Anglo-Americans, Mexican-Americans, and Puerto Ricans. The effects of income and culture are then considered in combination. The results show that income, as represented by the samples in this study, made a more modest difference than culture. In combination, income and culture were a sizable source of differences. Interestingly, income differences among Anglo-Americans had the least influence on psychological distance, whereas income differences among Puerto Ricans showed the greatest impact on distance.

Gender, age and other sociodemographic variables are considered to be potential sources of differences between people, affecting their worlds and their behavior. Our findings on the effects of cultural background may be surprising to many. Expectations and estimates have been disadvantaged by identifying culture by external indicators, such as language and surname. Ways of measuring its impact on people's worlds and behavior have been lacking as well.

The comparative results produced by imaging and mapping provide a solid foundation for drawing inferences about the relationship of Anglo-Americans and Hispanic-Americans. Culture was found to be the most important source of variation in psychological dispositions that shape behavior. These findings offer strong justification for considering cultural dispositions in investigations of factors affecting substance abuse and for tracing their role in the processes of acculturation and culture change, topics addressed in the next two chapters. It is important to note that, although we must consider the effects of culture on dispositions related to substance use, we cannot make the mistake of lumping all people of Hispanic

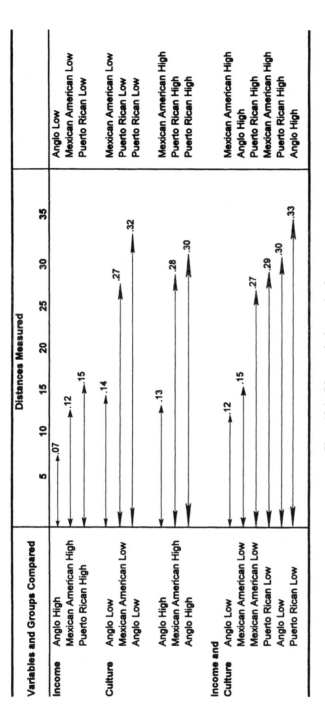

Figure 10.4. Distances by income level.

origin into one group, assuming they represent one culture. Although demographically they may be grouped under one label, they are more diverse than any other demographic group in the United States.

Additionally, our data suggest that within each Hispanic culture, there is more variability between subgroups than there are between comparable Anglo-American subgroups. For example, in previous studies gender and age had moderate effects on distance, at least when compared to the effects of culture. The distances between high- and low-income groups were also moderate. In all of these comparisons, Anglo-Americans showed the most homogeneity, and Puerto Ricans the least. That is, the distance between high-income and low-income Anglo-Americans or between male and female Anglo-Americans was consistently smaller than the distance between the comparable groups of Mexican-Americans or of Puerto Ricans.

Information on psychocultural distances between the various Hispanic and Anglo-American regional populations can be useful in the planning and development of educational and social service policies. The large body of research offers extensive details on the groups' views and attitudes. The detailed views and values of these Anglo, Mexican, and Puerto Rican populations have been presented in communication lexicons and culture guides (Szalay *et al.*, 1983; Szalay, Canino, *et al.*, 1993). The detailed information is necessary for the development and implementation of specific programs. They support the growing realization that success in so many fields, from mental health to personnel management, depends largely on taking people's dominant views and values into consideration.

MULTIDIMENSIONAL IMAGING AND MAPPING GIVES BROADER
UNDERSTANDING OF CULTURAL INFLUENCES

We have reviewed what cultural anthropology and cross-cultural psychology offer toward the understanding of culture and the role and nature of cultural factors in general. We have also considered the practical needs of health professionals, drug counselors, and prevention specialists to address the problems of the individual Hispanic clients or groups of clients. The need to address the Hispanic client who may or may not differ from other people in the Anglo-American environment is a challenge of fundamental practical importance and immense complexity. The most commonly used approach involves the administration of acculturation scales or questionnaires developed mostly by professionals of Hispanic-American background.

An alternative approach based on the imaging and cognitive mapping technology is the use of the cultural distance measure. The measure was originally developed as an analytic tool to trace and quantify similarities and differences between cultures and populations of different experiences and life conditions.

Newer alternative measures have been developed for specific applications, such as the measure of Vulnerability/Resistance designed to assess propensities for substance abuse. Our cultural distance findings indicate that acculturation is an important factor contributing to the diversity among Hispanic-Americans in this country. They support the importance of measuring acculturation as a prerequisite for providing services adapted to the characteristic dispositions of specific client populations.

The Distance measure offers a tool of high analytic sensitivity to identify cultural similarities and differences across many domains of life. At the same time the imaging and mapping method generates extensive details on specific perceptions and motivations that are useful in program development. The new measures inform on perceptual and motivational dispositions that shape people's choices and decisions. As the following chapters demonstrate, these insights are beyond the reach of direct questioning and scaling, and they are of special relevance in dealing with cultural factors and environmental influences that shape people's cognitions and semantic representations without their conscious awareness.

11

Acculturation—Its Impact on Substance Abuse
Puerto Ricans in New York

As noted in the previous chapter, there is more behind cultural differences than surname or skin color. What really matters is people's subjective world as shaped by their different backgrounds and experiences. As the findings here show, the differences between drug users and nonusers in Puerto Rico and in New York are indeed not just a question of language. The following investigations examined what happens to Puerto Ricans living in New York. In what particular ways did their world change under the influences of the American environment? How did they adapt to the new environment? How did their acculturation promote changes in their behavior? How did their dominant perceptions and attitudes change? In what way do these changes affect their vulnerabilities to use harmful substances? And how do these changes contribute to their soaring increase in drug use?

THE APPARENT PARADOX OF PUERTO RICAN DRUG USE

The following investigations examined how social influences shape the perceptions, motivations, and subjective world of Puerto Ricans living in a new cultural environment. How do Puerto Ricans who moved to New York change under the influences of the new environment? How do they acculture or adapt to the American environment? We are especially interested in how they cope in the new environment. Even more specifically, how does their acculturation affect their propensity to use harmful substances?

What happens to Puerto Ricans in New York is of broad interest for more than one reason. The upsurge of substance abuse is extraordinary, particularly in contrast to the low substance abuse in their original cultural environment of Puerto Rico. The explanations in the literature suggesting that acculturation leads to substance abuse appear to be at odds with our findings on Anglo-American and Hispanic-American distance. Clarification is essential because of their broad implications for understanding environmental influences and their role in substance abuse, and naturally a solution to the enigma is highly desirable from the angle of prevention.

The Cultural Distance measure, which has proven to be useful in gauging the relationship between cultural samples and changes in the relationship, offers a promising tool to clarify answers to these questions on a solid empirical foundation. Additionally, the Vulnerability measure can be used as an indicator of how changes in cultural distances relate to changes in propensities to use harmful substances.

The Contrast: Low Substance Abuse in Puerto Rico, Soaring Drug Statistics in New York

Epidemiological data show that experimentation with alcohol and other drugs, as well as rates of abuse, vary with ethnicity (Bettes, Dusenbury, Kerner, James-Ortiz, & Botrin 1990). Comparison of methodologically comparable surveys of adult populations conducted in the United States (Anthony & Helzer, 1991) and in Puerto Rico (Canino, Anthony, Freeman, Shrout, & Rubio-Stipec, 1993) show dramatic differences in prevalence rates of illicit drug abuse/dependence (7.3% in the United States vs. 1.2% in Puerto Rico). Similarly, school surveys of adolescents have found lower rates of drug use among the island Puerto Rican population (6%) (Robles, Moscoso, Colon et al., 1991) as compared with mainland Puerto Rican youths (28.4%) (Sokol-Katz & Ulbrich, 1992). In addition, a study of adult Hispanics within the mainland United States revealed that the highest lifetime drug use rates were found in Puerto Ricans aged 18 to 34 (Booth, Castro, & Anglin, 1990).

There is ample evidence to support the low estimated prevalence of substance abuse among island Puerto Ricans compared to their high level of substance abuse along the eastern shore of the United States. First, low rates of substance abuse are also found among other Hispanic groups living in their culture of origin, namely Mexicans and South Americans (Aguilar, Narvaez, & Samaniego, 1990; Almeida-Filho, Sousa Santana, Matos Pinto, & Carvalho-Neto, 1991). Second, there are lower rates of tobacco and alcohol use in island Puerto Rican children and adolescents as compared to those in the United States (Robles et al., 1991). Moreover, Hispanic adolescents begin using cigarettes and alcohol at a later age as well (Vega, Gil, & Zimmerman, 1993).

Family Cohesion and Social Values

The literature is rather extensive in observations and possible explanations related to the low prevalence of substance abuse among island Puerto Ricans as compared to their mainland counterparts. In Puerto Rico, close family attachments and responsibilities are fostered. The needs and objectives of the family as a group take precedence over individual goals and objectives (Hosftede, 1990; Triandis, Marin, Betancourt, Lisansky, & Chang, 1982). One generally finds strict family monitoring and close supervision of young people occurring within the context of a pervasive authoritarian orientation that fosters acquiescence to parents, teachers, close relatives, or significant societal institutions. It is generally believed that cultures, such as the prevailing culture in Puerto Rico, in which religious and family values are emphasized and in which children are closely supervised, have low rates of behavior problems and substance use (Robbins & Regier, 1991). One finds in Puerto Rican culture two strong elements that are traditionally associated with decreased risk of substance use problems in children: social control (Hirschi, 1969) based on strong family attachments (Hagan, 1989) and direct parental control based on strict discipline and coercion (Paterson, 1982).

The prevailing social and cultural context is different on the mainland United States, where there tends to exist a highly individualistic orientation, greater latitude in child rearing norms, more flexible disciplinary practices, and emphasis on the development of autonomy and self-sufficiency rather than acquiescence. Resettling in the United States mainland involves a change in social context that creates cultural conflict and exerts a push toward acculturation, including a shift from a collectivistic orientation to an individualistic one and a loosening of family networks and bonds (Rogler, 1994). This may explain the higher rates of substance use among mainland Hispanics as compared to island Puerto Ricans.

Gender Differences in Alcohol Use

Among adult Puerto Ricans the prevalence of alcohol abuse/dependence is very low among women (lifetime prevalence of 2%), whereas the prevalence for men is high (lifetime prevalence of 24%; Canino, Burnam, & Caetano, 1992). Culture influences dispositions in uniform ways in its members, yet it also can influence dispositions differently for different subgroups with the culture. For example, a very strong part of the impact of culture is the social and gender roles it prescribes. Gender differences are also expected inasmuch as societal mores prescribe different roles for each sex (Helzer & Canino, 1992). Although there is a wide variation in alcohol use among the different nations of Latin America from which come U.S. Hispanics, there is also some uniformity in its use. Drinking and drunkenness by men and by the young is more accepted than by women and by the elderly (Caetano, 1984). Cultural norms prescribe strong social disapproval of alcohol use and of misuse by women. Thus, it is expected that men and women in Hispanic cultures would have a different vulnerability or risk toward the use or abuse of alcohol, which results from their cultural or socialization patterns. Data from epidemiological surveys with Puerto Rican populations tend to confirm this hypothesis.

Drinking is usually a male activity in most Latin American countries (Caetano, 1984). Excessive drinking is also exhibited mostly by men, the great majority of women being either abstainers or very light drinkers.

Data from an epidemiological survey in Puerto Rico reflect these cultural patterns of drinking. Lifetime abstention rates among Puerto Rican women were 32% of the adult island population (Canino et al., 1992). Abstention rates by males in the Puerto Rican population were substantially lower (7.2%). Similar patterns of dramatic gender differences were observed for the prevalence of excessive drinking, intoxication, and alcohol abuse/dependence (Canino et al., 1992). Although alcohol use and abuse is predominantly a male activity in many parts of the world, differences are observed regarding sex ratios (Helzer & Canino, 1992). Among the more traditional societies (such as the Hispanic), the sex ratio tends to be much higher than in less traditional societies. Thus, U.S. data reveal that the prevalence of alcohol abuse/dependence among males in the U.S. is slightly more than among women, whereas in Puerto Rico it is 12 times more prevalent (Helzer & Canino, 1992).

Given the fact that societal cultural mores affect patterns of drinking, one would expect these patterns to change in the process of acculturation to the host country. The process of acculturation involves a change toward the host country's cultural values, habits, customs, and lifestyle, and this includes values toward drinking as well. U.S. family values tend to be more egalitarian, less restrictive toward drinking behavior among women, and stress less sex role differentiation compared to Hispanic values. Thus, it is not surprising that whatever imputted protection Hispanic women may have toward excessive drinking or alcohol abuse may diminish with increased exposure to the Anglo-American culture. Comparison between recent Mexican immigrants to the United States and native Mexican-Americans from Los Angeles have shown that in the latter group, women abstained from drinking only 6 times more than men and the sex ratio for alcoholism was 4:1, whereas in the former group abstention in women was 15 times more than in men and the sex ratio for alcoholism was 25:0 (Burnam, 1989). This is certainly what we found in our study of Puerto Ricans in New York and on the island (Szalay & Canino, 1991, Szalay Canino, & Vilov, 1993).

Old Reasoning vs. New Evidence about Acculturation and Substance Abuse

The increase from very low substance abuse in Puerto Rico to many-times-higher drug use in the U.S. environment led to a tendency to explain the increase in Puerto Rican drug use as a simple and direct consequence of their acculturation to the U.S. environment. In other words, the upsurge in Puerto Rican substance abuse was accepted as the result of shifting from Puerto Rican views and attitudes to American ones, thus adapting to the American culture. Based on the weight of drug statistics in New York and in Puerto Rico and on the results of acculturation survey conclusions drawn from stated preferences in favor of American entertainment, movies, food, and other items of consumption, such reasoning was compelling. Without systematic identification of dominant perceptions and motivations characteristic of Anglo-Americans compared to Puerto Ricans, without tracing the actual adaptation of Puerto Ricans to the American environment, and without differentiating between successful and unsuccessful acculturation and their behavioral consequences, it was indeed plausible to blame the substance abuse on acculturation.

The Hispanic cultural distance data presented in the previous chapter contradict such simple conclusions that ignore the critical difference between acculturation and other social influences that are disruptive and pathological. This distinction is addressed in the next chapter. The data on Hispanic and Anglo-American cultural distances indicate a pluralistic diversity in the relationship of Hispanic-American regional samples. The diversity among Hispanic-Americans is to a large extent a consequence of social influences in acculturation. The results consistently showed that Mexican-Americans have made the most progress in acculturation, reaching closest similarity to Anglo-Americans. Although the Mexican-Americans showed the highest degree of acculturation, their level of substance abuse did not soar in ways comparable to Puerto Ricans in New York. Their rate was generally lower than that of the American mainstream. The emerging picture is one of unexpected diversity among Hispanic regional samples parallel to their convergence with the U.S. mainstream. The ubiquity and power of the American influences promoting acculturation is impressive, but the most acculturated Mexican-American groups do not show increased vulnerabilities. The proposition that acculturation per se may promotes vulnerability requires closer examination.

In the framework of the Hispanic–Anglo-American distance data, the Puerto Rican samples offer the opportunity to examine the process of acculturation from two complementary angles. How do the influences of the new environment progress in shaping a new world in conformity with Anglo-Americans, and how does this progress build on or substitute for the original world of Puerto Ricans?

The distance data show that Puerto Ricans in New York did not change along a straight line, moving from Puerto Rican to American. Rather, they developed systems of perceptions and motivations that are different, characterized best as a triangle (see Figure 11.1). Considering the cultural distance between Americans in

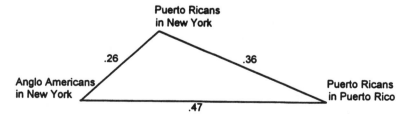

FIGURE 11.1. A triangular model of psychocultural distance.

New York and Puerto Ricans on the island (.47), Puerto Ricans in New York showed less distance from Anglo-Americans (.26) than they showed from their sisters and brothers on the island (.36). These measures suggest that the process of accultura- tion does not involve a straight line transition from the more traditional world of Puerto Ricans to the more modern, postindustrial world of the Americans. The new world of the Puerto Ricans is a product of interaction between old perceptions and motivations and those promoted by the new American environment.

As the previous chapters have shown, environmental influences are powerful forces elusive to direct assessment. The present findings demonstrate that envi- ronmental influences can work in opposing directions. They can promote vulner- abilities by eroding the defenses that protect people from involvement with harmful substances, and they can build resistance that strengthens existing protec- tions and coping mechanisms.

PUERTO RICAN DRUG USERS AND NONUSERS IN TWO CULTURAL ENVIRONMENTS

Imaging and mapping can be used to examine real-life settings, such as the social influences in the acculturation of Puerto Ricans, from several angles. How do so- cial influences promote the transition from the world of Puerto Ricans born in the more traditional cultural setting of the island? What does this process of transition involve from the angle of developing vulnerabilities to use harmful substance? How do these processes vary for Puerto Ricans who use drugs and for those who do not use drugs in the new host environment of the United States?

To examine differences in the psychological makeup of Puerto Rican youths, we tested both drug users and nonusers aged 17 or younger living in New York and in Puerto Rico. In New York we tested 93 Puerto Rican drug users and 100 nonusers. In Puerto Rico we tested comparable samples of drug users ($n = 98$) and nonusers ($n = 100$). American drug users ($n = 99$) and nonusers ($n = 100$) of com- parable sociodemographic background were also tested in New York. Nonuser samples were obtained through private and public schools, after-school programs, and youth organizations in New York and in San Juan, Puerto Rico. Drug user samples were obtained through drug treatment and rehabilitation centers in New York and in San Juan, Puerto Rico. School principals and program directors of the respective schools or treatment organizations contacted the participants, explained the purpose of the research, and elicited interest in participating in the study. Par- ticipation was voluntary and participants were paid for their participation. Whereas the majority of subjects were minors, parental permission was obtained. The norms for the native and for the host cultures were based on the responses of Anglo-American nonusers and Puerto Rican nonusers in Puerto Rico. *Accultura- tion* then was defined operationally as similarity to Anglo-American nonusers.

The data collection relied on three types of instruments:

1. *Demographic Measures.* Background data was elicited by a short questionnaire, which focused on important sociodemographic characteristics of the respondents. All of the participants answered questions on variables such as age, gender, education, and lifestyle or behavioral questions. For the Puerto Ricans, additional questions were also asked to determine family migration. For example, questions were asked regarding years of residence in the United States and/or Puerto Rico, parents' birthplace, number of relatives in the United States and Puerto Rico, and so forth. English speakers received the English version of this instrument and Spanish speakers received the Spanish version. If the respondents were bilingual, they were given the opportunity to decide which form they preferred.

2. *Questions on Preferences and Behaviors Relevant to Acculturation.* Based on scientific literature, a questionnaire was developed to assess cultural preferences and behaviors and how these influence psychological adaptation to the American environment. The questionnaire was administered to Puerto Ricans in New York and, in an adapted form, to Puerto Ricans in Puerto Rico. This instrument included a battery of questions and scales covering such topics as the use of English and Spanish in their daily lives, Hispanic versus American cultural preferences, and so forth. These questions and scales were comparable to conventional survey and scaling tasks discussed in Chapter 10, generally used in measuring acculturation.

3. *Measures on the Psychological Dimensions of Change.* AGA-based imaging and cognitive mapping measures relied on responses by the American and Puerto Rican users and nonusers to 40 stimulus themes selected to represent 10 domains, including family, friends, health, and substance abuse. The stimulus themes were selected in pretests to provide comparable, translation equivalent stimuli in English and Spanish.

The purpose of comparing the selected samples of Americans and Puerto Ricans was to identify cultural differences and their effects on drug use. Some of the main questions we examined were as follows: To what extent do Americans and Puerto Ricans differ in their dominant perceptions and motivations in general and regarding harmful substances in particular? How do Americans in New York and Puerto Ricans in Puerto Rico, users and nonusers, compare in their dominant perceptions and attitudes? Specifically in regard to acculturation, how do Puerto Ricans in New York compare to Puerto Ricans in Puerto Rico? What changes do Puerto Ricans show in the new environment, and to what extent do users and nonusers change differently? What do the differences show regarding their vulnerability to use harmful substances?

The investigations produced extensive findings both on Puerto Rican versus Anglo-American cultural dispositions as well as on the changes Puerto Ricans have shown under the influences of their new American environment. The tabular presentations of multigroup comparisons require too much space for presentation here. Selected findings have been published elsewhere (Szalay *et al.*, 1991; Szalay, Canino, & Vilov, 1993).

Acculturation Questionnaire Provides Relevant Details

The results based on imaging and mapping are supported by some of the responses to the acculturation questionnaire, whereas other results produced by the questionnaire are puzzling. Regarding Spanish language use, the results indicate that preference for the native language in various social settings, particularly at work, correlates negatively with psychological adaptation for both drug users and nonusers. Regarding the use of English, the more the nonusers reported to be at ease using English in various social settings, the more they have adapted to American perceptions and mental representations.

The popularity of various Hispanic and American sources of entertainment produced mixed results. The findings bring into question the broadly held view that mass media and American entertainment are major factors promoting American acculturation. American entertainment media may indeed be a potent source of cultural influences; however, these influences should not be automatically equated with those that promote psychological adaptation. The attraction of expensive cars, affluence, and leisure is wide and universal but shows little relationship to the integral acceptance of American social and political values. The results show that the stated preferences for American versus Hispanic cultural alternatives and lifestyles, which represent the main thrust of past acculturation studies, tell us relatively little about the deeper process of perceptual adaptation. Questions about cultural preferences provide gauges of the popularity or appeal of American products and the expectations attached to the American way of life. However, there are essential differences between influences based on the appeal of American products (e.g., American film, music, entertainment) and the propensity to adapt to American culture. This difference is of special weight and relevance to the task of promoting perceptual and motivational dimensions needed to cope with the social influences promoting substance abuse.

Mapping the Distance between Anglo-American and Puerto Rican Users and Nonusers

Our focus is on changes in the dominant perceptions and motivations of Puerto Ricans living in New York. The results of imaging and mapping indicate changes at various levels of cognitive–semantic representation. They show how Puerto Ricans in the United States develop images (of self, friends, drugs, etc.) under the influences of their new U.S. environment and how they adopt perspectives, motivations, and systems of mental representations similar to those of Americans. The comparison of Puerto Ricans in New York with the native and host norms informs on the effects of the accumulative learning processes that change the respondents' images more or less in conformity with images of people in the new American environment. The results on cultural images show that Puerto Ricans in New York assume an intermediary position between the native culture and the host culture.

Working across all of the themes and domains covered in this investigation, the transition from Puerto Rican to American cultural perspectives was traced along three main dimensions of psychological adaptation. A Priorities measure was used to assess the extent to which Puerto Ricans in New York approximate Americans in their dominant priorities. An Evaluation measure was used to assess how closely Puerto Ricans in New York approximate Americans in their attitudes/evaluations of what is positive or negative. The Evaluation measure indicated changes from native attitudes to those characteristic of the host environment. Finally, a measure of Perceptual Similarity was used to trace changes in the perceptual/representational dimension, showing how Puerto Ricans in New York have adopted American images, meanings, and perspectives characteristic of the host environment.

Discriminant function analyses based on these measures were used to examine the interrelationship of culture and drug use. In Figure 11.2 the distance

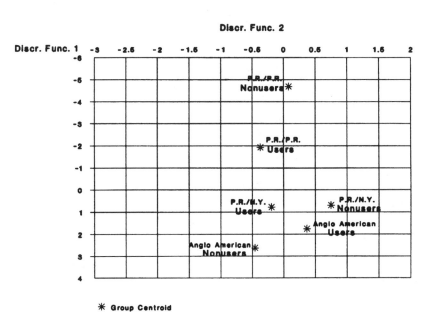

FIGURE 11.2. The interrelationship of culture and drug user/nonuser groups.

between the American and Puerto Rican culture groups (showing drug users and nonusers separately) are illustrated. The acculturation of Puerto Ricans in New York is revealed in their sizable distance from the native culture and growing closeness to the host culture.

We limit our presentation to the summary results across all of the themes used in mapping the worlds of the three cultural groups:

1. The Puerto Ricans in New York occupy an intermediary position between Puerto Ricans in Puerto Rico and Anglo-Americans in New York. Their position reflects a close approximation of the Americans compared to the marked distance they have developed from their native culture. This distance is particularly sizable when the Puerto Ricans in New York are compared to nonusers in Puerto Rico.

2. All three user groups cluster relatively closely together. The distance between Puerto Ricans in New York and Anglo-American users in New York is the closest, an indication that Puerto Ricans in New York may be influenced more by Anglo-American users than by a process of acculturation dominated by the culture of American nonusers.

3. Puerto Rican nonusers in Puerto Rico, Puerto Rican nonusers in New York, and Anglo-American nonusers in New York are the most distant from each other, forming a sort of external circle of people with three distinctly different subjective worlds. How these worlds differ in specifics is revealed by the more detailed comparative imaging analyses performed at lower levels of cognitive organization. In general, the findings show the progressive approximation of the Anglo-American world by Puerto Ricans in New York in all three main dimensions: priorities, attitudes, and perceptions.

Differences in Acculturation of Puerto Rican Users and Nonusers

There were distinct differences in the effects of the American environment on Puerto Rican users and nonusers. The differences registered across the 40 themes involve many details beyond the scope of this presentation. To provide a brief summary we may consider the correlation of changes registered along the three main dimensions of cognitive mapping: priorities, attitudes, and perceptual representations.

The Puerto Ricans who use drugs and those who do not use drugs differed markedly in their psychological adaptation in all three dimensions of the comparison. These differences are particularly informative when correlated with the amount of time the respondents have spent in the United States (see Figure 11.3). Contrary to past approaches that tacitly assumed that users and nonusers go through essentially the same process of acculturation, the findings show that this assumption was fallacious.

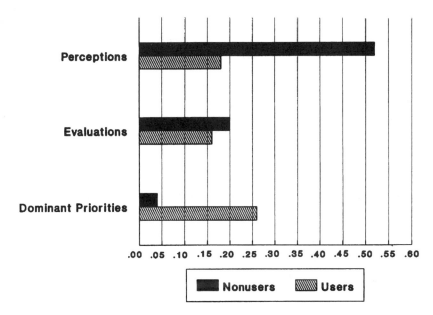

FIGURE 11.3. Psychological adaptation of New York Puerto Ricans in three dimensions: Correlations with time as the criterion.

Of particular importance here are the differences observed in the dimension of perceptual change. This analysis informs on the progress in the system of perceptual/semantic representation, that is, in the respondent's subjective world. The results obtained with the Perceptual Similarity measure show a particularly strong, significant relationship with time spent in the U.S. environment. The results indicate that Puerto Rican nonusers have made significant progress in adopting American views and perspectives, whereas drug users have not.

Adaptation to American attitudes and evaluations showed a weaker correlation with time. On these dimensions of secondary importance the differences measured between users and nonusers did not reach the level of significance.

Adaptation to American priorities showed moderate correlations with time as a criterion measure only for the users, indicating that this measure is less effective in capturing a critical parameter of the change produced by environmental influences. Nonetheless, the results suggest that drug users more readily accept certain American priorities (e.g., emphasis on wealth, freedom, and comfort) but fail to adopt deeper cultural views and perspectives.

In general, the findings show the special importance of perceptual similarity in the process of psychological adaptation. The other two dimensions, priorities and attitudes, are meaningful but less informative on the central process of adaptation whereby Puerto Ricans learn to view the world through American cultural perspectives.

Social Influences Promoting or Hampering Acculturation

The finding of more successful adaptation among nonusers than drug users deserves special attention. It shows the need to distinguish between appealing appearances and genuine changes of psychological adaptation. It is one thing to prefer American music, the free life, American cars, and affluence. It is another to internalize the American ideals and values of personal autonomy, privacy, achievement motivation, and democracy. The findings make these differences apparent. Whereas Puerto Rican nonusers progress in their adaptation to the new environment, the drug users are more affected by environmental influences of drug users. The nonusers progress toward the mainstream of the American nonusers, but the drug users do not really acculture; the changes are reminiscent more of influences of the American counter-culture of drug users.

Puerto Ricans in the Bronx under the influence of their immediate social environment are placed in a setting in which the environment promotes welfare dependence, instant gratification, and dependency. These social influences, unfortunate as they are, should not be confused with the American culture. The results of these influences certainly promote drug dependence, not as a process of acculturation but as a consequence of the influence of the immediate environment. Puerto Ricans who, despite the environmental influences, manage to become competitive and self-reliant can be shown to progress in their adaptation to psychological dispositions of the mainstream American culture. The adoption of these characteristics is the essence of acculturation.

The upsurge of drug abuse among Puerto Ricans who have settled in the United States comes from those who are rather blocked or delayed in their process of adapting to the world of mainstream American nonusers. Imaging and mapping help to recognize important differences between real acculturation in which immigrants, under the influences of their new environment, learn a new world, including its protective values and coping mechanisms that strengthen their resistance to social influences promoting drug use. In contrast, the Puerto Rican users block or delay the learning that would offer them the protection, the resistance essential to survive in the new environment, while social influences promoting vulnerability to substance abuse are particularly common and powerful.

The affinity between the Puerto Rican drug users in New York and the American drug users in New York indicates that it may be more appropriate to speak of acculturation to the local drug culture rather than to the American culture in general. There are those who are in the process of acculturing to the United States, but they are not those shown by the soaring drug statistics. It is important to distinguish clearly the environmental influences that promote American values and perspectives providing resistance and effective coping from environmental influences that promote vulnerability to substance abuse and delay successful acculturation.

The Difference between Those Who Acculture and Those Who Do Not

As the example of the Puerto Ricans in New York demonstrates, in developing resistance and in learning to cope with environmental influences promoting vulnerability, the relationship between the old and new environments is of exceptional importance. The triangular relationship reproduced for the distances between Anglo-Americans in New York, Puerto Ricans in New York, and Puerto Ricans in San Juan (Figure 11.1) illustrates that the socialization and learning in the new environment builds on the foundational conditions characteristic of the home environment.

The example of Puerto Ricans in New York presents a case where coping with environmental influences demands a clear awareness of cultural differences between the home culture and the host culture. The Puerto Rican nonusers in New York epitomize successful acculturation in which learning and socialization build resistance and effective coping skills by drawing on the protective forces of both the old and the new environments. In contrast, the Puerto Rican users exemplify the failure of acculturation promoted by strong cultural differences between the home culture and the host culture. The gross cultural differences are exacerbated by the intensive social influences promoted by the new environment. New York is well known as an urban environment exceptionally high in substance abuse.

The results show how migrants to a host environment can lose their native protective mechanisms before they develop resistance to cope with the influences of the new environment. Puerto Ricans in Puerto Rico who are not abusing alcohol or other drugs are protected by the strong cultural values and norms that consider substance abuse dysfunctional and socially unacceptable. Puerto Ricans who settle in the United States, in order to resist social influences that promote substance abuse in this new environment, are at first partially protected by their traditional values-based rejection of substance abuse. However, with time they must gradually shift to protective mechanisms of their new environment. In American society primary protective factors are not parental authority and traditional values but rather a practical recognition that substance abuse is dysfunctional and works against personal success and self-interests. Americans with these dominant values in the new environment can serve as role models of self-reliance and independence. The situation of the Puerto Ricans in New York is difficult and serious in many respects. Successful, healthy acculturation that provides protection and coping skills is in high demand indeed. To meet this demand and promote effective prevention requires recognizing the differences between those who succeed and those who fail. Rather than blaming acculturation as the source of substance abuse, we can learn a great deal from the ones who do acculture and who develop effective resistance to cope with adverse pathogenic influences. The drug users represent another rich source of information for focusing on variables that hinder successful adaptation.

The Phantom Power of
Environmental Influences

Comparisons of Anglo-American, Mexican-American and Puerto Rican college students, both users and nonusers, were used to examine the relationship between cultural factors and substance abuse. The findings support that nonusers exhibit high resistance, that is, successful coping and successful acculturation. In comparison, the Hispanic users develop vulnerabilities reflected by increased distance from their native culture as well as from their host culture. The increased vulnerability of users reflects intensive environmental influences. We also assessed the effects of high- and low-use environments on Anglo-American college students to again examine the impact of one's environment on vulnerability to substance abuse. The power of environmental influences is explicable by their ubiquity, multidimensionality, and unobservable, incipient nature.

CULTURAL INFLUENCES: COMPARISONS OF MEXICAN-AMERICAN AND PUERTO RICAN COLLEGE STUDENTS, USERS, AND NONUSERS, WITH ANGLO-AMERICANS

This chapter is organized to offer research-based answers to some fundamental questions about the role of culture and of environmental influences, considered separately and in combination. The first, most generic question is: How do college students of Anglo-American, Mexican-American and native Puerto Rican background stand in relation to each other in terms of their overall cultural distance? The next question is: How do these overall cultural distances change if substance abuse is taken into consideration by comparisons of frequent users and nonusers? Another question is: How different are frequent users and nonusers in their own cultural setting?

Our investigations performed on college samples provided the opportunity to compare Anglo-American, Mexican-American, and native Puerto Rican students in subsamples of frequent users and of nonusers. As previously described, frequent users were defined as students who reported daily drinking or binge drinking more than once a week, or any use of marijuana or other psychoactive drugs. Those who reported less frequent alcohol use were categorized as occasional drinkers and those who reported no use of alcohol or other drugs were categorized as nonusers. The Anglo-American samples included 400 frequent users and 400 nonusers; the Mexican-American and the native Puerto Rican samples each included about 200 students.

The students were asked to respond to 24 themes presented to them in random sequence in multiple free-response association tasks. The 24 themes were selected in the representation of 6 domains of life (Family/Self, Alcohol and Other Drugs, etc.). The thousands of spontaneous responses elicited from the students served as the foundation to reconstruct the students' dominant perceptions and attitudes and to map their subjective worlds in the domains related to substance abuse. Following the multiple-response elicitation task, the students completed a brief questionnaire on their sociodemographic background, academic performance, use of alcohol and other drugs, lifestyle, and so forth. The following results come from respondents identified from the background questionnaire as Mexican-American or as Puerto Rican.

The measures used in these analyses are described in the appendix. The AGA measure of cultural distance is the opposite of the Similarity measure, which is based on Pearson's product-moment correlation coefficient (r). Cultural distance ($1.00 - r$) has values ranging from 0 to 1. Low distance values mean high similarity, just as high distance values mean low similarity. The cultural distance values presented in the following on the cultural samples are average distances calculated on the basis of all 24 themes. Changes in distance reflect the results of processes such as acculturation or culture change promoted by environmental influences. The Distance measures offer opportunity to consider what happens internally—whether the change processes promote similarities in dominant perceptions and attitudes or whether they promote distance and differences.

Cultural Distances

The largest cultural distance measured was between Anglo-Americans in the United States and Puerto Ricans in Puerto Rico; the smallest distance was between Anglo-Americans and Mexican-Americans. The distance between the two Hispanic-American groups was slightly less than the distance between Anglo-Americans and Puerto Ricans, suggesting strong similarities between Anglo- and Mexican-Americans. The distances measured here between college student samples are similar to the distances measured in the four earlier investigations of regional Hispanic and Anglo-American samples presented in the previous two chapters. In the previous comparisons, Anglo-Americans and Mexican-Americans were consistently closer to each other than were other Hispanic samples to Anglo-Americans or to each other. These findings should not be taken as proof that all Mexican-Americans in the United States are accultured; they merely support that the acculturation of the Mexican-Americans in the United States is high.

Distances between Hispanic and Anglo-American Student Samples

Anglo-Americans & Mexican-Americans	Mexican-Americans & Puerto Ricans	Anglo-Americans & Puerto Ricans
.40	.70	.76

The results in Table 12.1 show the cultural distances between Anglo-American and Hispanic-American college students in subgroups of frequent users and of nonusers. The findings show the combined effects of culture and of substance abuse. The last column gives an indication of the proportion of differences measured between the frequent users and the nonusers in these three pairs of comparisons. In light of these results, cultural background appears to be the most influential factor affecting distance, as we compare Anglo-Americans with Mexican-Americans and Puerto Ricans in this sequential order. It may not have been anticipated that the nonuser cultural groups would be consistently closer to each other (left column) than the frequent user groups (right column). The distances, that is, their differences, progressively increase from the Anglo/Mexican to Anglo/Puerto Rican comparisons.

The distances measured between users and nonusers of the same cultural background provide the opportunity to examine how different experiences of use affect cultural distance, and also how cultural distance and substance abuse affect vulnerability to substance abuse. Table 12.2 shows the distances between users and nonusers in the six domains of life (24 themes).

As the mean distances indicate, the Anglo-American users and nonusers show the greatest distance, whereas the Puerto Rican users and nonusers show the least distance. Across the domains, the Distance measures show relatively little variation. They are highly consistent, however, in showing the higher Anglo-American versus lower Mexican-American and even lower Puerto Rican distances

TABLE 12.1. Distances between Anglo-American and Hispanic-American Frequent Users and Nonusers

	Cultural distances		
Groups compared	Nonusers	Users	(Differences)
Anglo-American and Mexican-Americans	.38	.42	.04
Mexican-Americans and Puerto Ricans	.62	.71	.09
Anglo-Americans and Puerto Ricans	.63	.79	.16

TABLE 12.2. Distances Between Frequent User and Nonuser Samples
of the Same Background

Domains	Anglo-Americans user-nonuser	Distance Mexican-Americans user-nonuser	Puerto Ricans user-nonuser
Family	.43	.42	.36
School	.42	.37	.35
Social	.40	.38	.34
Friends	.41	.37	.34
Drugs	.63	.47	.45
Problems	.39	.36	.39
Mean distance	.44	.39	.37

between users and nonusers. The Drugs domain shows the largest distance between users and nonusers, though this may be considered as only natural. What
could not be anticipated is the relatively large distance for Anglo-Americans,
showing the exceptional importance of the Drug domain in shaping the differences
between frequent users and nonusers in this mainstream culture. The foundation of
this difference in dominant perceptions and attitudes can naturally be traced to
particular images. A detailed identification of the perceptual and motivational dispositions characteristic of any of the Hispanic samples in this comparison would
lead us to specifics beyond the level of our present interest. The few specifics regarding Anglo-American and Hispanic images of marijuana (Chapter 10) may
serve to illustrate the nature and scope of these cultural differences.

We may generally conclude from these findings that the etiology of substance
abuse involves significant cultural variations and that the variations are empirically identifiable. Their recognition is desirable in the pursuit of culturally sensitive substance abuse prevention. This new knowledge is of practical value to
service providers and to drug counselors interested in how to approach and treat
clients of a particular cultural background. The distance data would indicate where
to expect more significant cultural differences, and then one could examine the
comparative imaging results to gain insights into the nature of these differences.

Ethnic–Cultural Variations in Alcohol Consumption Reported
and Vulnerability Measured

The self-reported alcohol use and the Vulnerability scores calculated for the
groups compared show some interesting differences (Table 12.3). The Anglo-
American users reported the highest level of alcohol use, and their Vulnerability
scores were also the highest. The Hispanic-American users reported less alcohol

TABLE 12.3. Reported Alcohol Use and Measured Vulnerability/Resistance

	US-Americans		Mexican		Puerto Rican	
	Users (400)	Nonusers (400)	Users (226)	Nonusers (211)	Users (203)	Nonusers (219)
Reported use: Average # drinks/week	10.9	0	6.1	0	6.5	0
Binge drinking (past 2 wks., 5+ drinks at a sitting)	6.1	0	2.4	0	2.5	0
Vulnerability/ resistance score	10.6	−9.6	5.0	−11.8	−1.1	−10.2

use and their calculated Vulnerability scores were proportionately lower as well. The findings on the nonusers are consistent with the above picture: The Hispanic-American nonusers show the highest Resistance scores; the Mexican-American nonusers show about the same resistance as the Puerto Rican nonusers. The Mexican-American users produced a much lower Vulnerability score (5), half of the Anglo-American score. The Vulnerability score of the Puerto Rican users is even lower (−1.1) and actually falls into the range of Resistance (scores below zero).

In general, the reported alcohol use data and the calculated Vulnerability scores show good agreement. These two data sets that are independent from each other in their foundation support the same conclusions. The Anglo-Americans show the highest alcohol use and the highest vulnerability. The Mexican-American and Puerto Rican samples of college students show higher resistance and lower levels of reported alcohol use. The three groups of nonusers had similar Vulnerability/Resistance scores, but the groups of frequent users showed substantial differences in their Vulnerabilities, ranging from 10.6 to −1.1. Although comparative statistics offer up-to-date information on reported use, the Vulnerability/Resistance measure provides a way to gain insights into the underlying psychocultural foundation of these differences in behavior.

Next, we may consider a few instances of substance use and lifestyle as they are linked to the vulnerabilities measured in the different cultural groups. The findings indicate the extent to which each culture group shows similar vulnerability in the context of specific behaviors.

Ethnic-Cultural Differences in Cigarette Smoking and Vulnerability

Students who choose not to drink or use other drugs also tend to be nonsmokers, with little cultural difference. Although about a third of each user group does not smoke, there are some noticeable differences in the proportionate distribution of smokers. Anglo-American users are the heaviest tobacco users, and Puerto Rican users are the least heavy smokers. The impact of cigarette use on Vulnerability is shown in Figure 12.1 as follows:

- Vulnerability increases as a simple direct function of the reported frequency of smoking.
- The difference between the Anglo-American and Mexican-American users is consistently less than between Anglo-American users and Puerto Rican users for all levels of smoking. The Mexican-Americans generally show less vulnerability than the Anglo-Americans.
- In all three nonuser samples the nonsmokers are similar in their level of resistance.

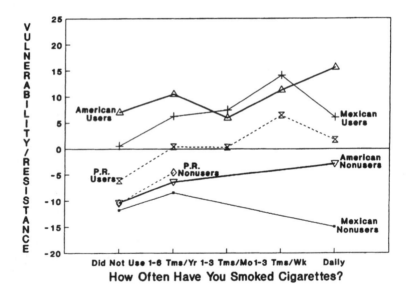

How Often Have You Smoked Cigarettes?

How Often Have You Smoked Cigarettes?	American Users (400)	American Nonusers (400)	Mex.Amer. Users (226)	Mex.Amer. Nonusers (211)	P.R. Users (203)	P.R. Nonusers (219)
Did Not Use	32%	89%	33%	90%	35%	95%
1-6 Times/Year	19%	3%	31%	5%	22%	5%
1-3 Times/Month	9%	2%	13%	0%	13%	0%
1-3 Times/Week	9%	2%	9%	0%	10%	0%
Daily/Almost Daily	31%	5%	13%	5%	19%	0%
Total	100%	100%	100%	100%	100%	100%

FIGURE 12.1. Cigarette smoking and vulnerability of three ethnic–cultural groups.

Ethnic–Cultural Differences in Marijuana Use and Vulnerability

The majority of Anglo-American users (68%) are marijuana users, in contrast to 58% of the Mexican-American users and only 39% of the island Puerto Rican users. Frequency of use is also lower among the Hispanic student groups. As can be seen in Figure 12.2, there is almost no difference in the vulnerability of three cultural groups of nonusers. The following trends were noted in the vulnerability of the user groups:

- Compared to the flat slope of increase in vulnerability measured in the context of smoking, the slope of vulnerability steepens sharply as a function of frequency of marijuana use.
- The Anglo-American users showed the greatest increase in vulnerability as a result of marijuana use. The smaller proportions of Mexican-Americans

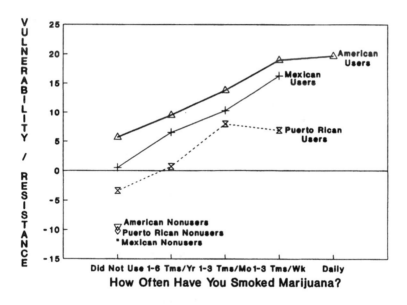

FIGURE 12.2. Marijuana use and vulnerability of three ethnic–cultural groups.

How Often Have You Smoked Marijuana?	American Users (400)	American Nonusers (400)	Mex.Amer. Users (226)	Mex.Amer. Nonusers (211)	P.R. Users (203)	P.R. Nonusers (219)
Never	32%	100%	42%	100%	61%	100%
Seldom	36%		42%		29%	
Sometimes	15%		11%		6%	
Often	12%		5%		3%	
A Lot	6%				1%	
Total	100%	100%	100%	100%	100%	100%

who use marijuana showed similar increases in vulnerability but lower than for Anglo-Americans.

- The Puerto Rican vulnerability measured in the context of marijuana use is consistently lower than for Mexican-Americans or for Anglo-Americans, and they showed less increase and a leveling off. The results suggest that marijuana use affects the Puerto Ricans' vulnerability differently from the Anglo-Americans or the Mexican-Americans.

Academic Achievement and Vulnerability of Anglo-American and Hispanic-American College Students

In addition to substance use, we examined the influence of other behavioral and lifestyle variables on the vulnerability of Anglo-American and Hispanic students. In the case of academic performance, the users showed lower academic perfor-

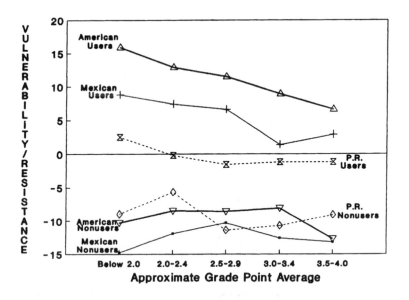

Approximate Grade Point Average?	American Users (400)	American Nonusers (400)	Mex.Amer. Users (226)	Mex.Amer. Nonusers (211)	P.R. Users (203)	P.R. Nonusers (219)
Below 2.0	3%	1%	3%	4%	2%	2%
2.0-2.4	19%	8%	21%	13%	19%	10%
2.5-2.9	36%	23%	38%	36%	38%	30%
3.0-3.4	28%	39%	29%	32%	32%	37%
3.5-3.9	14%	29%	10%	14%	10%	22%
Total	100%	100%	100%	100%	100%	100%

FIGURE 12.3. Academic achievement and vulnerability of three ethnic–cultural groups.

mance than the nonusers, regardless of cultural identity; the distinction was strongest between Anglo-American users and nonusers. Figure 12.3 shows the relationship between academic performance and psychological vulnerability to substance abuse for the three culture groups:

- The relationship between reported grade point average and the vulnerability of the users and nonusers was the simplest in the case of the Anglo-Americans. Users and nonusers were the furthest apart for this cultural group. They exhibited a similar decrease in vulnerability in conjunction with increasing GPA. The two lines are parallel, showing similar decreases.
- The Mexican-American users showed a similar drop in vulnerability with better grades. However, their level of vulnerability was lower than that of comparable Anglo-American users. Mexican-American nonusers showed the strongest resistance with little variation based on academic achievement.
- The Puerto Rican users started off at the lowest point of vulnerability of the three user groups and also showed the least drop in vulnerability with better academic performance. The Puerto Rican nonusers also showed relatively little change when GPA was 2.5 or higher. In general, the Puerto Rican users and nonusers showed the least difference in their vulnerabilities represented by the two generally parallel lines.

Religious Attendance of Anglo-American and Hispanic-American Students: Its Impact on Vulnerability as a Function of Frequency of Attendance

Another lifestyle variable that has been identified as a protective factor is attendance of religious services. As Figure 12.4 shows, religious attendance is much more frequent among the nonuser groups, particularly the Puerto Ricans. The following trends are observed regarding the impact of religious services on the vulnerability of Anglo-American and Hispanic-American students:

- Attending religious services made the greatest difference between users and nonusers in the case of the Anglo-Americans. These lines are the furthest apart and equidistant from each other.
- The nonuser groups were clustered together, indicating nonusers have a markedly lower vulnerability at all levels of religious involvement.
- Mexican-American users showed less vulnerability than their Anglo-American counterparts, but essentially the same trend of decreasing vulnerability with more regular attendance of religious services.
- This same trend held for the Puerto Rican users as well. The Puerto Rican users showed lower vulnerability than Anglo-American or Mexican-American users, but otherwise were affected in the same way as the other two groups.

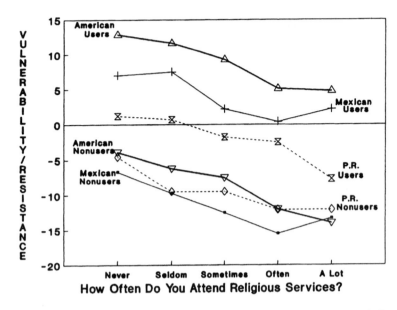

How Often Do You Attend Religious Services?	American Users (400)	American Nonusers (400)	Mex.Amer. Users (226)	Mex.Amer. Nonusers (211)	P.R. Users (203)	P.R. Nonusers (219)
Never	31%	18%	23%	10%	32%	14%
Seldom	35%	17%	34%	30%	24%	19%
Sometimes	17%	15%	17%	18%	19%	16%
Often	10%	18%	14%	19%	13%	19%
A Lot	6%	32%	12%	22%	11%	32%
Total	100%	100%	100%	100%	100%	100%

FIGURE 12.4. Religious attendance and vulnerability of three ethnic–cultural groups.

Anglo-American and Hispanic-American Trends in Substance Use, Lifestyle, and Vulnerabilities

We have examined the relationship between two indicators of alcohol use and vulnerability. Line graphs on cigarette and marijuana use show the relationship between the reported frequency of drug use and the level of vulnerability. The Anglo-American, Mexican-American, and Puerto Rican line graphs of cigarette use have shown similar slopes: vulnerability increases as cigarette use increases. Overall, the Anglo-American line graphs indicate higher vulnerabilities whereas the Puerto Rican line graphs indicate the lowest level of vulnerabilities. The data on marijuana use produced analogous results. The main difference is the steeper slope of vulnerability rising as reported use of marijuana increases. There were few Mexican-American and Puerto Rican frequent users of marijuana, but even for those who used it "seldom" and "sometimes," the increase in vulnerability was steep. Once again, Anglo-Americans start with a high level of vulnerability whereas Puerto Ricans start from the lowest level.

Of the two non-drug-related behaviors examined, academic achievement (GPA) showed a steep decrease in vulnerability for the users as grades improved. This steep decrease is particularly characteristic of the American users who at the lowest GPA showed the highest vulnerability. Vulnerability gradually decreased in sizeable increments with higher GPA values. All three nonuser groups are represented by flat lines in the range of resistance, indicating that academic achievement did not affect their vulnerability.

Attendance of religious services showed remarkably consistent trends for both users and for nonusers. There was a gradual increase in vulnerability as the frequency of attendance of religious services decreased. The Anglo-American users with low attendance showed the highest vulnerability and there was a decline in vulnerabilities as attendance increased. This trend was similar with Mexican-Americans and Puerto Ricans as well, only they started at a lower level of vulnerability and showed further decreases in vulnerability. Regarding nonusers, the trends were similar and the groups were much closer together than the user groups. The Mexican-American and the Puerto Rican users show similar slopes but at lower levels of vulnerability than Anglo-Americans.

In general, the findings on cultural differences in vulnerability and reported use are highly consistent. They show a close relationship between reported behavior and the vulnerability independently measured. We have found also important and sizeable cultural differences in reported drug use as well as in their vulnerability measured independently.

Converging Findings

The comparative analyses reported in this section converge on certain main conclusions:

1. The three groups of different cultural background have shown differences in cultural distances with a high degree of consistency. These findings reflect differences in psychological dispositions that inform on the foundation of cultural difference observed in the actual behavior of the groups. The consistently low distance measured between Anglo-Americans and Mexican-Americans could be rather readily explained as a generally higher level of acculturation for the Mexican-Americans compared to the consistently larger distance measured between Anglo-Americans and Puerto Ricans.

2. The distances between the three cultural samples showed a broad range, from .40 (Anglo-Americans and Mexican-Americans) to .76 (Anglo-

Americans and Puerto Ricans). The distances measured across culturally different nonuser groups and user groups ranged from .38 (Anglo-Americans and Mexican-Americans) to .79 (Anglo-Americans and Puerto Ricans). We have found that the distances measured between user groups and nonuser groups of the same cultural background show a narrower range, but they reflect measurable and identifiable dispositions characteristic of the culture groups examined. The user–nonuser distances were .37 for Puerto Ricans, .39 for Mexican-Americans, and .44 for Anglo-Americans. The distances between frequent users and nonusers were highly consistent within each cultural sample.

3. The relationship between the vulnerability measured and the behavior reported shows a close agreement in the context of alcohol use. The relationships reconstructed for Anglo-Americans, Mexican-Americans, and Puerto Ricans support the same close correspondence between reported alcohol use and the vulnerabilities calculated independently for these groups. (The differences appear to be reflections of genuine cultural differences in the use of alcohol.) This suggests that although the cultural characteristics of alcohol use do vary, the Vulnerability/Resistance scores indicating propensities toward use have similar validity in each cultural context.

4. The findings on the direct linear relationships between the frequencies of reported use of cigarettes and of marijuana and the increase in vulnerabilities again show consistent differences between the three cultural groups. These differences, for example, highest resistance among Puerto Rican nonusers and highest vulnerability among Anglo-American users, emerge consistently across all of the examples. The same holds for the findings on the direct linear relationship between the frequency of select lifestyles and the associated vulnerabilities. Whether we consider the findings on the inverse linear relationship between low vulnerability and high GPA or the frequency of attending religious services and vulnerability measured, the findings show similar differences in the three cultural groups compared.

Caveat

The finding that Mexican-Americans show little cultural distance from Anglo-Americans in contrast to native Puerto Ricans may create the impression of a fallacious generalization. In our many Hispanic-American comparative studies, Mexican-American samples were generally more similar to the Anglo-Americans. Because they live in the environment of the American society, it is safe to conclude that these relatively small cultural distances are due to some degree to acculturation. It is also possible that the Mexican culture is more similar to that of the

United States than is the Puerto Rican culture, so Mexican-Americans may come in already more similar to Anglo-Americans. Also, the Mexican-American college students cannot be taken to represent the diversity of the Mexican-American population in the United States. Although the samples were numerous and the number of Mexican-Americans reached several thousand, this should not be considered as a generalization that Mexican-Americans are all acculturated, whereas Puerto Ricans are not. There are obviously many Mexican-Americans, particularly among the new immigrants, who have progressed little in their acculturation. At the same time, there are Puerto Ricans who are second- or third-generation Americans who are highly acculturated. Our interest was exclusively in measuring the impact and conditions of the acculturation process rather than to sample Mexican-Americans or Puerto Ricans representatively in order to gain meaningless generalizations about their level of acculturation.

A second problem relates to our use of the word "acculturation." We tried to stick to a use where acculturation referred to the situation where people from a different culture move and settle into the environment of a new culture. Living in the new cultural environment, they gradually learn and adopt the culture of their new environment. This specific interpretation of acculturation left us with a limited vocabulary to describe changes by cultures under the influence of each other. For instance, we did not discuss changes in the island Puerto Rican culture due to influences of the American culture, which affect Puerto Ricans who do not migrate to the United States. Living in a world of shrinking dimensions, social and cultural influences are important, numerous, and of considerable relevance to substance abuse.

The following investigations address broad and important categories of social and cultural influences that may support or work against the process of acculturation.

SOCIAL–ENVIRONMENTAL INFLUENCES IN SUBSTANCE ABUSE

Various disciplines use different labels to describe social influences. Some speak of socialization or enculturation and other of acculturation, cultural adaptation, cultural assimilation, and culture change. Acculturation is frequently used in reference to processes whereby people from a different background adapt to a new host environment, for example, Puerto Ricans migrating to New York. It is a similar problem that large countries like the United States exert influences in smaller ones like Puerto Rico, producing effects frequently characterized as culture change. Naturally these circumstances are different and have different influences on substance abuse.

What is common to these two different circumstances is that each involves two types of learning. One is deliberate, purposeful learning that may require an intensive effort. For immigrants this could be learning a new language, traffic regulations, and all of the things one needs to know to navigate in the new environment. The other type of learning is less conscious or identifiable. Puerto Ricans, as immigrants in a new environment or as citizens of a small country flooded by communications (TV, films, books) from their big neighbor, are exposed to influences from a world different from their own. These environmental influences are usually slow and accumulative and can change people's perceptions and motivations without their conscious awareness. In this respect the changes occurring in acculturation, under the influences of the new host environment, are particularly illustrative and paradigmatic. The new settlers or immigrants can undergo a great deal of change in their subjective worlds as the result of slow accumulative influences. As we have shown in the case of Puerto Ricans in New York, or by the high degree of acculturation of Mexican-Americans, influences of the U.S. environment are indeed massive, both in depth and scope beyond expectation.

The impact of environmental influences on student behavior and on vulnerability, as demonstrated in the last chapters, stems from their hidden nature or phantomlike character. The effects of these environmental influences aggregate slowly and shape the world and the behavior of people without their awareness. The findings on cultural differences and their role in acculturation and culture change demonstrate the power of environmental influences in shaping psychological dispositions related to substance abuse.

The findings presented on the effects on different cultural environments are consistent with our findings on the effects of high-use and low-use college environments. As we have discussed in Chapters 7 to 9, high- and low-use environments differ in their influences on the vulnerabilities of students. Our findings show that environment is a powerful factor that shapes behavior in general and the use of substances in particular. One's environment can be a new country or culture, or it can be a new setting within one's culture. For example, when Anglo-American students enter college, they too enter into a new culture with its own set of norms, values, and expectations and they too are shaped by this new environment. We have examined the impact of the various college environments on the students who attend those institutions. The findings have similar implications not only in understanding substance abuse in different cultures but also in understanding our own societal domestic problems as well.

Socioenvironmental influences deserve special attention because they can be so readily overlooked due to their hidden, implicit nature. Their role has been demonstrated previously by our findings on the effects of the environment on vulnerability. The latest chapters were conclusive in showing the effects of socioenvironmental influences, behavior, and vulnerability in various Anglo-American and Hispanic-American environments. They have explanatory potential to help cope with the increase of substance abuse domestically as well as worldwide. Finally, we present findings that further support the conclusion that these influences may work as phantoms but they are undeniably real.

Influences of High- and Low-Use Environments on Vulnerability to Substance Abuse

The following analyses are based on comparisons of colleges selected to represent high-use and low-use environments. The selection was made from 43 colleges in our database at that time. In order to rank the colleges by level of substance abuse, students who reported daily or almost daily drinking or any illicit drug use were defined as *users,* and the colleges were then ranked from high to low, based on the proportion of users. Students from the top eight colleges were selected to represent a high-use campus environment and students from the bottom eight were selected to represent a low-use campus environment. The high-use environment sample included 2,947 students; the low-use sample included 3,027 students. Although the colleges selected are likely to differ on many characteristics, the dimension relevant to the present design is their level of substance abuse.

In the high-use environment, 62% of the students were heavy alcohol and/or drug users (binge drinking at least once a week, consuming an average of 10 or more drinks per week, daily alcohol use, or any use of illicit drugs); this is three times more than in the low-use environment. In the low-use environment 27% of the students reported no use of alcohol or other drug, compared to 6.5% in the high-use environment. All other students fell into the occasional user category: one third of the students in the low-use environment and one half of the students in the high-use environment.

Analyses focused on the degree to which vulnerability varied by such factors as personal characteristics (gender), behavior (marijuana and alcohol usage), and social environment ("high-use" vs. "low-use" college campuses). The effects of social environment are most clearly seen in the comparisons of the vulnerability of students with the same behavior patterns: for example, nonusers on "high-use" campuses versus nonusers on "low-use" campuses.

A three-way ANOVA was used to examine the effects of reported marijuana use and campus environment on the students' Vulnerability/Resistance scores. As expected, a main effect was obtained for self-reported marijuana use (F [4, 5763] = 305.11, $p < .001$), indicating that subjects who reported higher levels of marijuana use showed higher vulnerability (i.e., attitudes and perspectives more similar to frequent users) than those reporting little or no use. More important, a main effect was also obtained for campus environment (F [1, 5763] = 329.70, $p < .001$), showing that students at high-use colleges showed greater perceptual similarity to frequent users (high vulnerability) compared to students at the low-use colleges. This main effect is important because it suggests that even nonusers in a high-use environment are more vulnerable than nonusers in a low-use environment. Thus, we can see the impact of one's environment: on a high-use campus, even nonusers show perceptual similarities with the dominant high-use culture.

In general, the low-use campus environment is characterized by low Vulnerability scores ($M = -3.8$), and the high-use campus environment is characterized by higher vulnerabilities ($M = 7.8$). There is also a consistent linear trend that suggests that more frequent drinking patterns are associated with higher vulnerabilities. On low-use campuses, students with the same drinking patterns show consistently lower vulnerabilities.

It is important to keep in mind that underlying the global Vulnerability measure are a host of perceptual and attitudinal trends that differentiate users from nonusers. Analyses at this level (see Chapters 1 and 2) provide the detailed information that can be used to effectively reach students in prevention planning that takes into account the different ways users and nonusers view the world. When we simply ask people how much they use, we know that frequent users use more than nonusers. When we investigate their subjective views of the world, we begin to understand why.

High-use environments are sources of social influences that result from the myriad of social experiences and contribute to a social climate promoting vulnerability. The results on alcohol and marijuana indicate that higher use is accompanied by higher vulnerability to substance abuse, and at all levels of use students in the high-use campus environment have consistently higher vulnerabilities. The ANOVA results showed that the differences measured are not artifactual in the sense that higher vulnerability is simply a result of the fact that there are more users on high-use campuses than on low-use campuses. Had this been the case, we would not have expected to find a difference in vulnerability between nonusers at the various campuses. As shown in Figure 12.5, nonusers have a Vulnerability/Resistance level of -5.3 in the high-use campus environment and -10.1 in the low-use environment.

Social Environmental Influences—The Hidden Driving Force

The new evidence on the power of social influences that promote vulnerability in high-use environments deserves special attention. The various insights offered in the preceding chapters support two main points. Starting with our central subject of substance abuse, social influences emerge as a central explanation for the growth of drug use and drug dependence, domestic as well as global. Cultural factors, acculturation, and culture change play a role in promoting substance abuse and vulnerabilities. Although for those whose attention is focused on the situation in the United States the cultural perspectives of the drug problem may appear too far removed, the extended research findings stand to show cultural influences can and do promote vulnerabilities as well as resistance. They are indispensable to a broad understanding of those powerful and hidden processes that are the driving forces behind drug epidemics at home as well as overseas. The

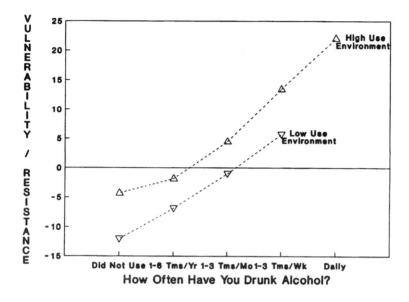

FIGURE 12.5. Alcohol use and vulnerability among students on high-use and low-use campuses.

findings on the differences in vulnerabilities of students in high-use and in low-use college environments illustrate the power and ubiquity of social influences in the same way that the findings on Puerto Rican or Mexican-American students who reported differences in drug use are in agreement with their differences in vulnerabilities measured.

A second main reason for elaborating on social and cultural sources of substance abuse rooted in hidden socioenvironmental influences is their practical implications for prevention. It is customary to recognize social influences in the relatively narrow context of questions addressing peer pressure. As illustrated by the present findings, environmental influences are broader and more influential than those identified in the context of peer pressure and they are often much more subtle. As much as they are powerful in promoting substance abuse, they offer similarly rich opportunities for promoting resistance to substance abuse. To take advantage of these opportunities requires that the psychological dispositions characteristic of particular populations be recognized. Then, prevention can be systematically planned to build resistance through positive, constructive social influences. A few such examples on the use of the new information in program development are discussed in the following chapters.

Program Development and Culturally Adapted Training

This chapter stands as a strong example of what could be done in more specifically targeted substance abuse prevention programs based on the imaging and mapping approach. The application stretches over 20 years of experience accumulated by the Center for the Improvement of Child Caring under the leadership of Dr. Alvy Kerby in Studio City, California. This program, characterized as the largest in the country, has focused on providing training for parents of minority background using the imaging and mapping-based cultural insights. The following chapters discuss the use of imaging and mapping by colleges interested in developing effective prevention programs on campus.

THE ANALYSIS OF CULTURE

Leading anthropologists of our century—Margaret Mead, Ruth Benedict, Edward T. Hall, Francis Hsu—have made us increasingly aware of how cultural differences are rooted in different worlds. These differences in people's subjective worlds, mostly inaccessible to direct observation, are the foundation of observable differences in their behavior. The literature on culture is extremely rich, and it intrigues professionals in many fields, ranging from cultural anthropology and psychological anthropology to cultural psychology and child development, from comparative politics and international relations to psychiatry and social work, and from comparative language studies and semantics to social problems and public policy.

The thousands of volumes written on related subjects, from the highly philosophical and theoretical to the highly empirical laboratory-based investigations, all face the dilemma that culture involves the whole person, and his or her natural behavior cannot be dissected and analyzed by ignoring its broad integrative nature.

The more abstract and theoretical the approach, the more it tends to lose its potential to explain the power of culture as a covert force that shapes behavior by organizing and representing it in close relationship to everyday life and existence.

The technology of imaging and cognitive mapping builds on the explanatory power of images as natural units of cognitive–semantic representations and shows the aggregate power of clusters of such images to shape behavior in a particular domain of life. We have already demonstrated how differences in the image of alcohol for drinkers and for nondrinkers or in the image of drugs for users and for nonusers of drugs offer insights into the psychological dispositions that explain differences in their behavioral choices. In this chapter we review differences in images between African-Americans and Caucasian-Americans and between Mexican-Americans of different income levels. We show how differences in images related to children and child rearing practices such as spanking are informative on differences in the behavior of these Caucasian-American, African-American, and Mexican-American parents toward their children. Though the differences are not directly discussed in relation to substance abuse, we use them to illustrate the same principles of how cultural images shape cultural behavior. More specifically, the examples suggest how information on clusters of images affecting behavior can be used in developing programs designed to change behavior that appears to be detrimental to the person or group under consideration.

TRACING AND USING CULTURAL DISPOSITIONS IN TRAINING

The use of the imaging and mapping technology to explore cultural differences in the child rearing views and practices does have implications for substance abuse prevention in the long range, but our immediate objective is to demonstrate experiences that bear on the use of imaging-based cultural insights in program development and training designed to overcome culturally rooted psychological dispositions shaping decisions and behavior.

Just as substance abuse is very much a problem area generated by the *Zeitgeist,* large-scale social problems of deep psychocultural foundation, the same is true about problems we encounter in child care and child rearing in the minority populations. In our contemporary postmodern sociocultural environment, adherence to traditional values and practices in child rearing appears to severely reduce chances for social and economic success. Traditional African-American and Mexican-American child rearing is characterized by authoritarian values, punitive practices, and strict rules designed to strengthen the parental control rather than encourage the autonomy of the child. These educational practices can be detrimental to the healthy development of the child. Children inculcated by values of authority, submissiveness, and obedience tend to be impaired in their self-confidence, inquisitiveness, self-reliance, and inventiveness. Such practices are naturally harmful to a child in a competitive social environment, such as the United States, where success is inseparable from using one's personal talent and assets to their full potential.

The Culturally Adapted Parent Training developed by Dr. Kerby Alvy, executive director of The Center for the Improvement of Child Caring (CICC) in Studio City, California, is an exceptional success story. The performance of the Center is impressive both in its scope and in its impact. It is the largest program of its type and has trained over 5,000 people. The success of the Center is all the more remarkable because it involves the complex and delicate subject of child care, with the bold objective to improve parental performance, to overcome deeply ingrained practices, and to modify traditional behavior based on empirical research findings. Since the late 1970s the CICC has relied on the AGA-based technique of imaging to reveal the cultural differences that require attention in designing their programs. This involves the introduction of changes in behavior in a context where parents' actions are based on culturally shaped habits rather than on a rationale supported by research evidence and advanced reasoning.

William Raspberry, in an article in *The Washington Post* (March 31, 1997) on parenting education, discussed at some length the CICC's culturally adapted training program. As he observes, "if only parents could be taught . . . the importance of making children feel loved and valued . . . modeling values . . . almost all the social problems that occupy us would be a lot easier to deal with."

The parents' approach in caring for their children and shaping their behavior is guided naturally by their best intentions. Differences in child rearing are widely discussed by anthropologists, psychologists, and educators. They show broad variations across cultures, and their implications are debated by social scientists as well as by popular authors. Despite the diverse views there is agreement on a few fundamentals. Child rearing is learned mostly from the social environment, without the parents being aware of how much their behavior is shaped by their culture and being even less aware of how their practices shape the development and the lives of their children.

BRIDGING CULTURAL DIFFERENCES IN CHILD REARING APPROACHES

The interest pursued by the CICC programs is not in the food the parents provide for their children or in the toilet training they implement. It is in social behavior and development. How do major ethnic/cultural populations of different socioeconomic background differ in the way they promote social values like obedience, compliance, independence, and autonomy in their children? In general, it is well recognized that the norms the parents follow usually reflect the norms of their social environment. This is one area of life where the impact of culture is the most powerful as well as the most covert.

The Diagnostic Identification of Cultural Dispositions

The Center's program is effective in showing the cultural dispositions that are at the foundation of differences found among African-American, Mexican-American and Caucasian-American parents in the way they treat their children. Using the AGA method of comparative imaging and mapping, the program has been effective in showing that child rearing values and practices of African-American and Mexican-American parents are different from those of many Caucasian-American parents. They are founded on cultural differences in perceptions and attitudes involving a more directive and more controlling role of African-American and Mexican-American parents compared to a more independent and self-regulating educational approach taken by the certain groups of Caucasian-American parents.

Using the imaging technique, the CICC gained insights into these cultural differences in perceptions and motivations. The research results showed group differences with a high degree of consistency. These cultural differences in outlook that resulted in differences in behavior emerged clearly from the diagnostic assessment. It revealed differences in perceptions and motivations in their images of the child, of raising children, of spanking and other methods, and of achieving various objectives of education and upbringing. For instance, fundamental differences emerged in the parents' approach and their goals in upbringing to establish control over the children, making them dependent on parental authority versus encouraging the children to make their own decisions and to promote their personal judgement and independent thinking.

Imaging offers insights into the foundation of different child rearing practices based on the underlying cultural views and assumptions that shape the parents' behavior in child rearing, as well as in other fields. The effectiveness of the imaging technology in revealing these previously hidden cultural forces underlying differences in observable behavior makes it became possible to address them systematically.

Use of the New Insights in Program Development

A second major achievement of the CICC programs was built on this first step of accurate diagnostic identification. Alvy and his associates concluded that if the new insights were critical in their own understanding of the role of cultural forces in shaping the parents' behavior, eventually they could prove useful in helping parents see the views that control their own behavior. These new insights would also show differences in their own views and the views of other cultural groups and how these different views result in different behaviors.

The CICC experience offers AGA-based cultural knowledge on perceptions, attitudes, and deep culturally based behavioral dispositions that make the difference between effective parenting and parenting practices that are punitive, dysfunctional, and harmful to children. The comparative analysis of parent populations representing various cultures and economic backgrounds (African-Americans, Mexican-Americans, and Caucasian-Americans) is used in a diagnostic phase to identify the hidden sources of parenting practices that unintentionally harm the children. The findings accumulated across these diverse populations by CICC and by our own research institute (ICS) show a high degree of correspondence.

Since the ICS is primarily a research organization with specialized interest in the assessment of psychological and socioenvironmental factors shaping human behavior in areas relevant to educational and mental health applications, the applied uses of the imaging data by the CICC are far ahead of our own. The CICC has already used the research findings in developing drug prevention programs for parents. Though program development has not been along the line of our specialized interest, we are strongly aware of such needs and of the demanding requirements to bring these powerful psychological dispositions and socioenvironmental factors effectively into program development. Therefore, the CICC's success is of considerable relevance and value from the angle of this broader venture.

CICC's Use of Cultural Experts

The cultural insights gained from imaging are built into the CICC training programs by using teams of cultural experts. The method of using experts on the African-American and on the Mexican-American culture deserves close attention. These experts have professional training in such relevant fields as psychology, anthropology, and sociology. As Dr. Alvy described the program development stage, the AGA data comparing family and parenting concepts across cultural and socioeconomic groups served a variety of purposes. The data was reviewed by each program's cultural advisory committee. These committees of well-respected and highly credentialed researchers and practitioners were responsible for making recommendations of what to emphasize in the culturally adapted parenting programs. The basis for these recommendations included a review and discussion of the AGA imaging and mapping methodology and results.

During the review of the comparative imaging data by the African-American and Latino communities several unexpected and fruitful events took place. The African-American committee, with several nationally known critics of traditional, culturally based research on ethnic minorities, was impressed by the cultural fairness of the AGA data. This made it easier for them to accept certain findings, especially concerning the strong association of whipping, spanking, hitting, and obedience in the low-income African-American images of disciplining children. These findings provided a culturally fair and empirical basis for including significant program sections on a form of discipline that had become common practice in many African-American communities, especially in inner city areas. This form has been referred to by African-American parenting authorities as "traditional Black discipline," which they contrasted with a more contemporary and positive concept of disciplining, referred to as "modern Black self-disciplining." These authorities usually have no research-based foundation to identify those dispositions which influence peoples' behavior, regarding such specifics as traditional Black discipline. The AGA data provided such support, and this made it easier for the African-American advisory committee to stress the importance of moving beyond the traditional slavery-generated approach and made it easier to include this pivotal matter in the program curriculum.

The curriculum writers included a presentation of the AGA data on disciplining children for discussion during the program. They also included an AGA exercise that gave the parents an opportunity to supply their own associations to the concept as a prelude to a discussion of the meaning and parenting implications of this data. The inclusion of both the research methodology and the findings has proven to be a very helpful instructional tool. The inclusion of a real-life example of the association of punitive child rearing with disciplining children, the presentation of group data, and a discussion of these phenomena within the context of the slavery experience and racist public policies have made it much easier for African-American parents, who have relied heavily on punitive practices, to learn and use more modern, nonpunitive practices, like those that are taught in the culturally adapted "Effective Black Parenting Program."

Integrating Research Findings with Expert Opinions

The key to the success of the CICC programs in using cultural experts is a clear differentiation between what is well founded and what is questionable. The cultural experts' attention is on the explanation of the responses of their culture group rather than on predicting and interpreting their behavior. Experts vary in their judgments of how important education is for contemporary Mexican-Americans. Competent experts familiar with their background know what *bien educado* means. *Bien educado* refers to the appropriate behavior of the child who follows the parents' norms and expectations, including good manners, obedience, respect for elders, and being pleasant and affectionate toward others. Since the imaging shows how middle-income and low-income Mexican-Americans vary along the important dimensions of *bien educado,* the experts could concentrate on their cultural experience rather than guess about internal changes that are inaccessible.

Alvy's experts came to a high degree of consensus about what the quality of *bien educado* implies regarding a child in general. This consensus was supported by the detailed results of comparative imaging (see Figures 13.5, 13.6, and 13.7 later in this chapter). It is only natural that cultural experts who live in different social and cultural environments have no magic insights about what is timely and dominant in the minds of specific populations. On the other hand, with the imaging results showing what are the dominant trends of perceptions and attitudes, they have a relatively simple task to interpret and explain the differences.

As the approach by Alvy demonstrates, a solution in which research findings and cultural expertise are used effectively in an integrated framework reinforces the complementary features and reduces the ambiguities that result from the incidental or tangential variations. This solution combines information on dominant perceptions and motivations that have timely relevance with cultural and social perspectives that have deep historic roots in their own rationale and have valuable explanatory power. The combination of several innovative solutions explains the success of the CICC program in a complex and demanding area that is of exceptional timely importance.

In summary, the program of culturally adapted child rearing is built on the recognition that success requires taking the trainees' world and their dominant perceptions and motivations into systematic consideration. From our interest in program development, three areas of experience deserve special attention:

1. The identification of low-income and middle-income African-American, Mexican-American, and Caucasian-American psychocultural dispositions shaping parenting practices that determine the effectiveness of parental care (Diagnostics).
2. Program development based on the results of timely diagnostic assessment, including the use of the findings to develop a coherent set of principles, as well as examples to show parents the nature and sources of their problematic behavior and help them adopt new practices to improve their effectiveness.
3. Implementation of culturally sensitive, effective program alternatives for major cultural and socioeconomic populations of parents using timely research findings integrated with broad cultural perspectives.

Identification of Cultural Dispositions Shaping Behavior

In the diagnostic assessment, the CICC programs rely on the multiple free-response association task using word themes like *family, children, raising children* and *disciplining children.* The response elicitation to these stimulus themes is in the parents' native language, as described in the appendix. The most widely used cultural groups are African-Americans, Mexican-Americans, and Caucasian-Americans of various socioeconomic levels selected on the basis of the characteristics of particular program populations, that is, the background and economic conditions of the parents receiving the training.

The following example is based on the comparative imaging of low-income and middle-income African-American, Mexican-American and Caucasian-American groups (Alvy, 1994). The excerpts are from the description of the diagnostic results. The semantographs show the main perceptual and attitudinal components of the images of the groups compared. The length of the bars indicate each component's proportion of the total image or meaning for one group compared to that of the other group. This visual representation is a simple device to convey how an image like *disciplining* encompasses proportionately different perceptual and attitudinal components for the groups compared.

Images by Black Head Start and White Higher-Income Parents

Responding to the multiple free-response elicitation task used by AGA, members of the Black Head Start group and of the Higher-Income White group produced hundreds of responses to each theme used as a stimulus word. We begin by comparing their reactions to FAMILY.

Figure 13.1 contains the superimposed semantographs of the Black Head Start and White Higher-Income groups regarding their worldviews of the concept of FAMILY. As can be seen, the components of "Immediate Family, "Love/Psychological Caregiving," and "Togetherness" were the most dominant for both groups. There is also a substantial overlap throughout the semantograph, indicating that the groups are very similar. This similarity is further confirmed in the correlation coefficient that was calculated between the two groups in terms of the percentages of weighted responses for each component of meaning. As is indicated in the key of the semantograph, $r = .93$ which is highly significant statistically ($p < .01$). This provides further evidence that these two groups are really quite similar in their worldviews regarding the idea of family, despite their cultural and class differences.

The worldview of the Black Head Start group regarding FAMILY revealed a greater emphasis on "Togetherness," which led to the program's adoption of a "family unity" rationale for teaching and explaining family rules. For example, in helping parents to motivate their children to follow family rules, the program asks parents to provide children with good reasons why they should follow the rules, rather than telling their children to follow the rules "just because I told you." One of the main appeals that parents are taught to employ as they discuss rules with their children is that rules help to keep the family unified and together. This type of program strategy ("appealing to their minds and not their behinds") was influenced by the Head Start parents' associations to the concept of FAMILY.

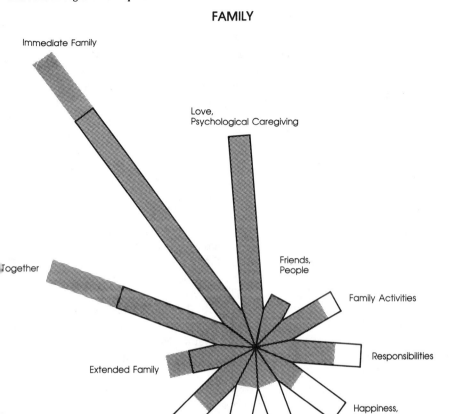

FAMILY

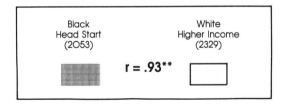

FIGURE 13.1. Semantograph of FAMILY comparing Black Head Start (BHS) and White High-Income (WHI) parent groups. [The size of each meaning component of the semantograph is the percentage of responses (weighted associations) for the components. The total weighted associations or concept score is in the key.]

Figure 13.2 displays the semantographic comparisons between the Black Head Start and White Higher-Income groups in terms of their worldviews for the family process concept of RAISING CHILDREN. Here there is much less overlap and the groups are very different, with a small and statistically insignificant positive correlation. While "Love" is a dominant component for both groups, there is slightly more emphasis on loving children as a part of raising them for the Black Head Start parents, and this emphasis was capitalized upon in the program by appealing to the parents' love of their children as the main reason for taking the time and effort to learn and to use the program skills. The strong emphasis on "Teach/Educate" by the Black Head Start parents also led the program creators to refer to child rearing as being an issue of "teaching" children. In order to build a Pyramid of Success for Black Children, parents are oriented to model and *teach* various qualities. The Black parents' emphasis on "Discipline" as a main component for RAISING CHILDREN reinforced the need to place special emphasis on this phenomena in the program.

Figure 13.3 reveals even greater differences between these groups in terms of their frame of reference on DISCIPLINING children. Here the differences are so great that the low and statistically insignificant correlation is a negative one. Three of the dominant components of DISCIPLINING for the Black parents are "Punishment," "Spank/Whip and Obedience/Respect." This triad of important meanings was understood as empirical substantiation of what the Black parenting scholars called "traditional Black discipline" and indicated that this orientation was still present in some African-American communities.

Because such an attitude is likely to be strongly challenged by the program's emphasis on the use of nonviolent disciplinary approaches, and because it is likely to be so firmly entrenched in the minds and histories of many parents, the program creators decided to use the word association method as a program-teaching technique for bringing this orientation out in the open so that it could be more carefully examined. Thus, parents in the program are asked to give their associations to the idea of disciplining and their associations are compared to those of the Head Start parents. The dominance of associations of punishment and spanking and whipping is related back to the slavery experience, and the ideas of the Black Parenting scholars about the influence of slavery are discussed. Parents then have a new or different perspective on the origins of this approach to discipline in African-American communities and therefore are more likely to be receptive to learning other disciplinary approaches.

The program then capitalizes on the fact that the Head Start parents also emphasized "Love and Understanding, "Talking," and "Explaining and Teaching" as part of their DISCIPLINING worldview to draw the parents' attention to the Black scholars' comments about a different approach. Here the program introduces its major disciplinary strategy, The Modern Black Self-Discipline Strategy, which is grounded in the ideas of the Black parenting scholars and offers a clear alternative to traditional Black discipline.

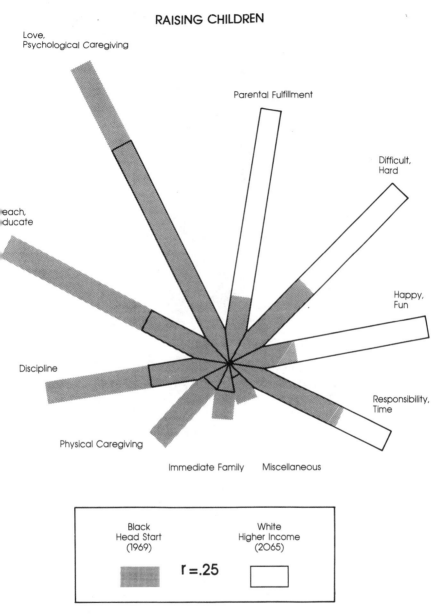

RAISING CHILDREN

Love,
Psychological Caregiving

Parental Fulfillment

Difficult,
Hard

Teach,
Educate

Happy,
Fun

Discipline

Responsibility,
Time

Physical Caregiving

Immediate Family   Miscellaneous

Black Head Start (1969)	White Higher Income (2065)
r =.25	

FIGURE 13.2. Semantograph of RAISING CHILDREN comparing Black Head Start (BHS) and White High-Income (WHI) parent groups. [The size of each meaning component of the semantograph is the percentage of responses (weighted associations) for the components. The total weighted associations or concept score is in the key.]

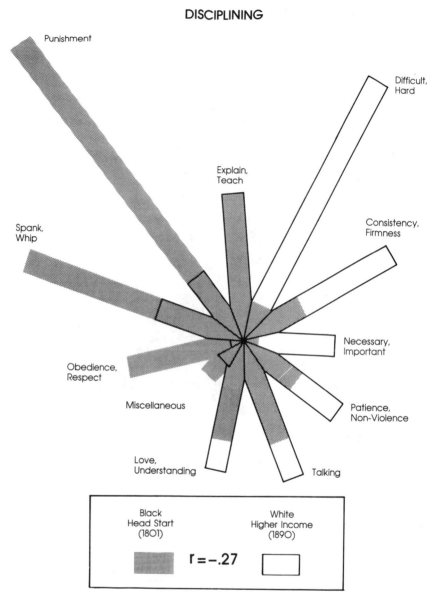

FIGURE 13.3. Semantograph of DISCIPLINING comparing Black Head Start (BHS) and White High-Income (WHI) parent groups. [The size of each meaning component of the semantograph is the percentage of responses (weighted associations) for the components. The total weighted associations or concept score is in the key.]

The program also made use of the fact that obedience and respect were more salient aspects of the Black Head Start parents' worldview on disciplining (associations of this nature were almost nonexistent in the worldview of the White Higher-Income parents). The Black Head Start parents' emphasis on respect contributed to the decision to refer to those child behaviors that parents would like to increase as being respectful behaviors, and to refer to those they would prefer to decrease as being disrespectful behaviors (in contrast to such similar behaviors being termed appropriate or inappropriate in the original Confident Parenting Program). This cultural accommodation was also in line with the program's desire to acknowledge and utilize colloquial and Ebonic expressions. By referring to the child behaviors that the parents would like to decrease as being *dis*respectful behaviors, the program reinforces and is evocative of a cultural expression for showing disrespect, i.e., "dissin." For Black communities where this type of Ebonics expression is prevalent, calling unacceptable or inappropriate child behaviors disrespectful strikes a very responsive chord and helps make the program resonate with the linguistic culture of the community. The program also refers to using drugs as disrespectful behavior, where the drug user is "dissin" his or her own body.

The data on the parents' actual practices with their children in a variety of typical child rearing situations (the objective level of culture) also had an influence on what was taught and emphasized in the program. Figure 13.4 contains a graph of the type of practices that the Black Head Start and White Low- and Higher-Income parents used when their children complied with parental requests or did what they said. The fact that 24% of the Black Head Start parents did not say anything positive when their children were cooperative alerted the program creators to emphasize the need to be responsive when children are behaving respectfully and to orient parents that it was important to "catch the children being good." The fact that relatively few of the Black Head Start parents who were responsive actually praised the specific behaviors of their children was also a reason to stress the need for parents to acknowledge the actual behaviors that are praiseworthy.

Images by Mexican-American Low- and Middle-Income Parents

As Alvy observes, the enormous challenge of creating a parenting program for Latino parents that would have appeal to all Latinos is reflected in the diversity existing within these Mexican American low and middle income groups. Although they share a common ancestry, they differ widely in terms of socioeconomic and educational backgrounds, language abilities and preferences, generational levels, and types of ethnic identifications. This challenge could be met by creating different programs for different groups of Latino parents, but that was not a practical solution. Instead, the cicc chose to work on creating a generic program that would be geared more toward poverty-level Latino parents who were more likely to be

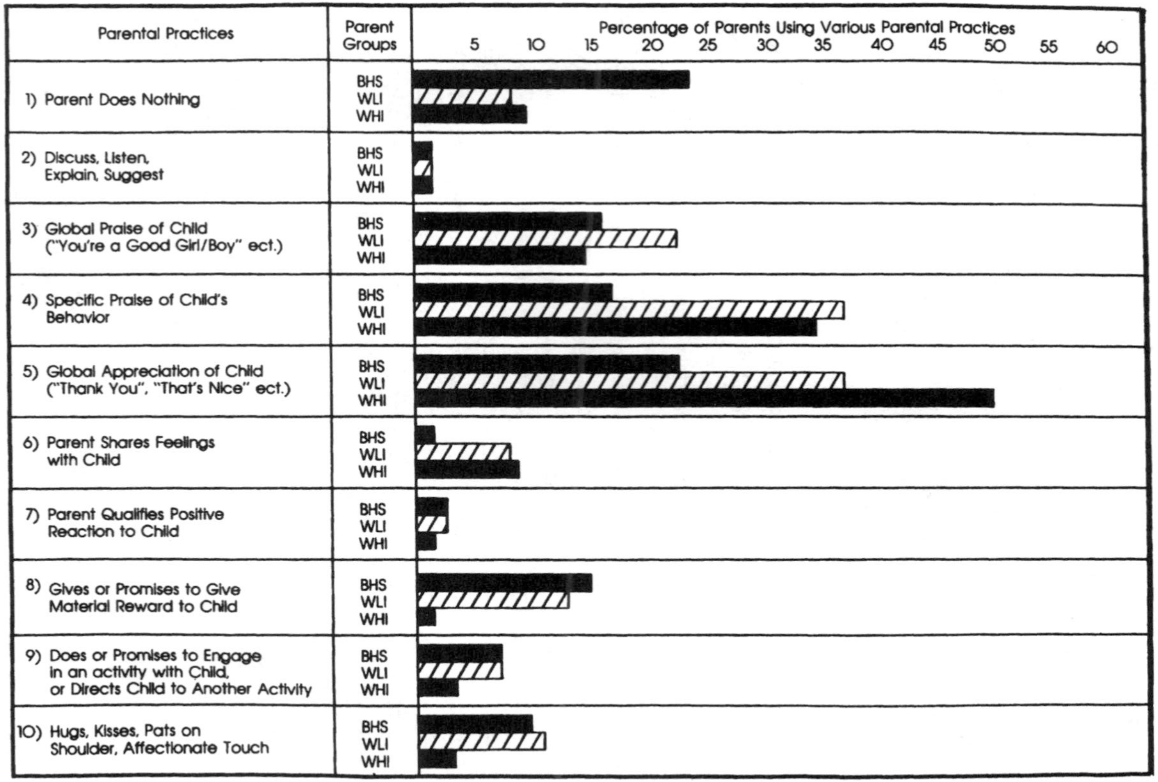

FIGURE 13.4. Percentage of Black Head Start (BHS), White Low-Income (WLI) and White Higher-Income (WHI) parents who used various types of parental practices in response to their preschool children doing what they say ($N = 100$ parents per group). [Percentages total more than 100% because some parents used more than one practice.]

newly immigrated. Thus, the CICC placed more emphasis on the results for the for-eign-born parent group (MAL) in framing and designing the program. Particular interest was shown in the results regarding the worldviews of each group.

The Figure 13.5 semantograph displays the superimposed worldviews of the two groups regarding CHILDREN, which shows a great deal of overlap and similar-ity, including a highly significant correlation between the percentages of weighted associations of the components of meaning ($r = .79$, $p < .01$). Children being en-joyable and playful carried a dominant meaning for both groups, with the middle-income group showing more emphasis in this area. "Love and Psychological Caregiving" was also a dominant aspect of both groups' worldview, and here the middle-income parents were more dominant. Two other components were more fa-vored by the low-income group, "Learn/Teach" and "Obedience/Respect." Here we begin to get a sense of what turns out to be the major discriminator between these two Latino groups, an emphasis on a particular type of social education in the newly immigrated parent group.

Figure 13.6 indicates that the idea or process of RAISING CHILDREN also is heav-ily instilled with "Love and Psychological Caregiving" for both groups with al-most equal frequency. However, the groups differ greatly on their overall view of raising children, as reflected in the low and statistically insignificant correlation. These differences are due mainly to the fact that the lower-class parents' view of raising children is so heavily suffused with the practical issues of teaching, edu-cating, and learning, including a moral focus on teaching right and wrong. Of particular significance is the fact that for the lower-income parents, the word "edu-cating" was the strongest single association to RAISING CHILDREN.

These results for the lower-income, newly immigrated parents pointed out the importance of a particular child rearing value that the Latino scholars had dis-cussed, the value of raising children to be *bien educados,* which encompasses a child's appreciation of respect for elders as well as maintaining certain understood social graces. This value appeared to be much more salient for the low-income par-ents, as reflected in the dominance and content of the "Teach/Educate" component.

The value was also understood to play a major differentiating influence in the groups' worldviews regarding DISCIPLINING children (see Figure 13.7). Here the two Latino parent groups, who share a common ancestry and language, are apprecia-bly different in their cultural frames of reference for disciplining, as the low and statistically insignificant correlation attests. The two most dominant components of meaning for the low-income parents are "Teach/Educate" and "Obedience/ Respect," echoing worldview results from previous semantographs.

The consistency of emphasis on worldview associations among the lower-in-come group seemed to reflect an underlying desire to raise children to become *bien educados.* This trend, coupled with the Latino scholars' writings and dis-cussions about the centrality of respect (*respeto*) and about becoming *bien educa-dos,* led the CICC to decide to frame the teaching of the entire culturally adapted

CHILDREN

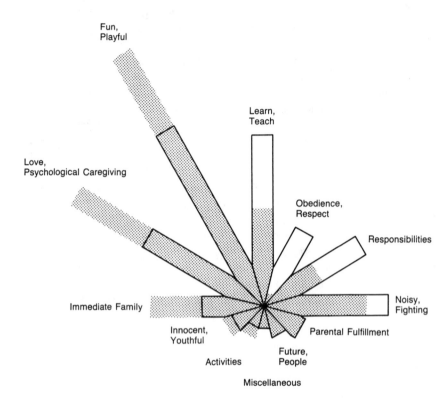

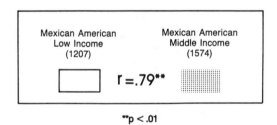

**p < .01

FIGURE 13.5. Semantograph of CHILDREN comparing Mexican-American Low-Income (MAL) and Mexican-American Middle-Income (MAM) parent groups. [The size of each meaning component of the semantograph is the percentage of responses (weighted associations) for the components. The total weighted associations or concept score is in the key.]

RAISING CHILDREN

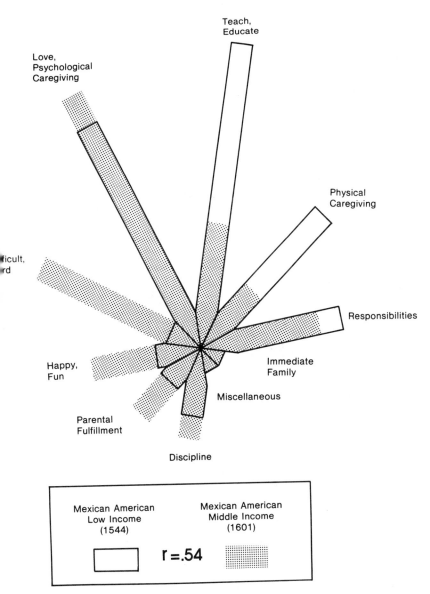

FIGURE 13.6. Semantograph of RAISING CHILDREN comparing Mexican-American Low-Income (MAL) and Mexican-American Middle-Income (MAM) parent groups. [The size of each meaning component of the semantograph is the percentage of responses (weighted associations) for the components. The total weighted associations or concept score is in the key.]

DISCIPLINING

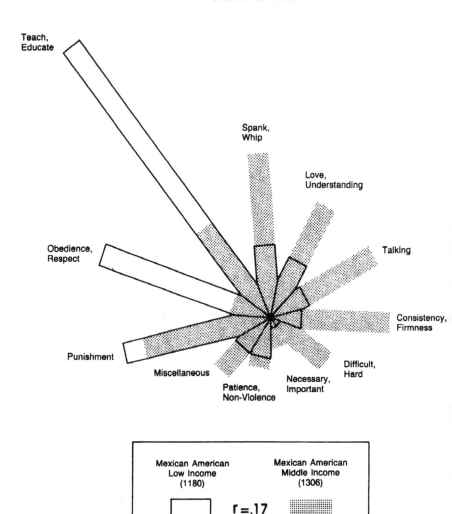

FIGURE 13.7. Semantograph of DISCIPLINING comparing Mexican-American Low-Income (MAL) and Mexican-American Middle-Income (MAM) parent groups. [The size of each meaning component of the semantograph is the percentage of responses (weighted associations) for the components. The total weighted associations or concept score is in the key.]

program around the value of raising children to be *bien educados*. Eventually that value became the name of the program, Los Niños Bien Educados.

The CICC also came to realize, on the basis of the worldview data and on the basis of the writings and research of Latino scholars, that there would be many varieties of commitment, appreciation, and even knowledge of this value among various Latino parent groups. Indeed, it did not seem to be particularly salient for the middle-income, first-generation parent in the study group. Their appreciation for "education" had more of an academic flavor as opposed to a social flavor to it. And undoubtably other groups of Latinos of Mexican descent, or of Cuban or Puerto Rican or Central or South American descent, would have somewhat different appreciations. Thus, it could not be assumed that all Latinos would be equally committed to this value, although all probably were exposed to it by their parents, grandparents, or great grandparents.

CONCLUSIONS SUPPORTED BY THE CULTURE-ADAPTED TRAINING EXPERIENCE

The programs developed and implemented by the CICC in the training of African-American (Alvy, 1987), Mexican-American (Spiwak, 1982) and Caucasian-American groups of various socioeconomic backgrounds support several conclusions. Of most immediate relevance to our present interest is the success of the CICC programs to build effective training based on the imaging findings produced by the AGA method. The CICC program experiences indicate that the diagnostic method of imaging offers timely information on cultural differences. This information is not only consistent with the experiences of cultural experts but also provides a way to guide and focus the expertise on select areas of cultural characteristics that are useful in explaining differences in behavior.

The emerging cultural insights and knowledge provided a solid foundation for developing programs designed to train members of various cultural groups to modify their behavior in order to achieve certain desired objectives, such as promoting the independence, autonomy, and self-reliance of their children and recognizing how these qualities are essential to help their offspring to be competitive in a cultural environment where these qualities are essential to their success.

As the CICC experiences since the late 1970s demonstrate, the imaging data are useful not only to gain cultural insights but also to present these insights to the trainees in ways that their implications are clear and compelling in supporting the desired behavior change as the ultimate training objective. The CICC experience is similarly relevant and useful in offering exemplary educational solutions for integrating cultural findings with cultural expertise in order to promote behavior change in the broader context of the people's cultural experience and the essential needs emerging from it. This approach can help to demonstrate, for instance, how a past history of slavery has created strong propensities for obedience and dependency and how the advantages of a free competitive environment make it indispensable to become competitive and self-reliant.

BREAKING THE CHAIN OF DEPENDENCY AND DESTITUTION

The objective of helping parents raise their children in ways that they become truly competitive and successful in our contemporary social environment is gaining support through new perspectives. In the past this need has been recognized in the context of ethnic minorities that have been historically excluded in every possible way—politically, socially, economically—from the American mainstream. Although many of the political and legal barriers have been abolished, other social and psychological barriers remain. Social changes and welfare legislation resulting in changes in the very nature and functioning of the American family have produced new developments.

Senator Daniel Patrick Moynihan has been a sensitive and acute observer registering these developments. He is also uniquely prepared to place the changes in proper social and historic perspectives. As early as in 1965 he was saying that our society is moving into an era in which destitution in childhood, relatively independent of economic forces, will be the principal social problem. As he put it at that time: "A community that allows a large number of young men to grow up in broken families, dominated by women, never acquiring any stable relationship to male authority, never acquiring any rational expectation about the future—that community asks for and gets chaos."

In 1991, the Commission chaired by Senator John D. Rockefeller concluded: "Too many of today's children and adolescents will reach adulthood unhealthy, illiterate, unemployable, lacking moral direction and a vision of a secure future." This commission reported a five-fold increase in the number of unwed mothers in less than twenty years. In the *Congressional Record* (September 12, 1991) Senator Moynihan published the percentages of unwed mothers by states, Washington, D.C. leading the list with 62.7%, supporting the Rockefeller Commission's conclusion:

> "We must begin today to place children and their families at the top of our national agenda. . . . Many young people believe they have little to lose by dropping out of school, having a baby as an unmarried teenager, using and selling dangerous drugs, and committing crimes."

The statistics presented more recently by Moynihan (*Washington Post,* January 28, 1997) show that from the teenage illegitimate birth ratio has grown from 15% in 1960 to 76% by 1994. In the District of Columbia it has reached 96%. The soaring teen pregnancy rate is indicative of a historically unparalleled process whereby the traditional family in which two adults share intensive involvement to assure the optimal psychological and physical development of their children is substituted by a teen-headed new type of family in which the socialization, the upbringing, and the promotion of mental and physical development of one or more infants becomes the task of one teenager, a part-time parent who may be expected to be the wage-earning provider as well. This situation is described as the "children raising children" paradigm. The economic absurdity of this paradigm may be more readily recognized as abject poverty by those who are forced to face it. Along this line, "destitute" conveys a strong meaning, though predominantly an economic one. When Senator Moynihan uses the term in this context, he refers predominantly to the psychological and mental correlates of present teen parenting, where the dominant agent of socialization is TV.

It is possible that Dr. Alvy would reject out-of-hand the proposition that requires not just modifying elements of parenting that have become dysfunctional in a postmodern social environment but building parenting from scratch. Nonetheless, if he would want to try, he could certainly have many new trainees.

The technology of comparative imaging and mapping can provide a solid foundation upon which to build this new paradigm. The first step is to gain an understanding of the worldviews of the people—the parents and the teenagers from many different socioeconomic and cultural backgrounds. The next step is to take into consideration the social environment that is shaping those subjective worldviews. Then, through integration of the insights offered by the imaging and mapping and by contemporary social and cultural expertise, new community-based educational and training programs can be developed that build bridges between what is the current reality and what every parent would wish to transmit to the next generation and the next beyond that one.

Part V

Applications: Diagnostics, Program Planning, and Evaluation

14

An Early Warning System

Assessment of Risks by Measuring
Vulnerability/Resistance

Risk assessment is a widely recognized need in prevention. It bears on decisions about who needs attention as well as about how the program should be focused. Imaging and mapping extend risk assessment beyond statistical probabilities to risks based on psychological dispositions and on environmental influences. Early identification of vulnerabilities can be particularly beneficial in offering the advantages of truly proactive programs. The Vulnerability data show which students to target and the image data show how to reach them.

The core of effective prevention is identifying the factors that make people vulnerable to substance abuse. Until now, risk factors have been based primarily on probabilities derived from demographic information, but with our imaging and mapping techniques we can supplement the traditional approaches with the identification of key psychological and social environmental factors. Our Vulnerability-based risk assessment not only reveals the level of risk but also provides a substantial understanding of the underlying psychological dispositions and, in some cases, social environmental influences that create the risk. Moreover, the imaging and mapping technology can identify psychological vulnerabilities at the early stages of development. This information is clearly relevant to the task of planning and targeting prevention programs.

The concept of *risk* is just as important in the field of substance abuse prevention as it is in any large scale venture in education, health care, or in other kinds of social intervention because the planners must form a clear idea of who the people are who can benefit the most from being served by the program. Our measure of an individual's vulnerability or resistance to substance abuse differs from other risk measures in that it not only indicates who shows the greatest likelihood of becoming involved, but also provides insights into why they are at increased risk.

THE DEMOGRAPHIC BASIS OF RISK ASSESSMENT

In early work, risk assessment was based on rather simple identification of those groups that had significantly higher or lower rates of substance abuse than average. We have known for quite some time that being male (Berkowitz & Perkins, 1987; Maney, 1990), engaging in criminal behavior (R. Jessor & Jessor, 1977), having friends that use (Brook, Cohen, Whiteman, & Gordon, 1992; Newcomb & Felix-Ortiz, 1992), and alienated social status (Brunswick *et al.,* 1992; R. Jessor & Jessor, 1973; Thompson, Smith-DiJulio, & Matthews, 1982) are all risk factors associated with higher levels of substance abuse.

Recently, however, researchers have begun to address the inadequacies inherent in this type of demographic risk factor. Pentz (1994) argued that although observable categories are easy to use, the categories themselves are not risk factors. By using categories such as ethnicity or gender to define risk, we are in jeopardy of designing and implementing prevention programs based more on social stereotypes than on the actual contributing factors. Likewise, Pickens and Svikis (1991) argued that these categories or groups are too broad to be informative. To say simply that men differ from women or that African-Americans differ from Caucasians leaves open several possible sources of those differences, including socialization, genetics, environmental differences, and social roles. It has become popular to report "sex differences" in a number of areas of scientific study, including persuasion (Eagly, 1987), aggression (Eagly & Steffen, 1986; Hyde, 1984), and leadership (Eagly & Johnson, 1990). However, several have argued that variables such as gender (McHugh, Koeske, & Frieze, 1986) and race (Yee *et al.,* 1993) are actually proxies for some other causal variable or variables. The presence of group differences does suggest that some aspect of group membership is important. The very idea that Hispanics or African-Americans or males or females have different psychological propensities for substance abuse or for other problematic behavior has probably been the underlying motivator for studying group differences.

In other health-related areas such as coronary heart disease, concentrated research into the process and immediate causation of the problem has revealed a number of factors that contribute to the development of the condition. We know that individuals are at risk who are under a great deal of stress, particularly if they have a Type A personality. Diet, lack of exercise, and smoking also contribute to the conditions from which coronary heart disease is likely to develop. As a result, though they cannot change their gender, men and women can take steps to reduce their risk by reducing their stress and their smoking, increasing their amount of exercise, and changing their diet. So it is with alcohol and drug prevention: once we discover the attitudes, expectations, goals, and beliefs that make some people more vulnerable to substance abuse than others, those elements become natural targets for prevention efforts. It is the identification and measurement of these dispositions that separates our research on vulnerability and resistance from traditional risk assessment data.

VULNERABILITY ASSESSMENT REACHES BEYOND UNIDIMENSIONAL DEMOGRAPHICS

As theory and research methodology in the substance use field have developed in recent years, researchers are beginning to move beyond demographic-based group identification toward the identification of specific intrapersonal and interpersonal variables that place certain people at higher risk. Pickens and Svikis (1991) have termed these variables "risk mechanisms" (as opposed to "risk factors"), whereas we have written about and discussed them in terms of "vulnerability." Although the terms sound similar, there are important differences between risk (or risk factors) and vulnerability. The most important one is that risk assessment aims primarily to identify who is at risk; vulnerability assessment, supported by imaging, aims to explain the foundation of the risk and how to address it. Demographic risk points the prevention specialist to groups who need the most attention but provides little guidance regarding the type of attention to be given. Once we identify the psychological dispositions that make one vulnerable, however, we then know not only who needs the most help but also how we can best provide it.

When we speak of vulnerability, we speak of psychological factors within the individual (attitudes, beliefs, expectations, etc.), even before the onset of substance use, that make that individual more likely to move to abusive use. These contributing factors represent various sources of psychological, environmental, biological, and social risk. One current conceptualization of substance abuse is that of a problem that can be approached via different paths. Some of those may involve more biogenetic factors, others may involve psychopathology-related factors, and still others may involve psychosocial factors. Additionally, each path is not necessarily marked by one single dominant risk factor but may contain a constellation of factors that increase one's vulnerability. Mausner and Kramer (1985) use the term "web of causation" to describe this perspective. The data we have presented in this volume clearly capture and map a significant part of this web. Our data are elaborate, lengthy, and complex because we are mapping one's dispositional makeup as it relates to substance-using behavior. Although previous research has done so, we do not focus on a single specific group membership nor are we content simply to look at a few personality characteristics.

In many conceptualizations (e.g., Brook *et al.,* 1992), an individual's vulnerability increases as the number of risk factors present increases. Although our Vulnerability measure is expressed as a single number, it is not a reflection of a single unitary risk factor. Rather, by assessing the degree to which an individual person or group shares the subjective world of users, it represents a complex, multidimensional measure of risk. It is the result of a multidimensional assessment that gauges the perceptual and attitudinal dispositions of the respondent in comparison with those of a reference group of habitual users. In this process, the dominant perceptual and motivational priorities of the respondent are compared with those of the reference group along its main dimensions.

The Vulnerability measure goes beyond the assessment of prevalence rates. For example, our results indicate not only that men use more than women, but that men see the world in ways similar to that of frequent users, even if they themselves are not frequent users: they share the frequent users' lack of fear for personal safety; they do not attend parties with hopes of socializing, but with expectations of beer and sex; and they are more cynical and mistrusting of social institutions (Doherty & Szalay, 1996). These are some of the reasons why men are more vulnerable, and these are the factors we must target when trying to reach this "at-risk" population.

TESTING THEORIES ABOUT CAUSATION AND CONTRIBUTING FACTORS

As stated above, researchers in substance use prevention are now beginning to investigate what some of the causal variables associated with demographic group membership might be. They are developing theories that go beyond demographics and are proposing models that address underlying causal variables. For example, low socioeconomic status is considered to be a risk factor for inner-city African-Americans. But moving beyond group identification to the underlying causal variables, theories now incorporate factors such as social roles and status. As we discussed in Chapter 7, many inner-city African-Americans experience delays in assuming adult roles (e.g., unemployment rates are higher, marriage rates are lower), and their marginalized social status leads to a lack of these protective factors; this places them at higher risk than higher-economic status others (Black or White; Brunswick *et al.,* 1992). Here, then, it is proposed that a lack of opportunities for socio-economic success and marginalization from mainstream society are what leave inner-city African-Americans vulnerable to engaging in substance abuse, a behavior that is counter to the norms and values in mainstream society. Thus, opening successful employment opportunities and creating a connection between these youths and the larger society would seem to be necessary features of any prevention program.

Although theories such as the Role-Conflict model are an encouraging improvement over simple identification of group differences, given the limitations of traditional survey research, we are still faced with the problem of providing solid evidence for these theories. Although it is true that the theory can explain the descriptive data, we are left with assumptions as to causation. We may assume that inner-city African-Americans, for example, who use drugs and alcohol do so because of this alienation from traditional roles and norms of the larger society, but we need evidence to confirm if this is indeed so. The AGA method allows us to examine evidence that may support or refute such assumptions by analyzing the responses to themes such as authority, government, and responsibility.

Thus, findings such as those described in the previous chapters shed light on the mechanisms underlying demographic group differences in vulnerability to substance use. As we have explored, we have found that though specific mechanisms have some correlation with group membership, they are as likely to cut across group membership. For example, users, as a group, tend to be cynical and mistrusting of social values and institutions. This is true for both White and Black users, male and female. Such alienation may be more common among certain socioeconomic and demographic groups, but it is the alienation, not the group membership, that predisposes these individuals to use alcohol or other drugs.

The AGA method provides keys that open the doors to the information that prevention personnel need in order to discover factors that underlie propensities for use or for non-use of harmful substances.

ANTICIPATING ALCOHOL AND DRUG PROBLEMS

The Time Factor

Substance abuse, as a source of many behavioral and health problems, is a result of existing behavioral dispositions. Once experimentation starts and chemical dependency grows, the debilitating medical and psychological consequences become apparent. The goal of prevention is to arrest this process as early as possible, which means finding ways to detect vulnerability and build resistance before the process advances too far.

The practical need for early detection follows from the logic of prevention. Our imaging and mapping technology extends the frontiers of risk assessment and prevention into the sphere of hidden psychological dispositions and takes the critical dimension of time into consideration.

Vulnerability and Age

Vulnerability to substance abuse may have some genetic components and certainly can involve dispositions rooted in one's family history. However, our results show that vulnerability has its primary foundation in psychological dispositions and that age is a critical factor, as we have discussed earlier in Chapter 7.

Our studies with different age groups show clearly that by junior high school, the psychological distance between students who have experimented with drugs and alcohol and those who have not is already distinct and that junior high users' reactions to the standard stimulus concepts already reflect many of the same patterns that are characteristic of adult users. The findings in Figure 14.1 come from an earlier study when the Vulnerability measure was not available; the Distance measure we used is described in the appendix. The consistently larger distance measured between users and nonusers (black bars) as compared to the distance between nonusers of different age/grade levels (shaded bars) shows the comparative effects of age and drug use. The effects of both variables emerge with a high degree of consistency. The age differences show additive effects: the larger the age difference, the larger the distance. It is indicative that the difference between use and no use is greatest at the elementary and junior high school level. Bearing in mind that the stimuli include family and self-images as well as alcohol and drug images, the dramatic shift in the perceptions and attitudes of such young children invite our attention to that age group as a focus for prevention activities.

Variation in Vulnerability at Specific Levels of Substance Use

Regarding individual, personal development, the concept of "early warning" has a somewhat different meaning. For an individual, successful prevention of substance abuse depends on how early it is possible to detect vulnerability. The more effective early detection can be, the better our chances are to target the incipient psychological dispositions before the perceptions and attitudes coalesce into a strong propensity for substance abuse. In this context, "early" does not refer to age or time but to personal susceptibility. Although susceptibility may evolve as chronological age increases, it can be affected dramatically by personal experiences, social environment, and institutional climate.

Although we already know that increased drinking increases vulnerability to substance abuse, students at the same level of drinking may show varying levels of vulnerability, depending on other influences in their lives, such as the environment in which they live. As an example, Figure 14.2 shows the distribution of Vulnerability scores for students at one particular high-use college campus (College #73) who reported various levels of alcohol consumption. Clearly, as the number of drinks per week went up, vulnerability rose (though there is nothing in the makeup of the Vulnerability score which is directly related to substance abuse behavior). At this school, students at all levels of consumption displayed higher vulnerability than did the comparable subgroups of students in the total population of 30,000 students, although the general relationship between alcohol consumption and Vulnerability score holds for the larger group as well. Students drinking one to four drinks on this particular campus are already exhibiting a

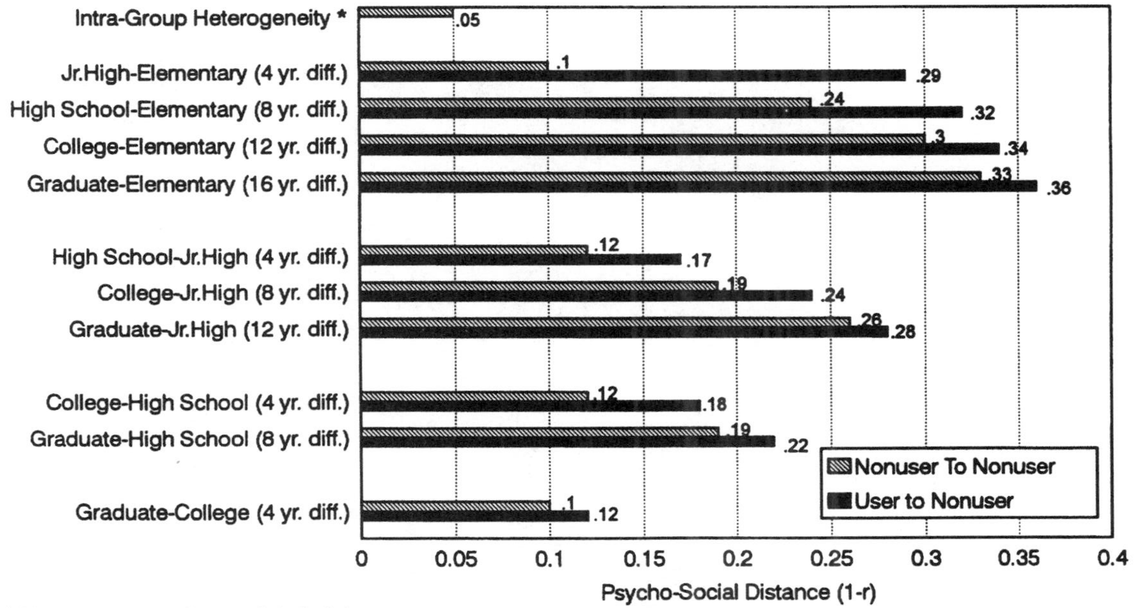

Intra-Group Heterogeneity *
Jr.High-Elementary (4 yr. diff.)
High School-Elementary (8 yr. diff.)
College-Elementary (12 yr. diff.)
Graduate-Elementary (16 yr. diff.)
High School-Jr.High (4 yr. diff.)
College-Jr.High (8 yr. diff.)
Graduate-Jr.High (12 yr. diff.)
College-High School (4 yr. diff.)
Graduate-High School (8 yr. diff.)
Graduate-College (4 yr. diff.)
.05
.1
.29
.24
.32
.3
.34
.33
.36
.12
.17
.19
.24
.26
.28
.12
.18
.19
.22
.1
.12
Nonuser To Nonuser
User to Nonuser
0
0.05
0.1
0.15
0.2
0.25
0.3
0.35
0.4
Psycho-Social Distance (1-r)

*** Distance=1-r (coefficient of similarity)**
Distance is conceived to include intragroup heterogeneity measured at .05.

FIGURE 14.1. Psychological distance between students as a function of age and substance abuse. [The data were based on 200 subjects in each group except for the Jr. High users (n=86) and the Graduate users (n=84).]

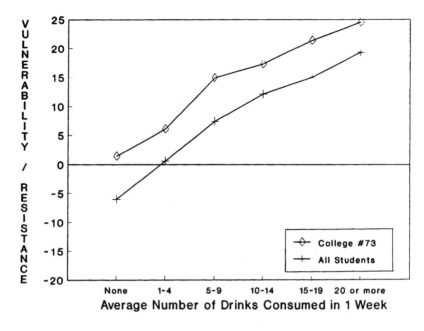

FIGURE 14.2. Weekly alcohol consumption and Vulnerability/Resistance at a high-use college.

Average # of Drinks Consumed in 1 Week	College #73 (345)	All Students (21,991)
None	15%	37%
1-4	22%	32%
5-9	15%	12%
10-14	14%	8%
15-19	6%	3%
20 or more	28%	8%
Total	100%	100%

higher degree of vulnerability generally associated with up to nine drinks per week in the general student population. Within each context, the different levels of behavior provide meaningful reference points so that one can readily see how much a change in behavior (e.g., alcohol consumption) is accompanied by measurable changes in vulnerability.

The Impact of Social Environment on Vulnerability

Students living in some environments are not at increased risk of substance abuse. The importance of a particular campus environment can clearly be seen as we track the vulnerability of students by class year at the same college shown in Figure 14.3. Figure 14.3 presents the Vulnerability scores of freshmen, sophomores, juniors, and seniors at the same campus (#73) along with the scores for the overall sample. Across all schools, there are virtually no differences in vulnerability from first through fourth year, but students at campus #73 show a distinct increase in vulnerability over the first three years before dropping somewhat during their senior year. The results reflect the culture of acceptance that is present within this particular college environment and underscore the need to understand the context within which a given individual or group is being assessed.

To know how a college stands regarding substance abuse, it is desirable to know not only the mean Vulnerability score of the college's own students but also the comparable data from other high- and low-use colleges as well. How the college environment makes a difference may be seen in broader perspectives in

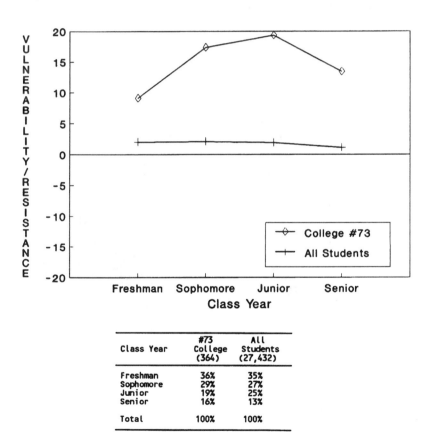

Class Year	#73 College (364)	All Students (27,432)
Freshman	36%	35%
Sophomore	29%	27%
Junior	19%	25%
Senior	16%	13%
Total	100%	100%

FIGURE 14.3. Vulnerability/Resistance by class year at a high-use college.

Figure 14.4 where 49 colleges are ranked from low Vulnerability to high Vulnerability. The college Vulnerability scores, ranging from −11 to +14, are means based on 400 to 800 students at each college. The numerical score for a particular college becomes more meaningful when it can be seen in relation to the scores of other colleges, or to scores of its own student subpopulations (e.g., fraternity/sorority/independent, male/female, etc.). The ability to place a college student body or other group of students into a larger framework provides a useful perspective for evaluating the magnitude of the alcohol and drug problem in various social cohorts and institutional settings.

Early prevention requires early detection of vulnerability. Whether "early" refers to a young age or to a previous point in time or to another level of vulnerability, what is essential is that differences in propensities for substance abuse can be detected based on empirically quantified results similar to an MRI or an X-ray revealing internal states or processes. The reference points help to place changes in proper perspective over time where the analogy of "early warning system" holds rather literally.

Resistance and vulnerability represent reciprocal views of the same continuum: as resistance decreases, vulnerability grows. The central objectives of prevention, then, are to strengthen and maintain the students' position within the region of resistance and to move students from the region of vulnerability toward and into the region of resistance. Our imaging and mapping results show the detail

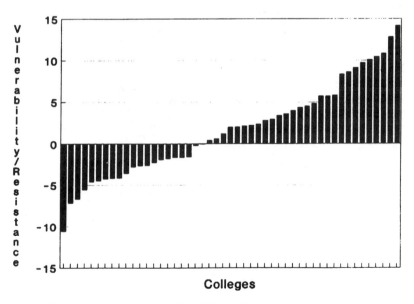

FIGURE 14.4. Range of mean Vulnerability/Resistance scores at 49 colleges.

underlying the perceptual and attitudinal dispositions that characterize both vulnerability and resistance, and that information can be a solid foundation for prevention program planning that will help students build the psychological resistance that will enable them to maintain drug-free lifestyles, even under adverse social-environmental influences.

Planning and Targeting Programs Based on Imaging and Mapping

The AGA-based diagnostic assessment offers planners and educators up-to-date research findings on their students' internal dispositions and on their propensities for using alcohol and other drugs. The assessment focuses on perceptual and motivational dispositions identified as the most dominant in shaping the student's choices to use or not use harmful substances. This knowledge offers program planners and educators a research-based foundation for developing prevention programs (activities, curriculum material, and communications) targeted on the psychological dispositions shaping the choices of the population under consideration.

DATA-BASED PROGRAM DEVELOPMENT

Most prevention programs are action oriented. In most instances they are based on various theories of human behavior or on general theories of substance abuse, as exemplified in the preceding chapter. Their theoretical foundation is rational and reputable and yet the broad diversity of programs suggests that their relevance and practical utility to substance abuse prevention remains open to debate. Empirical data necessary to decide their relevance are generally lacking. Nevertheless, success depends on developing programs that take into consideration the students' dispositions, which may vary from person to person and from group to group.

Compared to the customary theory-based program planning, the AGA diagnostic assessment has the advantage of program planning based on current research findings. Rather than proceeding from a theory of undetermined relevance, the imaging and mapping approach provides program developers and educators research findings on the dominant perceptual and motivational dispositions that promote vulnerability and on those that promote resistance in the case of particular population samples relevant to their interest.

The AGA technology identifies the dispositions that shape the decisions of particular groups regarding their use of alcohol and other drugs. Identification on a group-by-group basis provides timely information on the students' vulnerability/resistance, and the results of this diagnostic assessment are the foundation of systematic program development. Planning and building activities and communications can be focused on the variables identified as potentially the most influential in reducing the vulnerabilities and building the resistance of the group under consideration.

Input from Imaging

The psychological dispositions identified through the reconstruction of select images show that alcohol and other drug use has a broad foundation rooted in many domains of life. The images in the Alcohol and Drug domain showed the greatest perceptual and attitudinal differences between users and nonusers. These consistent differences revealed the powerful influences shaping contrasting choices in the use of harmful substances (Chapter 1). Images of Friends and Entertainment emerged as the second most influential domain (Chapter 2). The data suggest that users and nonusers are guided by different ideas about friends, fun, and parties. Other domains—Self and Family, Problems, Social Institutions—revealed further differences that shape substance abuse (Chapter 2). Although the role of the latter domains is more limited, they are still informative on the broad foundation of the users' and the nonusers' differences in behavior, perceptions, and motivation.

Presentation of findings on a particular population of interest is accompanied by findings on comparable samples of users and of nonusers. This serves several purposes. The user and nonuser responses and their scores provide useful reference points for the program planner. Two comparisons are of special relevance here. The difference between users and nonusers shows how important particular perceptions are and how much they contribute to the contrasting behaviors (use vs. no use). Comparison of the target population responses with the user and the nonuser responses shows in which ways their perceptions or motivations are similar to those of the reference groups.

The consistency of observations—for example, to what extent the prevention population reveals positive or negative attitudes toward alcohol, how similar or different they are from the users—offers insights relevant to program development. The program developer can see where the prevention population stands and how influential particular perceptions and motivations are in shaping the group's present behavior. The simplicity and clarity of the image data offer up-to-date information on the group's perspectives and how they shape behavior regarding substance abuse. They provide a solid foundation for developing program strategies as well as program elements by targeting activities and communications on perceptual and motivational dispositions identified as the most dominant and influential in shaping the group's behavior.

The differences in the images of users and of nonusers and of the specific prevention population offer practical details relevant to program development:

1. They demonstrate the relationship between the dominant perceptions/motivations identified by imaging and by the behavior reported.
2. They show which perceptions and attitudes are most influential in shaping the behavior of the target population.
3. They suggest alternatives in how to reduce vulnerability and how to promote resistance by developing programs that promote perceptions and attitudes that are most suitable to achieve the desired effects.

Input from Cognitive Mapping

Imaging offers insights into dominant perceptions and attitudes that form the respondent's world. Cognitive mapping involves reproduction of the respondent's world along selected dimensions, such as the relative propensity for use or for no use. The diagnostic assessment of propensities for use is of special relevance to substance abuse prevention. It can not only show the extent to which a person or group is psychologically vulnerable or resistant to substance abuse, but it can also show what is at the foundation of the vulnerability or resistance, in terms of dominant trends of perceptions and motivations.

Cognitive mapping, particularly the Vulnerability/Resistance measure, can be used to assess the impact of any particular program or policy alternative on behavioral dispositions, susceptibility to social influences, and the proclivity to engage in experimentation. These characteristics were previously beyond empirical assessment and are clearly relevant to a person's decision to use harmful substances.

EXAMPLES FROM COLLEGE APPLICATIONS

Whether interests lie in developing drug-free leisure activities, effective prevention curricula, posters, or any other communication, program developers and educators face similar needs and requirements. Their success depends on a capability to reach their students by addressing their dominant priorities and interests. To be effective, programs, activities, and communications have to be geared to the students' understanding of the world and its problems as the students see them.

The planning of any human activity, any goal-oriented performance, usually raises two fundamental questions: what to do and how to do it. Planning prevention programs on the college campus tacitly or explicitly involves these two types of decisions. The mapping results can help planners decide which targets to pursue in order to promote a drug-free lifestyle and environment. Regarding how to do it, the results of comparative imaging provide a wealth of up-to-date information that allows them to take into systematic consideration the dominant psychological dispositions of the students.

As we have worked with educators and program managers from dozens of schools, it has been our experience that the imaging results showing how users and nonusers have different outlooks on life have been readily accepted. Demonstrating that different outlooks result in different behavior, use or no use, helps them to appreciate how the dispositions of students shape their behavior. In turn, it was relatively easy to communicate the recognition that by gaining insights into these dispositions, we can get a practical handle on those perceptions and attitudes that make the difference in the students' current behavior. At the level of images, it was relatively easy to demonstrate the importance of these insights and to communicate their practical value. This helped to reinforce a commonsense recognition that the student's perceptions and attitudes are important in shaping their behavior. There was a natural readiness to recognize that the students' world is based on their subjective images and that successful prevention requires taking these differences into consideration. This indicates that the comparative imaging data are simple, easy to understand, and easy to use. They have been available from the beginning of our college-level prevention studies. Much of the work up to this point has focused on the use of the image data. This is the level of application discussed in *Rethinking the campus environment* (Goree & Szalay, 1996).

Practitioners can use information about images with no more than a careful review of the results from a campus population in relation to the reference groups of users and nonusers. Through a simple review of how the response distributions compare, it becomes apparent which psychological dispositions are dominant in promoting substance abuse and which ones strengthen resistance. The colleges that participated in the initial research received in-depth assessments of the psychological dispositions of their own students in relation to the reference groups of users and nonusers. In their case, it was easy to apply the insights according to their specific campus goals and interests. The campus planners looked at how their own students responded to the key themes in order to assess how relevant these dispositions were to the problems on their own campus. The review of images for contrasting dispositions offers specific insights into how to develop activities, curriculum material, and social marketing that take the students' psychological dispositions into consideration. In other words, it gives an indication of how to promote nonuser perceptions and motivations and how to counterbalance user dispositions.

The growing research evidence suggests that the secret of effective prevention lies in knowing what makes certain people prone to use harmful substances and what the dispositions are that help others to resist and avoid experimentation. The comparative imaging data show how users and nonusers see things differently, how these differences influence their behavior, and how perceptions and motivations can be hidden sources of vulnerability that promote experimentation and use. These results served as the basis for the development of diverse activities and programs.

Curriculum Infusion Promoting Alcohol and Drug Awareness

The image data on the students' perceptions of alcohol and other drugs provide a quantitative basis for concluding that users and nonusers differ sharply in the degree to which they perceive the use of alcohol and drugs as personally or socially harmful. Using these insights, colleges have built their staff training, Alcohol Awareness Weeks, and resistance training in ways that reinforce the students' desire to take charge of their lives and assert their freedom from dependencies. Colleges have begun to incorporate these findings into their alcohol and drug education components; they are developing materials for curriculum infusion to emphasize consequences that the imaging analyses indicate users tend to overlook or minimize.

Planning Alcohol-Free Entertainment Opportunities

Recognizing the importance of the social and entertainment dimensions of college life, some of the colleges in our studies have focused on the user–nonuser differences found in their images of friends, fun, and parties. Attempts are being made to weaken the association between entertainment and alcohol/drugs that is so strong among the users, as quantified by the comparative imaging analyses. Colleges have capitalized on the nonusers' perspectives on friends and social gatherings and reorganized elements of their entertainment programming. Planners are organizing alcohol-free entertainment opportunities centered around specific celebrations such as birthdays in recognition of the life achievements of members of student groups. A review of the imaging results helped to identify which occasions and themes were important to the students. For example, from their images of fun and parties we know that users are interested in the drinks and nonusers are interested in the food to be served at social gatherings. Making efforts to make the refreshments more appealing may be a minor but important shift that would support the nonuser dispositions without sending a message of deprivation to the users/ drinkers. Some institutions are providing the imaging materials as resources for their residential life staff who are responsible for organizing and encouraging alcohol-free social events.

Developing Leisure Activities That Build Resistance

Recognizing the important distinction that nonusers view a much broader diversity of activities as fun and entertaining, campus programmers are promoting more leisure activities that help to expand the Users' perception of fun and entertainment beyond their linkage to alcohol. They are offering more opportunities to engage in physical fitness activities and a variety of athletic activities such as golf, tennis, jogging, and team-building exercises.

Programs Designed to Deepen Friendships and Social Relations

The nonusers' interest in deeper and more meaningful social rapport makes a natural target for programming and training efforts. From the imaging data, we know that low-risk users and abstainers prefer smaller, more intimate gatherings rather than large, boisterous parties. Campus planners are looking for ways to promote social gatherings that are conducive to developing social relationships that are more personally supportive and enduring. Providing opportunities for small group interactions—for example, arranging individualized floor parties in the residence halls—is one way of encouraging and affirming the nonuser dispositions and making the nondrinkers more visible on campus.

Working through the Student Government

One of the distinguishing characteristics of users that emerges across a number of images is their skepticism and mistrust surrounding issues of authority and discipline. Planning programs that help to build trust in the external systems can be expected to counterbalance this aspect of the users' frame of reference. Setting clear campus policies with consistent enforcement of boundaries is one such approach. Also, activities that aim to instill a greater sense of self-discipline and personal authority may help to empower the students and strengthen their resistance to substance abuse.

Building Resistance through Volunteering

The findings on the Vulnerability/Resistance of student volunteers suggest that volunteers tend to be similar to nonusers in their dispositions and in their ways of looking at the world, thereby providing empirical support to the protective benefits of volunteerism. Reliance on student-to-student interaction, as in peer counseling, has the advantage of counterbalancing some of the characteristic user dispositions to be skeptical and distrustful toward older people in authority positions (teachers, administrators), to resist "scare tactics," to discount potential risks, and so forth. This natural channel of communications can also be instrumental in building lasting social relations among students who are not inclined to participate in organized group activities.

The Vulnerability/Resistance data, which are more recent in origin, are generally intellectually appreciated by scholars but have been less widely used in systematic planning. The greatest potential advantages can come from the combined use of imaging and mapping, with the mapping-based Vulnerability/Resistance data directing targeting decisions and the imaging data supporting the development of programs designed to reach the students with programs, curricula, and special marketing. Such uses are now on the drawing board at some colleges and will require some time to settle into the level of routine application.

EXPERIENCES FROM COLLEGE APPLICATIONS

What Have We Learned from Mapping?

Our findings and experiences since the late 1980s support the conclusion that the most critical requirement of program planning is to identify the dominant propensities that shape the students' behavior and to develop programs that address the dispositions that offer the best opportunity to reduce vulnerability and promote resistance to substance abuse. Although these conclusions are broad and rather universal, their practical implementation requires solutions that vary from group to group.

The intrinsically hidden nature of psychological dispositions is certainly a major reason why contemporary prevention programs take such widely different approaches. It may also explain at least partially why there are so many conflicting theoretical positions. Up-to-date research results identifying the dominant perceptual and attitudinal dispositions that promote or cause one to resist experimentation with alcohol and other drugs suggest here a viable alternative. As demonstrated in the Chapter 3 discussion of the system of mental representation, its influence on the organization of behavior, and the role of its key parameters, particularly Vulnerability/Resistance, the cognitive mapping strategy and the Vulnerability/Resistance measures provide useful support to program planning on the critical question of targeting programs. More specifically, mapping and the resulting data on vulnerability/resistance offer opportunities to answer the following questions about the populations under consideration:

What is the level of their vulnerability/resistance? A general sense for the proportions of the alcohol/drug problem on a particular campus can be obtained by measuring the students' overall level of Vulnerability/Resistance. It provides an indication of the general campus drug climate, placed in perspective by comparisons with high-, medium-, and low-use colleges and with the national reference norms for comparable student subpopulations.

What are the dominant propensities that promote vulnerability and that support resistance to substance abuse? An assessment might show that students on a particular campus share the users' perception of alcohol as fun and that they do not pay much attention to the dangers of drinking and driving compared to nonusers. This finding reveals the need to broaden the students' ideas of entertainment and find ways to raise their awareness of the consequences of alcohol and other drug use.

How are these propensities distributed across subsamples by background, gender, age, and so forth? Comparison of Vulnerability/Resistance scores within a campus population and in relation to established reference norms helps to place their levels of vulnerability into perspective in identifying which groups on campus are most at risk and which ones are most resistant to substance abuse.

How is the students' vulnerability/resistance shaped by environmental factors, lifestyle, group affiliation, and other relevant variables? The effects of combinations of factors can be calculated and the Vulnerability/Resistance levels can be compared for fraternity members in high- and in low-use environments, for example, or for any other group affiliation on campus. The proportion of students fitting these profiles can provide guidelines for decisions as to where to focus attention in prevention. As our experiences have shown, the results of the mapping-based diagnostics provide abundant details for program planning. Considering then the important situational characteristics that vary from campus to campus, program planners are in the position to make solid decisions.

What Have We Learned from Imaging?

The research findings obtained from comparative imaging covering the six domains of life were presented and discussed in the first few chapters. They exemplify the detailed information that comparative imaging offers for understanding the contrasting perceptions and attitudes of frequent users and nonusers of alcohol and other drugs. From the angle of program development, imaging provides program planners information of dual use.

First, it offers insights into their students' dominant perceptual and attitudinal dispositions that were found to be most influential in shaping their decisions and behavior related to substance abuse. We use the contrasting presentation of user versus nonuser images so that the reader can readily identify the perceptual and motivational differences that are involved in shaping use and in shaping no use. This information offers simple insights into what matters, which views promote use, and which ones build resistance. For example, from this information planners and educators can determine whether the student subpopulations they want to reach are characterized by high vulnerability, are generally more resistant, or are thoroughly mixed. The figures presenting Vulnerability/Resistance results have shown how colleges vary in their student compositions. As we have shown in part I, if planners are dealing with populations of high vulnerability, they cannot count on the students' awareness of risk and harm and must find ways to build such an awareness. If they are dealing with students who have relatively low vulnerability, the program developers and educators can decide how to build resistance by addressing the students' concern with being independent and maintaining control over their own lives. This deeper understanding is essential in order to recognize the sources of differences in the students' behavior and their foundation in the students' inner world.

Second, this information is key to program development adapted to the frame of reference of specific student populations. It offers insights into how to develop programs and communications in such a way that they tie in closely with the views and beliefs of the students they want to reach. In dealing with the more vulnerable groups, the focus may be on how to build the students' awareness of harm and consequences, or on how to relate to their strong interest in entertainment. In the case of low-vulnerability groups, program developers can build resistance by capitalizing on the broader meaning of entertainment for them, on their desire for social contacts of a more personal and lasting nature, or on their strong sense of responsibility and discipline.

Again, imaging data obtained on the planner's campus population is a rich resource for finding ways to reach the students. The information can serve as the foundation of communications that build on the student's subjective world, his or her subjective meanings, priorities, and frame of reference. The scope of the information is extensive; nonetheless, practitioners can focus on themes and domains that are especially relevant to their own objectives and selected targets. In training others to use this new information effectively, it may be useful to refer once again to the analogy of maps—the reconstruction of the student's mental map that directs his or her behavior. Like land maps, the imaging and mapping approach provides guidance into the students' worlds, and helps the planner to address the world of the students as the students themselves see and understand it.

THE COMPLEMENTARY USE OF IMAGING AND MAPPING

In the first chapters we discussed how the users and the nonusers have different images, and we described the method we use to reconstruct those images. In the chapters that followed we elaborated on the worlds of the users and of the nonusers built on the different images. We have shown that the worlds differ in their organization and amount to two contrasting systems of mental representation. We described how these systemic differences can be assessed by cognitive mapping. Our use of the terms *imaging* and *mapping* may convey the impression that we are talking about two distinctly different processes. This impression would be wrong because both aim to reflect people's subjective representation of their environment. In the case of imaging, we are describing the elementary units of these systems, whereas in the higher levels of mapping we are describing the organization of the system that holds the images together and shapes behavior through its systemic influences.

In the case of imaging, the reader can see how the images are reproduced and how they bear on people's subjective world in a very concrete, simple way. In the case of cognitive mapping, advanced, computer-assisted analyses produce clear, conclusive results but the procedure by which they are derived cannot be so readily seen or understood. To some, the concept of cognitive mapping may seem abstract and confusing, but by seeing where the imaging data come from and what they are based on, it is easier to see the connection. These two categories of information come from the same source, and their combined use offers the best way to get the most practical use of this new information on psychological dispositions affecting substance abuse.

For program planning, the distinction of imaging and cognitive mapping is useful because it bears on practical utility. As conveyed by the model of cognitive–semantic representations described in Chapter 3, imaging is centered on the specifics of select images. The insights are useful in developing focused strategies and communications. For example, in searching for ways to address the dispositions of users to overlook harm and consequences, the detailed image data become invaluable.

In the interests of planning what general strategy may work best in facing a particular student population, it is naturally compelling to start with diagnostic assessments that rely on the Vulnerability/Resistance measure. The Vulnerability/Resistance scores will indicate which segments of the population are most vulnerable or most resistant, and in that way help to target students at risk or to enlist the social power of students who are already exhibiting strong resistance to substance abuse. The focus may shift many times within one planning task, yet the fact remains that high-level analysis calls for a mapping of prevailing propensities. Once the population targets have been identified, program implementation requires the specifics offered by imaging. The diagnostic assessment and the use of the findings in program development are two separate but closely related tasks that can ideally complement each other.

Perceived Harm—An Example

In a world scared and confused about substance abuse, the surveys conducted by the Institute of Social Research (ISR) at the University of Michigan since the late 1970s are exceptionally conclusive and informative. The results of this survey show with consistency a close, inverse relationship between drug use and perceived harm. An increasing awareness of the harms associated with drug use accompanied a decrease in use of practically all substances between 1981 and 1990. This was followed by a reversal in the early 1990s. Since then there has been a continuous increase in substance abuse along with a similarly continuous decrease in the students' perception of harm. The ISR's finding that when students perceive drugs and alcohol as harmful, substance use and abuse decrease naturally has important implications for prevention.

Using different samples, a different method, and cross-sectional rather than longitudinal comparisons, we obtained similar results: students who do not perceive harm in alcohol/drug use show high vulnerability and tend to use alcohol and drugs; those who are aware of and preoccupied with harmful consequences are resistant to experimentation and risk taking. Our findings, based on 30,000 students tested nationwide, support the University of Michigan's ISR surveys in two main contexts of special relevance to prevention. The students' recognition of harm and their perception of drug use as personally and socially unacceptable behavior emerged from our research, as they did in the Michigan survey, as two of the most important factors distinguishing nonusers from users across all of the thousands of students tested.

The simplicity and conclusiveness of the ISR findings based on thousands of students suggest that the psychological disposition of recognizing harm associated with alcohol and other drug use is eventually the single most critical factor shaping the student's propensity to use harmful substances. The ISR surveys offer a history of two decades demonstrating how long-range trends in substance abuse can be traced to changes in the drug climate and in the social environment supporting or weakening the students' awareness of harm. The benchmark findings of the ISR surveys help place our findings in perspective.

Program Planning Based on Cognitive Mapping

The Vulnerability/Resistance results on propensities to use or not to use harmful substances are comparable to the prevalence findings of drug surveys, with some important differences. Rather than relying on the students' self-reports of their drug behavior (which substances, extent of use, frequency), the Vulnerability/Resistance data indicate how the students' behavior depends on dominant trends of perceptions and attitudes resulting in aggregate propensities for use or for no use.

This assessment offers insights into the students' behavior based on the psychological dispositions that are at the foundation of their choices. These insights can help planners reconstruct, beyond self-report, the dominant variables that are behind the students' decisions. In the context of perceived harm, cognitive mapping shows what the dominant perceptions and attitudes characteristic of the nonusers are that make them resistant and what the qualities are that make the users vulnerable to use.

This new information shows not only what the students do regarding alcohol and other drug use but also how particular student populations, including subgroups by age, sex, ethnicity/culture, lifestyle, and campus environment, vary in their propensities. In other words, the mapping-based diagnostics tell the planner what the dominant perceptual and motivational dispositions are that make the nonusers resistant and the users vulnerable. Unlike traditional survey results, cognitive mapping reveals the students' level of psychological vulnerability or resistance to substance abuse. Regarding perceived harm, the findings show not only how influential this disposition to recognize harm is but also how important it is in shaping the students' vulnerability/resistance to substance abuse.

Program Targeting Based on Imaging

Equipped with this new knowledge drawn from cognitive mapping, educators and program developers are in the position to develop programs built systematically on the dominant dispositions of their student population. In developing and implementing their plans, the findings from imaging offer useful details. In this respect we may use again the findings on the students' dispositions related to their awareness of harm. We will consider how the findings on perceived harm can be useful in building programs designed to increase an awareness of harm associated with substance abuse. This task takes on special importance as shown by the ISR data as well as from our findings.

The comparison of user and nonuser perceptions of harm indicates particularly wide differences; nevertheless, building awareness of harm is an immense and delicate task. In the case of resistant groups, the question of harm can be addressed directly. Students with a natural tendency to stay in charge of their own lives will be receptive to programs that discuss risks and harm. In the case of vulnerable groups, program developers and educators face a more difficult and challenging situation. This challenge increases with the level of dependence or vulnerability of the students under consideration. When risk and harm have little meaning for the students, educators cannot easily build on the students' experience because references to harm are likely to elicit the negative connotation of scare tactics, as extensively discussed in the literature. Under such conditions it is essential that the planners take the world of their vulnerable students into careful consideration.

In this respect, effective program development requires more than describing the harm and building on fears using matter-of-fact information. Building awareness of harm by expanding the students' scope of experiences regarding consequences requires special attention when the students have strong dispositions for selective perceptions, denial, or for lack of trust. The comparative image data offers opportunities for gradually, systematically building awareness of consequences. Such a process can help increase awareness of risks and harm linked to drug use by taking the characteristic dispositions of vulnerable students into consideration. Examining the world of the vulnerable students, as reflected by the image data, offers educators a way to identify the priorities and concerns to which these students pay attention. These are different from those derived from the "straight" thinking of the nonusers, and they can be just as effective to command attention. Reviewing the subjective images, we found that vulnerable students show some preoccupation with the future, particularly with the possibility of failure and being a loser. They are concerned with personal rapport, friendships, and social relationships. There are indications that their preoccupation with fun, parties, and noisy entertainment may be a reflection of a desire for more enduring relationships. Their ambivalent feelings about parents, friends, and school may reflect not so much a lack of interest as a dissatisfaction with the actual state of affairs, including their own insecurities, confusion, and performance.

On the basis of these characteristic psychological dispositions, planners can develop more effective programs by building awareness of consequences that bear on the vulnerable students' subjective world, priorities, and interests. Having peers who can speak about the consequences of substance abuse in their own lives—the impact on family, relationships, job and career, health—helps to avoid the frequent users' skepticism about adult authorities exaggerating the dangers of drinking and drug use. Rather than speaking directly about harm to a high-risk audience, it is important to find ways to build their experiences and to expand their awareness of consequences in areas of their lives that are important to them, such as their social life—friendships, entertainment, leisure—as well as job and career opportunities. The users' generally greater attention to AIDS, death, pregnancy, violence, and guns may indicate that they engage in behaviors that put them at risk of such outcomes. Thus, preventing these behaviors should be part of substance abuse prevention programs as well. Programs that offer tools to increase the students' confidence in facing the future can also reduce vulnerability.

The findings suggest a variety of opportunities to reach students by taking their world into consideration. For example, by relying on volunteers and peer counselors who are beyond suspicion of representing the establishment, it is possible to reap multiple benefits. Volunteering was found to promote resistance not only in the students counseled but also in the students doing the counseling. Other findings support the use of select activities, lifestyles, group membership, and environmental conditions identified as effective in promoting resistance and reducing vulnerabilities.

The magnitude of the task of developing effective prevention programs that can reach students with various degrees of vulnerability is apparent to educators and specialists as well as to the millions of parents facing individual problems related to drug use. The growing empirical evidence of the importance of psychological and social-environmental factors shaping substance abuse supports the need for a major paradigm shift in prevention: from *what* is being used to *who* is using and *why*. The diagnostic assessment of Vulnerability/Resistance offers a solid foundation for systematic planning. The image data offer the details necessary to develop programs specifically designed to address the needs of particular student populations.

The experiences with using AGA-based information on the psychological dispositions of users and nonusers suggest that program development can benefit from approaching the task of prevention based on the students' dominant perceptions and attitudes and on their vulnerabilities and resistance. The evidence supports that research-based program planning and development has a great deal to offer by reducing the uncertainties characteristic of programs built on the theoretical foundation of questionable relevance to the group under consideration. Based on our experiences in the context of college-based prevention, comparative imaging and cognitive mapping make different contributions. Mapping offers information particularly relevant to planning, whereas comparative imaging offers information useful in developing programs that take the students' perceptions, attitudes, and subjective worlds into consideration. Although the imaging based knowledge is readily applicable, the use of mapping-based insights is a much more demanding task. It requires more systematic training in the use of the information than was possible in the scope of the work done on the college campuses. Fortunately, other AGA-based applications of longer duration than the 2-year campus programs have provided relevant experience (Chapter 13).

16

Program Evaluation, Feedback by Measuring Vulnerability/Resistance

The difficulties of measuring program success in prevention are well known. They are major contributors to the general uncertainties surrounding substance abuse prevention. The sensitivity of the noninvasive, inferential imaging and mapping-based assessment has been tested in diverse tasks of program evaluation. Two main applications are discussed: assessing changes in campus climate and measuring the impact of selected program activities. Both offer feedback on program effects.

THE EVALUATION DILEMMA IN PREVENTION

It is customary to differentiate between outcome evaluation and process evaluation. When the focus of attention is the quality and characteristics of the end-results and how well they meet certain criteria, we speak of outcome evaluation. When the focus is the effectiveness, design, and time requirements of the process, we speak of process evaluation. In the case of primary alcohol or drug prevention, both of these conventional categories of evaluation are problematic. When the goal is to prevent experimentation and involvement with drugs, success means nonoccurrence. The lack of conclusive outcomes and the demanding design requirements to evaluate nonoccurrence make outcome evaluation impractical. The second route, process evaluation, requires monitoring internal changes produced step-by-step. Such monitoring and feedback has not been available in the past.

The difficulties intrinsic to the task of prevention evaluation contribute to the present uncertainties and confusion surrounding substance abuse prevention: despite the large number of different programs, those that make useful contributions cannot be conclusively separated from those that have little or no positive effects.

We present a few examples in this chapter to illustrate new alternatives offered by the AGA measures. The solutions are based on the capability to measure changes in relevant perceptions and attitudes, changes that reflect program impact. The first example illustrates this analytic capability in the framework of a therapeutic community-based treatment program. Program effects were measured along several relevant dimensions and domains of life. The controlled setting of a therapeutic community provided an opportunity to relate the changes to the outcome of the rehabilitation process.

The other examples come from prevention evaluation and demonstrate changes in dominant psychological dispositions and in the students' overall propensity to use or not to use harmful substances. The Vulnerability/Resistance measures are useful not only to assess the main direction and pace of change but also to provide relevant reference points for outcome evaluation.

Measuring Internal Changes Affecting Behavior

The use of our imaging and mapping techniques in evaluating the impact of alcohol and drug programs is built on experiences accumulated over a quarter of a century. More than a decade ago, Kelly (1985) described in *Evaluation Review* the sensitivity and flexibility of the AGA-based imaging and mapping method in the measurement of changes beyond the reach of traditional survey methods. Because these changes occur gradually and accumulatively and are not accessible through introspection, they have limited opportunity to emerge from the respondent's answers to direct questions. Kelly concluded that the imaging and mapping approach "permits an intensive, in-depth empirical assessment where previous assessment necessarily was either highly qualitative or cursory and partial" (p. 44). She reviewed several applications in measuring social changes, such as those involved in acculturation. One study measured the adaptation of Korean students to their new environment in the United States (Kelly & Szalay, 1972) and another assessed the acculturation of Filipino men in the U.S. Navy (Szalay & Bryson, 1977). In the latter study we traced the process of culture change and adoption of American images and meanings as a function of time spent in the United States. Our more recent study of Puerto Rican acculturation is a classic example of such changes, with implications for both mental health and substance abuse (Szalay, Canino, & Vilov, 1993).

Evaluation of Changes in Psychological Dispositions Affecting Program Success

Up to this point, we have focused on the measurement of the psychological dispositions of college students as an indication of their vulnerability or resistance to substance abuse. We can also capitalize on research that has shown that such dispositions are mutable: they are subject to change as attitudes and understanding change, and therefore they can provide a viable index of a person's current status with respect to alcohol and drugs. This is key to the whole concept of early identification, intervention, and prevention. It is also key to evaluating a program's ability to change people's dispositions and, in so doing, change their behavior.

In this chapter we begin our discussion of program evaluation not in the content of prevention but at the other extreme—the treatment of addiction. A treatment program naturally represents a much more controlled setting than we have encountered in the campus environment, and our research in the treatment field broadens the base of experience with this new technology.

MEASURING CHANGES PRODUCED BY TREATMENT

Reconstruction of the Recovery Process

With the support of NIMH, NIDA, and NIJ, we explored the extent to which selected long-term and short-term residential treatment programs produced changes in the clients' attitudes and perceptions as well as in their behavior. We used AGA-based mapping to reconstruct the recovery process as the client regained control over his or her life. Our interest was in the changes that are promoted for effective treatment. We have used imaging and cognitive mapping in several comparative studies within different treatment settings (Szalay, 1994; Szalay, Bovasso, Vilov, & Williams, 1992; Szalay, Carroll, & Tims, 1993). We compared pretreatment and posttreatment groups and examined how changes in the client's psychological dispositions progress during the process of treatment as he or she moves from acute drug dependence to a drug-free life.

The program evaluation described here involved a group of clients in a large, New York-based Therapeutic Community (TC; Szalay, 1994). TC treatment is designed to use the power of social influences—the internal dynamics of close community settings where the clients live together and share their problems. It draws upon the experiences of recovering addicts who have overcome their dependence and committed themselves to helping others become drug free. A major objective of such treatment programs is to promote a new outlook on life that is conducive to coping with the problems of life and to developing a drug-free lifestyle. The behavioral changes in this controlled setting were related to changes in the clients' perceptions and attitudes as measured by comparative imaging so that we could see the main areas and scope of change.

In contrast to our student samples, where we had to rely on the student's personal statement about his or her drug behavior, the populations in treatment fit into well-defined categories: pretreatment addicts and successfully rehabilitated clients. With an average 18 month participation in the program, the clients achieved a drug-free status considered sufficiently stable by the treatment criteria for release from the program. Recovering drug addicts who had successfully completed treatment and maintained a drug-free status were compared with a matching sample of addicts tested at the beginning of their treatment. The pretreatment group consisted of 200 habitual drug users at the beginning of their treatment in the TC program. The posttreatment group included 200 residents at the same TC who had successfully reached a drug-free status and were in the final stages of their rehabilitation program. These clients had spent 18 months of their time at the treatment center under strict regulation and control. They were judged to be successful in their treatment by the following criteria: they maintained a drug-free status over many months; they assumed increasingly demanding jobs and responsibilities within the TC and later in normal job settings; and they made plans, held to schedules, and developed personal ties. About 75% of each group were males and 50% were minorities.

The AGA method of imaging we administered to the two samples included 40 image themes in such life domains as Self-Concept, Drug Abuse, Interpersonal and Social Relations, Work, and Future. Participation was voluntary and we assured the anonymity of the participants through a coding system.

Priorities: Life Became More Meaningful

To chart changes in *priorities* reflected by differences in the subjective importance or meaningfulness of the themes examined, we calculated Dominance scores based on the number of responses given to each theme by each respondent in the pretreatment and posttreatment groups. All themes had greater meaningfulness to the posttreatment respondents, suggesting more engagement in life activities and more attention to the task at hand. Greater priority to understanding, to their relationship to father, to self-identity, and to motivational and educational goals appear to be the most significant indicators of treatment success. Discriminant function analysis of individual Dominance scores resulted in correct classification of 77% of the pretreatment clients and 73% of the posttreatment clients.

Perceptions: Views of Self and Future Showed Greatest Shifts

To assess the overall distance or change in the *subjective meanings and perceptions* held by the pretreatment and posttreatment groups in the different domains of life, we calculated the correlation of response distributions of the 40 themes before and after treatment. Most agreement ($r = .93$) was found in their perceptions of addiction and drugs and least agreement (i.e., most change) was found in their perceptions of self ($r = .76$ for me, $r = .64$ for I am), achievement/hopes ($r = .86$), and interpersonal relations (love/trust; $r = .87$).

Attitudes: Clients Became More Positive toward Self and Their Problems

To measure changes in *attitudes* or *evaluations,* we calculated the client's Evaluation scores for each of the 40 themes. Client attitudes and evaluations were inferred from their rating of each image theme on a 7-point scale from very negative (–3) to very positive (+3). Comparison of the pretreatment and posttreatment groups' Evaluation scores suggests that client attitudes toward self as well as toward their specific problems (addiction, cure, problems) are the strongest indicators of treatment success. Discriminant function analysis of individual evaluations resulted in correct classification of 75% of the pretreatment clients and 80% of the posttreatment clients.

Program Impact on Selected Images and Domains of Life

Alcohol/Drugs: Changes Less Than Anticipated. One might expect the most changes in clients' perceptions and attitudes toward alcohol and other drugs over the course of treatment. Although no significant changes were noted in their subjective image of drugs, there was somewhat less emotional intensity (e.g., love/hate responses) and somewhat more recognition of the destructive consequences of substance abuse (e.g., death, disease). On the other hand, there were substantial changes in their views regarding alcohol (see Figure 16.1). Pretreatment addicts paid more attention to drinking a variety of alcoholic beverages and linked it with stronger pleasurable sensations. After treatment (which was predominantly for cocaine addiction), there was much greater awareness of harmful consequences (car accident, death), potential violence, and legal problems. Also, they associated alcohol more with negative emotional states (anger, fear, loneliness).

Self/Friends: Deeper Interpersonal Relations. Perceptions of self and friends provided a measure of the self-esteem and confidence of the treatment groups. Changes in self-image can be seen in Figure 16.2. The pretreatment group revealed a very low level of satisfaction with themselves, whereas the posttreatment group expressed much more confidence and self-worth. These self-perceptions are reflected in their opinion of friends and friendship. The pretreatment clients showed a deeper sense of loneliness than the posttreatment clients. They mentioned the absence of friends in their lives. They were preoccupied with negative aspects of both themselves and of their friends, such as hurting, hate, and badness. They had low self-esteem and very mixed feeling about friends. The posttreatment clients expressed more faith and confidence in themselves and in friends. They were happier with themselves and with their friends and perceived both as more caring and loving, honest, and trustworthy than did the pretreatment clients. Apparently they had been helped by their friends and them as supportive.

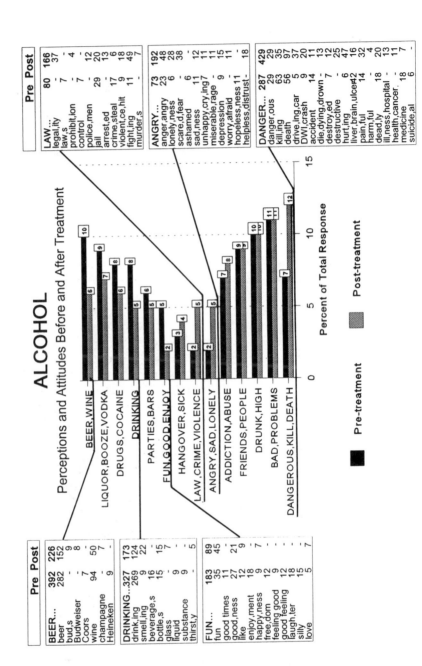

FIGURE 16.1. The image of ALCOHOL before and after treatment.

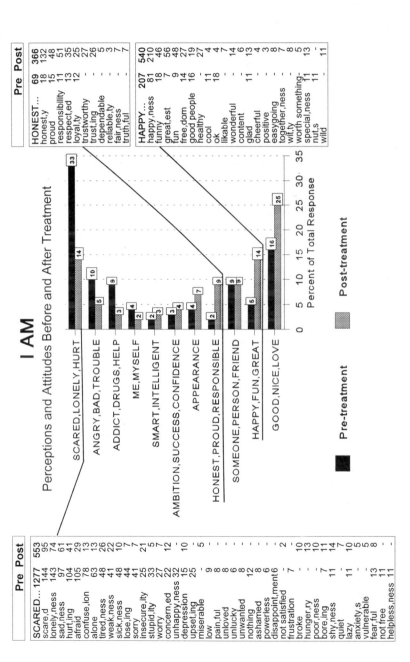

FIGURE 16.2. The image of I AM before and after treatment.

The friendships experienced in the TC seem to have had a positive effect on the clients' self-esteem and on their ability to trust and rely on others.

Problems: Stronger Coping Skills Noted.   In their images of problems, worries, and loneliness, the pretreatment clients referred to themselves more frequently than the posttreatment clients, revealing a more negative self-image and greater awareness of having emotional problems. They also tended to view personal and familial relationships as a predominant problem. The posttreatment clients were more outwardly oriented. They showed more apprehension about money and success. Anticipating their departure from the TC, they were concerned with work, jobs, and school. It seems that these clients had come to better terms with themselves and had greater confidence in their ability to find solutions to problems as they moved back into the world. After treatment they also showed more sensitivity to pain and hurt, health, and illness, particularly.

Changes Measured by Responses to Pictures

Similar trends differentiating pretreatment and posttreatment clients were noted in studies that included visual images. In another therapeutic community setting, pictures were included in the comparison of perceptions and attitudes of 100 clients before and after treatment (Szalay, Carroll, & Tims, 1993). Although one might expect that the same picture conveys the same meaning to everyone, Figure 16.3 demonstrates that this is not the case. The participants wrote down whatever came to mind upon viewing the specific picture, and their responses were analyzed to assess the main trends of perception. Pretreatment clients saw the two men in Figure 16.3 as unemployed and looking for work, and they referred more to the physical surroundings; posttreatment clients tended to see the two men as friends having problems but also seeking help and support.

The comparison of the pretreatment and the posttreatment clients' responses to 30 visual images shows in what ways their experiences in the course of the treatment program influenced how they viewed the outer world. The pretreatment clients registered more specific details and focused on what is directly observable: people, objects, and events. They took note of the actions without evaluating them and mentioned the people without going into the relationships between them. The posttreatment group went beyond the observable and tried to understand what was going in the picture. Posttreatment clients expressed more emotions, both positive ones like love and care and negative ones such as pain, confusion, and loneliness. They showed also more preoccupation with drugs where the people and events reminded them of drugs. When drug or alcohol use was more explicit, the pretreatment clients mentioned it more, probably reflecting their tendency to view the pictures more in terms of concrete observable details. When the posttreatment clients associated the people in the picture with

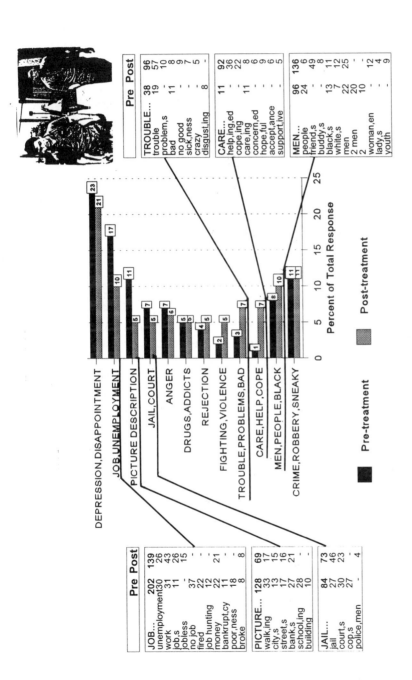

FIGURE 16.3. The perceptions of a picture before and after treatment.

drug use, they reacted more negatively. They characterized them as dumb, crazy, and bad. In response to pictures that showed people who were troubled or depressed, the posttreatment clients thought more of helping, talking, and understanding. They also thought more of friends, indicating the tendency to view friends as instrumental in solving or coping with personal problems; they may rely on friends more for support. The posttreatment clients had a more sophisticated view of drugs. They had a more negative opinion of drugs and were critical of the potential role of drugs in their lives.

In general, compared to pretreatment addicts whose thoughts were more limited to the concrete and visible, the posttreatment group showed an increased ability to look beyond the concrete details for deeper meaning involving human feelings and interpersonal relationships. The results suggest that the treatment program had an impact on the way in which these people looked at life events and on how they attempted to cope with them.

Successful Treatment Modifies Behavior Mediated by Changes in Psychological Dispositions

The findings obtained in prevention research demonstrated the close relationship between the students' psychological dispositions and their actual behavior. In that context nonusers represented the point of departure, and the findings showed that the more students perceive alcohol, entertainment, friends, and society in the same way as students who reported frequent use of alcohol and other drugs, the more they are predisposed toward substance abuse. The various projects in treatment research offered the opportunity to examine the relationship between dispositions and behavior from a contrasting line of progression, from use to non-use, starting with the addict who has just entered treatment and following the process that led the client back to a drug-free status.

The results presented here show how the treatment experiences effectively promote new perceptions and attitudes, new images of self and of others, new perspectives, and new priorities. They are informative on the resocialization of addicts who successfully completed the program and became drug-free. The results did show changes in their outlook and in their subjective world. The perceptions and attitudes on which posttreatment clients differed the most from pretreatment addicts reveal key psychological dispositions found to be the most instrumental in promoting program success. The global measures of priorities, attitudes, and perceptions place changes in broad perspective. They show where the largest changes occurred, what was the relative scope of change, and so forth. The details of perceptual mosaics found in the imaging process offer insights into the nature and content of the change and offer the basis for gauging the clients' progress toward perceptions and attitudes characteristic of those who are successfully maintaining a drug-free status.

Measuring Changes in Campus Climate

Because our primary focus is on prevention, in this volume we have only briefly touched upon treatment in the evaluation of changes in psychological dispositions accompanying changes in behavior toward a drug-free status. The use of the imaging and mapping technology for evaluating the effectiveness of treatment programs has much in common with the task of evaluating prevention programs. From our work in treatment evaluation we were able to demonstrate that effective treatment involves changes not only in behavior (becoming substance free) but also in perceptions, attitudes, and psychological dispositions. By developing an assessment system that identifies the dispositions differentiating users and nonusers, we are able to trace the process by which an individual's perceptions and attitudes change over the course of a prevention program in ways that make a critical difference in the outcome.

Building on our experiences gained in the task of treatment evaluation, we have made progress in developing a feedback system for use in prevention. Prevention practitioners, at least on the college campuses, are experimenting with a broad variety of programs, and it is essential that we be able to measure the effectiveness of them. We have examined two strategies: a global assessment of campus climate and its changes over time and an assessment of the impact of specific activities intended to support the campus prevention program.

At first we focused on the campus as a whole, administering our instrument to sizable student samples ($N = 400$) at the beginning and at the end of the 1- or 2-year program period. We conducted these "environmental assessments" at 57 colleges and universities that had received funding from the U.S. Department of Education (FIPSE) for their postsecondary alcohol and drug abuse prevention programs between 1989 and 1997. The primary purpose of the analysis was to assess the social climate on campus in relation to substance abuse and to identify key psychological and environmental factors that deserve attention in proactive prevention.

We assessed the dominant trends of perceptions and attitudes characteristic of students on each campus and compared the campus trends with those found among known alcohol/drug users and nonusers (the 400 users and nonusers described in part I). Through the detailed analysis of the students' images, we identified in what particular ways changes had occurred in the students' attitudes, perception of harm, perceptions of alcohol and other drugs, their relationship to their social environment, their concern with drinking, smoking, and so forth. As global indicators of drug climate, we calculated the students' overall psychological vulnerability/resistance in comparison with their self-reports of alcohol and other drug use. Comparing the results obtained 1 to 2 years apart, we looked at stability and change in campus climate regarding reported use and at how each campus stood in relation to high-use and low-use colleges selected as reference points. The imaging and mapping approach thus provided the colleges feedback not only on changes in their students' vulnerability but also on the specific perceptual and attitudinal changes involved in the shift in vulnerability/resistance.

TABLE 16.1. Changes in Vulnerability/Resistance and Reported Drinks
on 11 College Campuses

College ID number	Vulnerability		Average number of drinks consumed in 1 week	
	Year 1	Year 2	Year 1	Year 2
50	8.8	10.7	8	8
42	5.3	−1.1	5	2
55	4.2	7.2	7	7
31	2.9	6.0	-	3
60	2.8	4.0	5	4
36	2.3	3.3	-	8
57	1.5	−3.4	4	3
64	−3.3	.3	2	2
30	−5.6	−2.8	-	2
32	−5.2	1.7	-	4
37	−5.9	−1.5	-	2

Table 16.1 gives an overview of findings from these campus studies. Of the
57 colleges, we had test-retest results on 30 of them. When we used multiple re-
gression analysis to control for sampling differences (age, gender, ethnicity, class
year, campus residence), we found significant changes in vulnerability/resistance
on 11 campuses. Vulnerability actually increased on 9 of the 11 campuses, which
means that over time the students were generally thinking more like frequent users
than they had before. Drinking levels on all campuses either stayed the same or decreased somewhat. In many cases, vulnerability and reported drinking results
showed changes in the same direction. Because the colleges sampled their 400 students to be generally representative of the campus population rather than as participants in their campus prevention programs, it would be difficult to attribute the
changes in campus attitudes and perceptions to the program more than to any of
the other social influences on campus.

MEASURING THE EFFECTS OF SELECT PROGRAM ACTIVITIES

Although the global approach provided feedback regarding the changing health of
the campus environment as a whole, it did not provide any specific information on
the impact of the prevention programs themselves. Recognizing this, we began to
pursue psychological dispositions and environmental conditions within particular
campus program activities. Each college selected for evaluation one of its prevention-related program activities. These activities varied in the number of participants and in their scope and intensity, from a single alcohol-free social event to a
2 semester alcohol and drug education course. Some activities were ad hoc and
others required considerable advance planning.

For these initial assessments when it was considered desirable to keep testing time brief, we developed a short version that could be administered in about 20 minutes. The abbreviated evaluation tool was half the size of the original 24-word instrument used to test the 30,000 students. We were able to use our available database to focus on elements most effective for differentiating user and nonuser perceptual and attitudinal dispositions without a serious drop in analytic sensitivity. This feedback instrument requires about 20 minutes for each testing, one scheduled just before the start of the activity program and the other following completion of the activity. The characteristics of the two instruments are basically the same:

- Both the original version and the short version of the instrument are based on identification of the dominant perceptions and attitudes that differentiate frequent users and nonusers.
- Both are based on assessment of Vulnerability/Resistance as part of a system of contrasting trends of psychological dispositions that create propensities for using or not using harmful substances.
- Both rely on a two-pronged imaging and mapping approach involving the complementary use of detailed information on specific dispositions relevant to program development and the vulnerability/resistance of a person or group as indicated by a single score.

We examined the validity of the shortened measure by comparing it to the original measure and checking for internal consistency in the results obtained. We tested the two versions on a combined five-college sample of 1,778 students. For each student, we calculated the Vulnerability/Resistance scores for both versions and then computed the correlation between the two elements of each pair. The resulting coefficient ($r = .92$) was very high. With the original version, we found that we can predict whether an individual is a user or a nonuser with 80% accuracy. Our analyses showed that the shortened form shows similarly strong correlations between psychological vulnerability and behavior (see Table 16.2).

We have consistently obtained significant correlations between an individual's Vulnerability score and various measures of self-reported use. Comparison of the two instruments for several types of usage showed that the short form produced

TABLE 16.2. Consistency of Long-Form and Short-Form Vulnerability Measures in Relation to Self-Reported Use (**$p < .001$)

Self-reported use	24-Word version	12-Word version
Frequency of alcohol use	.48**	.47**
Average number drinks/week-self	.47**	.46**
Binge drinking	.42**	.42**
Marijuana use	.54**	.50**
Combined measure of use	.50**	.47**

Vulnerability/Resistance scores similar to those of the original long form in all five of the differing college applications. There was only a small drop in precision.

Postprogram Changes in Vulnerability/Resistance

Table 16.3 shows the vulnerability/resistance of students participating in prevention-related activities of varying length at the five colleges. Two of the activities were semester-length courses, one was a briefer course, and the remaining two activities involved the students in volunteer activities for different periods of time. In three cases (the Chemical Dependency course, Substance Abuse course, and Peer Counseling Training), the activities had the desired effect of increasing psychological resistance to substance abuse. However, the students who chose to participate in these activities had higher initial Resistance scores than did the general student population at their colleges. For the Chemical Dependency course, we found a greater drop in the vulnerability of the male students than of the female students. The students participating in the student government/leadership activities began with higher than average Vulnerability for that campus, and it *increased* over the 6-month time period.

TABLE 16.3. Changes in Vulnerability/Resistance Associated with
Prevention-Related Activities

	All students	Males	Females	Nonusers	Occas. drinkers	Binge/drinkers drug users
Chemical Dependency Course (4 months)						
Pretest (n = 64)	-.4	7.9	-6.4	–	-8.8	4.1
Posttest (n = 58)	-1.9	2.2	-4.6	–	-5.2	-0.0
Campus sample (N = 388)	0.3	3.6	-1.9	-7.4	-5.3	2.4
Peer Counseling (3 months)						
Pretest (n = 38)	-2.6	2.2	-4.8	-5.0	-5.4	-0.7
Posttest (n = 39)	-3.4	1.1	-6.3	-12.0	-11.1	1.4
Campus sample (N = 372)	2.9	5.7	0.6	-6.6	-3.7	6.1
Student Government (6 months)						
Pretest (n = 49)	1.4	1.6	1.4	-1.6	-5.1	6.4
Posttest (n = 48)	3.5	3.3	3.6	1.0	-2.1	6.3
Campus sample (N = 400)	-0.1	2.3	-1.8	-6.4	-5.8	3.0
Substance Abuse Course (5 months)						
Pretest (n = 32)	-5.6	-7.0	-4.6	-9.2	-9.0	-0.5
Posttest (n = 24)	-7.5	-8.4	-7.0	-9.5	-5.8	-8.3
Campus sample (N = 400)	-3.3	-0.2	-4.0	-10.3	-6.2	0.8
Social Values Course (2 months)						
Pretest (n = 132)	-1.5	2.8	-3.6	-11.5	-8.6	2.0
Posttest (n = 117)	-0.8	2.8	-2.6	-11.4	-5.1	1.9
Campus sample (N = 218)	-2.1	1.0	-3.8	-11.0	-6.4	1.9

Table 16.3 includes results for students in specific subcategories of use of alcohol and other drugs (nonusers, occasional drinkers, and binge drinkers/drug users). Resistance among the occasional drinkers was weaker after participating in four of the five activities, indicating that they were thinking and perceiving their world in ways more similar to known users than they were at the earlier time of testing. Students categorized as binge drinkers/drug users showed lower vulnerability in the posttests in the same four activities.

Postprogram Changes in Students' Perceptions and Attitudes

In addition to the overall Vulnerability/Resistance indicators of change over the course of the selected prevention-related activity, the nature of the shifts became clear in the comparative imaging analysis of students' perceptions and evaluations. When we reviewed the Chemical Dependency course, for example, we found the following trends:

- Prior to the course, the students generally exhibited a high tolerance of alcohol and other drugs on campus, particularly at parties and other social gatherings. After taking the course the linkage between FRIENDS and ALCOHOL/DRUGS was weaker, there was stronger disapproval of drugs and getting high (but not of alcohol), and there was greater awareness of the variety of substances and their physiological effects.
- FRIENDS and social ENTERTAINMENT were not as strongly linked to the presence of alcohol and other drugs in the posttest. FUN and PARTY took on broader meanings, including a greater variety of activities.
- In the sphere of self, society, and values, their view of school improved, with more references to fun and fewer to work.
- Their very negative view of SOCIETY, a user disposition, remained strong. Nevertheless, after the course the students did pay greater attention to the rules, norms, and values of society, a nonuser tendency.

These results suggest that the Chemical Dependency course had a desired impact beyond the transmission of academic information on the physical nature of alcohol and other drugs. There were noticeable changes in the students' views and attitudes toward at least the harder drugs, if not alcohol. Their dispositions in the posttest showed greater similarities to the dispositions characteristic of nonusers.

On the basis of these findings and others in this new endeavor, we are confident that the technology promises to be a simple and sensitive analytic tool for assessing the psychological impact of activities and programs developed to support the objectives of prevention. This can be achieved through the shortened version of our broader assessment instrument that has an administration time of about 20 minutes.

In the context of program planning and systematic targeting of activities and other program elements, the instrument provides a quick feedback mechanism that can be used at the end of each program period or periodically during the course of sustained program efforts. The feedback produced by this evaluation can be helpful for improving program impact, based on achievements as well as on expectations that are unrealized. This tool offers special promise by moving the strategy of prevention from preoccupation with vulnerability to program development focused on strengthening resistance.

The Three Applications in Perspective

The three applications discussed in this chapter illustrate how the imaging and mapping approach can provide feedback in a variety of different settings.

Changes Registered in Controlled Treatment Settings

We noted sizeable changes in dominant trends of perceptions that offer insights into the psychological impact of the treatment experience. The changes may be described as the product of intensive rehabilitation programs that put the participants under heavy pressure. The changes affected various domains of life differently. The treatment process through which the patients achieved a stable, drug-free status is accompanied by internal changes in perceptions and motivations that were considered to be inaccessible, hidden parameters of the treatment experience. The changes measured with the imaging and mapping strategy were frequently sizeable and readily identifiable. Though some of the changes in psychological dispositions could not have been anticipated, *post factum* they make good sense and show a high degree of internal consistency.

Evaluation of Changes in Campus Climate

Compared to the magnitude of change noted in the treatment evaluations, the changes in overall campus climate measured on a campus-wide basis were relatively small yet generally identifiable. Although the changes registered in specific images were small, the statistical measures showed high internal consistency and stability. Vulnerability/Resistance proved to be a sensitive and reliable measure of propensities for substance abuse and their changes over time.

Feedback on the Effects of Select Program Activities

In a few high-impact programs we found sizeable changes in perceptions and attitudes as valid indicators of the impact of select activity programs. Whereas the image data provided details of the changes, the Vulnerability/Resistance measure provided a useful overall indicator of program effects in terms of changes in propensities to use or not use harmful substances.

In the treatment setting, the person is placed in a new environment designed to promote change. Our measures were sensitive enough to trace the changes taking place in this controlled setting. In contrast, the campus includes a large population of students, many of whom may be unaware of the campus prevention program and few with direct exposure to the program itself. In this context there was a distinct interest in the extent to which the prevention program did affect the campus climate. The changes we measured were in some cases substantive; however, to what extent they may have been the result of the program or of some other variables remained uncertain. The third application involved specific activities (curriculum development, Resident Assistant training, etc.). The evaluation focused on a select group of people tested before and after their participation. Changes in their perceptions and attitudes and psychological vulnerability were measured. In each application, the vulnerability/resistance and other AGA instruments proved to offer sensitive measures of changes in psychological dispositions.

Part VI

The Latest Developments
and Future Perspectives

Some of the Well-Known Approaches to Drug Prevention

There is a rich diversity of approaches to drug prevention backed by extensive discussions of theoretical considerations. We tried to spare the reader from a lengthy discussion of theories, but now that we have presented our approach, it may be helpful to discuss briefly some of the most well-known alternatives. The literature, as well as our findings, show that variables affecting substance use are many. Also, the role of these variables in shaping decisions related to drug use varies greatly. Rather than searching for some magic approach of universal applicability, it is our reasoning that prevention requires an assessment of what makes a particular population vulnerable and a means of targeting them effectively.

Now that we have presented what we are doing, we offer a brief discussion of some of the major theoretical approaches in the field of prevention. We feel that this small deviation from our intention to be application-oriented may be relevant to those interested in how our approach fits in with others used by the many professionals working in this field.

In order to prevent the occurrence of any unwanted behavior, we need to understand the underlying causes of that behavior. Once we understand what causes it, we can take steps to avoid conditions that start the causal chain, or perhaps even interrupt the causal sequence before the undesirable outcome emerges. Substance abuse prevention is no different. Once we know why people seek out alcohol and other drugs, we can effectively prevent their abuse and addiction to them. For several decades now, researchers from many fields have attempted to uncover those critical factors that lead to substance abuse. One look at scientific journals devoted to alcohol and other drugs will demonstrate that researchers have not been at a loss for ideas. In fact, a 1980 NIDA research monograph (Lettieri, Sayers, & Pearson,

1980) presented 43 different theories of substance use! Certainly the number has grown even higher since then. And yet, in many ways, progress in the area of substance abuse prevention has been quite slow.

Recently, researchers have suggested that the problem is not a lack of theories but perhaps too many of them (e.g., Petraitis, Flay, & Miller, 1995). The theories seem to emerge from a wide range of perspectives, including biogenetic, interpersonal, sociological, and cognitive. Within each perspective there are a number of well-defined theories with considerable data to back up each one. However, if we were to begin to try to sort through all of the theories, we would quickly discover that we have lost the forest for the trees. Each theory seems to exist within its dominant perspective, but in isolation from theories of other perspectives. For example, those from the physiological approach may examine sensitivity to ethanol or certain dopamine receptors, and those from the family systems approach may examine parent–child interactions, but what is not studied is the relationship between these two domains. Do stressful family interactions influence sensitivity to ethanol, which leads to substance abuse, in which case ethanol sensitivity is a mediating variable? Do stressful family interactions lead to the use of alcohol as a coping mechanism only for those who are already highly sensitive to its effects, making sensitivity a moderating variable? Or do these two factors operate independently of one another and thus have an additive effect on vulnerability? Indeed we have a puzzle of many pieces, but few seem to be focusing their energies on putting the puzzle together. Instead, researchers seem determined to simply create more pieces.

Although the frameworks may be fragmented, each theory does contribute an important piece to the puzzle. With this information, prevention programs can be designed more effectively. Certainly there is no single cause of substance abuse, but many different factors from different domains contribute to decisions to use or not use alcohol or other drugs. Although it is beyond the scope of this volume to derive an over-reaching, all-encompassing model of vulnerability to substance use that will answer all questions, it may be helpful to examine the current state of knowledge in substance abuse etiology, in order to put the current work into a theoretical context. We begin with models that focus on indirect, or what some have termed "distal" (R. Jessor & Jessor, 1977; Petraitis et al., 1995) causes of substance abuse—factors that seem to increase risk through their effects on other factors—and move increasingly closer to more direct or "proximal" factors.

THE BIOGENETIC APPROACH

Biological and physiological researchers in the field concern themselves with understanding the physiological factors related to substance abuse and dependency. Research in this area has examined genetic predispositions as well as differences in physiological responses to substances that indicate a vulnerability to addiction.

For example, Newlin and others (Newlin, 1994; Newlin & Thompson, 1990) have measured sensitivity to ethanol as a predictor of substance abuse. They suggest that individuals with a family history of alcoholism are more sensitive to the positive effects that alcohol has on one's mood, but are less sensitive to the negative physical and emotional effects associated with the subsequent rebound from use. They believe it is this genetically transmitted fundamental difference in the physiological response to alcohol that leaves those with a family history of alcoholism more vulnerable to addiction to it.

While these types of vulnerability factors may not be amenable to change through prevention programming, theories and research along these lines do allow prevention personnel to identify those who may be most vulnerable. Biological researchers are quick to emphasize that biological causes alone cannot explain substance-using behavior, and that we must also look to personal and environmental causes that may interact with biological predispositions. For example, an individual who also suffers from depression or from low self-esteem may be at even greater risk for substance abuse if they are also physiologically more sensitive to the positive mood effects of alcohol. Thus, when taken in conjunction with other theories of vulnerability, biological evidence can assist prevention by allowing personnel to channel their efforts to those in the greatest need. This kind of evidence can also be used in educating those at risk about their increased vulnerability. Many individuals, especially adolescents, who are thinking about using substances or who have already begun experimenting, often tell themselves that they won't get hooked. Clear evidence of physiological differences in response to alcohol may help dispel this "myth of invulnerability" in those who are at greatest risk.

SOCIOLOGICAL MODELS

When looking for environmental factors associated with substance use, one can define "environment" very narrowly or very broadly. Sociological models examine a broader definition—cultural norms, traditional values, and institutional policies regarding substance use. The cultural context in which an individual lives, as well as one's affinity or commitment to that culture, are two important factors that influence not only substance use, but participation in other behaviors defined as deviant by that culture (R. Jessor & Jessor, 1977).

There is ample evidence that individuals who have low academic achievement (Forman & Linney, 1991; Kellam, Stevenson, & Rubin, 1982; Kumpfer, 1989), do not attend church (Bachman, Johnston, & O'Malley, 1991; Schlegel & Sandborn, 1979), and engage in criminal behavior (Forman and Linney, 1991; Kandel, 1980, 1982) are also more likely to use alcohol and other drugs. Several theorists (e.g., Problem Behavior Theory [R. Jessor & Jessor, 1977], discussed in the following text) have incorporated these findings into models which emphasize the level of commitment one has to traditional values of the culture. Some models such as Social Control Theory (Elliott, Huizinga, & Menard, 1989) go even further and examine how socioenvironmental conditions such as crime rates, poverty, unemployment, and family discord may lead to disillusionment and a failure to "buy into" the traditional values and norms of the general culture. To the extent that one feels an attachment to the general social structure and its institutions, one is likely to regulate one's own behavior accordingly. Conversely, those who lack such attachment may engage in a variety of "deviant" behaviors in order to rebel against the larger culture.

These theories and supporting evidence give prevention personnel a unique set of opportunities to prevent substance use. Although laws against substance use are necessary to convey cultural values, clearly they are not enough to prevent use for those who place little value on adhering to those laws. Programs that enhance the individual's feeling of inclusion into the larger social system may also increase resistance to substance use through the internalization of the cultural norms against it. Thus, programs designed to increase academic performance, decrease truancy, strengthen the family, improve neighborhoods, and reduce crime and unemployment, while addressing these other important social problems, may also have an indirect effect of reducing substance abuse.

DISPOSITIONAL THEORIES

Biological and sociological factors discussed previously may impact substance abuse through their effects on more intermediate factors such as one's personality and one's more immediate social network of family and peers. We will address personality theories here and social and interpersonal models in the next section.

There have been a wide variety of personality traits and affective states associated with substance abuse. For example, substance abuse has been associated with impulsivity (Sher, 1994), sensation seeking (Segal, 1977), aggressiveness (Patterson, 1986), depression (Deykin, Levy, & Wells, 1987; Helzer & Pryzbeck, 1988), neurosis (Martin & Sher, 1994), an external locus of control (Botvin, 1983; Wright, 1985), poor coping skills (Cooper, Russell, Skinner, Frone, & Mudar, 1992), and low self-esteem (Kaplan, 1975). Several theories have focused primarily on an individual's personality as a primary cause of substance abuse.

For example, Sher (1994) has examined how clusters of personality traits and states might influence substance abuse, particularly as those individual-level factors might be influenced by genetic predispositions in those with a family history of alcoholism. In his model of vulnerability, Sher theorizes that the majority of person factors that have been associated with substance abuse may all have an underlying biological basis due to alcoholism in the family. For example, he proposes that difficulties in coping ability may be a cognitive deficit associated with being a child of an alcoholic. Thus, according to his model, the relationship between a family history of alcoholism and subsequent alcohol use is mediated by personality traits and affective states that result from both the genetic and environmental effects of parental alcoholism.

A particular person factor that has received considerable attention is one's self-esteem. Many theories have postulated a link between low self-esteem and substance use. One such theory is Self-Derogation Theory (Kaplan, 1980). According to Kaplan, many factors associated with substance use, such as academic failure, parenting deficits, poor social skills, and poor coping skills, are mediated by self-esteem. Failure to gain approval from important others in the social network can lead to negative self-evaluations, or to low self-esteem. This in turn lowers the individual's motivation to conform to norms and expectations of those others, because previous attempts have led to negative consequences. Thus, according to Kaplan, the individual engages in deviant behavior, including substance use, to avoid meeting with further failure, and begins to seek out alternative social networks where approval can be met. In this model, self-esteem has a direct or proximal effect on substance use.

Although Kaplan's theory and other theories that focus on self-esteem sound plausible, the available research evidence suggests that the effect of low self-esteem on substance use is indirect, rather than direct, or mediated by other factors, such as personal goals and attitudes. Regardless of whether the effects are direct or indirect, however, self-esteem and other personality traits and affective states are associated with substance use. In terms of prevention, this presents several possibilities. To the extent that certain personality traits are biologically determined, this data allows us to identify those at risk. For certain traits, such as sensation seeking, prevention may consist of teaching young people different, more healthy ways to fulfill this desire. Additionally, if we can identify those factors that mediate the effects of these personality traits, we can target these more proximal factors for the at-risk populations. For instance, low self-esteem may increase the likelihood that an individual will experience emotional distress and utilize poor coping strategies. These two variables may be the more proximal factors that influence expectations and decisions regarding substance use (Sher, 1994). To the extent that affective states, dominant coping strategies, and some personality characteristics are amenable to change, prevention personnel can work to change them—increase self-esteem, teach coping skills, and enhance one's ability to delay gratification.

INTERPERSONAL THEORIES

Clearly the majority of research and theories in substance abuse etiology and prevention has focused on how one's behavior is influenced by his or her immediate social environment. Peer pressure and social modeling have received considerable empirical and theoretical attention. Adolescents who associate with substance using peers are more likely to themselves engage in substance use than those who do not (Black, 1991; Kandel, 1982, 1985; Single, Kandel, & Faust, 1974). Likewise, stressful relations with parents (poor parenting, childhood abuse, or parental substance abuse Jacob & Leonard, 1994) is also associated with increased substance abuse for adolescents. Interpersonal theories examine the more proximal effects of one's immediate social environment on decisions to use or not to use alcohol or other drugs.

Social Learning Theory

Perhaps the most well-known model of social influence is Albert Bandura's Social Learning Theory (Bandura, 1973; 1977). Like R. Jessor and Jessor's Problem Behavior Theory, Social Learning Theory was developed to explain a broad range of behaviors. The theory originated from Bandura's work on aggression. In his now-classic "Bobo-doll" studies, Bandura found that children imitated the aggressive behavior of adults (Bandura, D. Ross, & Ross, 1961). His theory has been expanded to explain a variety of behaviors including helping, prejudice, and substance abuse. According to Social Learning Theory, people observe the behavior of important others (called role models) and imitate that behavior. They then receive positive reinforcement for imitating it and this positive reinforcement leads to a continuance of the behavior. Specifically applied to substance abuse, an adolescent may observe his parents or peers using alcohol or other drugs. The individual then imitates that behavior. Positive reinforcement can come in many forms. The models themselves may actively reward the individual for the behavior through praise, acceptance, or inclusion in future substance-using activity. Alternatively, reinforcement may come intrinsically from a person's sense of achievement at being "just like" one's role model. Unlike many other behaviors that we may imitate, however, positive reinforcement for substance use may also come in a physiological form. The positive affective effects of substance use can also serve to reinforce the behavior. Thus, these three sources of positive consequences may serve as strong reinforcers which continue the behavior.

Social Cognitive Theory

Bandura later formulated Social Cognitive Theory (1986; 1992) that was similar to Social Learning Theory but focused more on how cognitive processes are influenced by the social modeling and social consequences that occur from one's environment. Bandura placed particular emphasis on how affective responses of others serve as signals for self-regulation.

When an individual finds himself or herself in an ambiguous situation, he or she may look to others for information on how to respond. This process begins in infancy, as infants learn that affective responses from their parents are informative when encountering new objects or people. Typically, when one's mother, for example, expresses positive feelings toward a new person, via smiles, gestures, and tone of voice, infants will approach the person, but expressions of fear will lead to avoidance. According to Bandura, this social referencing behavior—using affective responses of others to guide one's own behavior—continues throughout the lifespan.

At the most basic level, such social referencing serves this vicarious arousal function. When we observe others expressing a given emotion, it activates a similar emotional response in us. However, such social modeling has an even greater impact. It also serves what Bandura termed a *vicarious acquisition function*, where the individual adopts the attitudes of the model. Through social modeling, we may learn to like what the model likes, dislike what the model dislikes, and fear what the model fears. One common example is a youngster who decides that he or she does not like peas because an older sister, aunt, or other role model does not like peas. Likewise, when we adopt the attitudes of important models, we would then regulate our own behavior accordingly in response to those attitude objects. This is what Bandura termed the *predictive regulatory function.* If we observe a model engage in a particular behavior that brings about a desired outcome, we regulate our own behavior in light of the similar outcomes that we anticipate. A related function is the *self-efficacy and controllability function,* where observation of models' coping strategies used in response to a given situation can lead the observer to adopt similar coping strategies. If we observe the model successfully dealing with a given situation, our own self-efficacy—or belief that we too can effectively cope—is increased. We will have acquired some information as to the likelihood that outcomes in similar situations can be controlled and that given coping strategies will be successful.

It is this variable of self-efficacy that takes on a more central role in Bandura's revision of Social Learning Theory. Self-efficacy, or the belief that one possesses the ability to meet the demands of the current situation, is considered an important moderator of social referencing. To the extent that one has a high level of general self-efficacy, he or she will be more likely to utilize social referencing in ambiguous situations. Beyond that, however, Bandura (1992) states:

> People's judgements of their personal efficacy influence what course of action they choose to pursue, how much effort they will mobilize in an endeavor, how long they will persevere in the face of difficulties, whether their thought patterns are self-hindering or self-aiding, and their emotional reactions in taxing or threatening situations. (p. 179)

As with Social Learning Theory, Social Cognitive Theory is designed to explain a broad variety of human behavior. Let us give a specific example of how it might apply to substance use. At some point, the adolescent encounters his or her first opportunity to use or not use alcohol or other drugs. This situation may contain contradictory messages from the environment. The messages from society (parent, laws, etc.) state that substance use is bad. However, the individuals present in the current situation (typically peers) express just the opposite attitude. If our teen possesses a high level of general self-efficacy—a belief that he or she can handle himself or herself in many situations—he or she may be less likely to engage in social referencing. However, if social referencing does occur due to the ambiguous nature of the situation, he or she will look to models—people whom he or she has learned to trust as informative models—typically close friends, perhaps parents. If his or her friends respond to this situation in a calm and relaxed manner, he or she is likely to experience similar emotional arousal. Such social referencing may even lead him or her to adopt the same attitudes. In this and future situations, he or she will regulate his or her own behavior accordingly. Thus, if he or she believes that using alcohol and other drugs will lead to positive outcomes, because that is what his or her models believe, then he or she will be more likely to follow suit. Having observed a trusted model cope with the situation by engaging in substance use, our teen may also now have increased self-efficacy in his or her own ability to use them. Of course, the same processes could lead to continued abstinence if the model refuses to drink or to use other drugs. Having observed a trusted peer successfully refuse can model not only what an appropriate coping strategy might be, but can also boost the observers self-efficacy in his or her own ability to do the same thing.

The Social Developmental Model

Other theories focus more attention on the nature of one's relationships with others, especially one's parents. For example, the Social Developmental Model, proposed by Hawkins & his colleagues (Hawkins, Abbott, Catalano, & Gillmore, 1991; Hawkins & Weis, 1985) stresses how the primary source of social influence changes as an individual moves from childhood to adolescence. In early childhood, one's primary source of social influence is one's parents. Very young children adopt the same attitudes, values, and understanding of right and wrong that their parents have. As they grow older, they are exposed to other adults role models, particularly teachers. During the late childhood years, teachers become a source of social influence, as children are motivated to seek the teachers' approval. With the onset of adolescence, however, one's peers become the dominant social influence in one's life. In adolescence, friends take on an ever-increasing role in shaping one's attitudes and values. During this developmental stage, the teen is trying to achieve his or her own identity separate from that of his or her parents'. According to this model, teens are more likely to interact with peers who use alcohol and other drugs if they did not develop positive bonds with parents and teachers during earlier stages of development. As with the sociological theories, the focus here is on a lack of commitment to and internalization of the values and standards of conventional society. However, the difference between the Social Developmental Model and more sociologically based theories is that here it is believed that this lack of connectedness comes from deficiencies in specific interpersonal relationships rather than more environmental-based causes.

Each of the previous three theories would seem to suggest that effective substance abuse prevention consists of strengthening a teen's bonds to specific adults—parents and teachers—who convey an attitude that they disapprove of substance use. Note that both of these elements are critical. If adults are clearly opposed to substance use, teens will not respond to that message unless they see these adults as trusted and respected role models. Conversely, if adults who are trusted and respected role models do not present a clear abstinence-based attitude, then teens may not adopt that attitude either. In fact, Hawkins, Catalano, and their colleagues (Hawkins *et al.*, 1991) specifically include instructional skills training for teachers, especially at the elementary level, when children are still likely to look to teachers as role models. As with some of the sociological interventions, prevention efforts here can address substance abuse directly or indirectly. For example, the previously mentioned teacher training included various classroom techniques designed to heighten students' engagement in and positive attitudes toward school and school-related activities. Thus, increasing attachment to role models who convey traditional societal values in terms of academic achievement can have an indirect effect on substance use prevention.

Cognitive Theories

Even more proximal than one's social relations are the thoughts that immediately precede the decision to use or not use harmful substances. Each time an individual is faced with a choice to use, he or she must make the decision either to do so or to abstain. It is these thoughts and this decision-making process that are the most proximal factors of vulnerability, and they are often more tied to the individual's subjective reality than to any objective reality. Theories that are cognitive in nature focus on the individual's understanding and expectations about substance use and how they influence using-related decisions. For example, after a lengthy prevention program, an adolescent may be able to recite the statistics on the number of teens killed each year from alcohol-related traffic accidents. However, those who approach substance use from the cognitive perspective know that it is not this objective data that will influence the decision to drink and drive as much as one's subjective view—to what degree does the teen actually believe it will or won't happen to him or to her? Accordingly, a teen may know that a certain percentage of people die from alcohol overdose, but if he or she believes it is unlikely to happen to him or to her, or if he or she believes that ingesting a large quantity of alcohol will gain him or her acceptance in a desirable peer group, he or she is likely to make the decision to binge rather than to abstain. According to cognitive theories, it is these and related cognitions that are the most immediate and direct precursors to substance use.

The Theory of Reasoned Action

Like several theories already discussed, the Theory of Reasoned Action was developed to explain and predict a wide variety of human behaviors, from the choice of grocery products to the use of birth control. According to this theory, behavior results from a reasoned decision to engage in that behavior. Intentions are the most important predictor of behavior as they are the driving force behind decisions to act. As explained by this model, the decision to act in a certain manner is influenced by expectations about consequences of the behavior and the value that one places on those consequences (Franzoi, 1996). For example, a decision whether to wear one's seatbelt depends on both beliefs regarding the consequences of wearing or not wearing it, as well as the value that one places on those expected outcomes. If one believes that wearing a seatbelt will save a life in an accident and if that person also values his or her life, then we would expect to see the individual make a decision to wear the seatbelt.

This theory also emphasizes the importance of beliefs about social norms and one's motivation to comply with those norms. Social norms can influence the expected outcome of a behavior (approval vs. disapproval). Certainly, it is reasonable to expect that behavior that conforms to social norms will be met with approval, whereas behavior that violates norms will not be well received. This same model can also be applied to substance use. A key factor here would be one's perceptions of the social norms regarding substance use. A belief that use is common can imply that there is a social norm which condones and perhaps even encourages use.

The Theory of Planned Behavior

The Theory of Planned Behavior is another general behavior theory that can be applied to substance using behavior. It is similar to Reasoned Action in that it identifies intentions as the strongest guide to behavior. According to this model, however, intentions are determined by three things: one's attitudes, normative beliefs, and self-efficacy. People will be more likely to engage in behavior to the extent that they have a positive attitude toward that behavior or they have a positive attitude toward the expected outcome of that behavior. Social norms can greatly influence our attitudes toward certain behaviors or outcomes. We are more likely to have positive attitudes toward behaviors that we believe others also favor and engage in. The third element is self-efficacy or control. An individual is likely to develop an intention to engage in a behavior that he or she believes he or she is capable of performing or that he or she can control (Franzoi, 1996).

We can apply this model to substance-using behavior as well as to abstinence. For example, a child may develop an intention to remain abstinent from alcohol and other drugs if he or she has a positive attitude toward being drug free, or if he or she positively values the expected outcomes of being drug free, such as receiving praise from his parents, maintaining eligibility to participate in school-based activities, and so forth. On the other hand, to the extent that he or she positively values expected outcomes of use—acceptance from peers, enhanced fun, feeling and acting "grown up"—he or she may develop a positive attitude towards use. Several other models have already identified the role of social norms, or perceived social norms in influencing attitudes and decisions related to substance use. For example, if we perceive that many of our friends believe that being drug free is a good thing, and if we perceive that they themselves are drug free, we are more likely to have a positive attitude toward abstinence. To the contrary, if we perceive that many of our peers are using substances and thus approve of using them, this may influence our attitude in the opposite direction (e.g., Bachman *et al.,* 1988). Finally, intentions to remain chemically abstinent will develop to the extent that the youth believes he or she has the ability to do so. One important set of behaviors involved in remaining chemical free are refusal skills—saying "no" to peers, perhaps in pressure-filled situations. Likewise, intentions to use substances will develop if one is confident that one has the ability to successfully use them. We may wonder what kinds of factors are important to drug-related self-efficacy. The questions the youth can ask may be many—Can I get it? Do I know how to use it? Can I smoke a joint without coughing? Can I get drunk without throwing up or making a fool of myself?

This theory may explain why the use of "gateway drugs" such as alcohol, tobacco and "lookalikes" (caffeine pills designed to look like speed) increase one's vulnerability to substance abuse. Take cigarettes as an example. Research suggests that youths who smoke cigarettes are more likely to use marijuana than those who do not smoke (Botvin, 1983). One possible reason for the increased vulnerability may be that smoking cigarettes provides one with self-efficacy. Certainly, when attempting to smoke anything in front of one's peers, we would want to be sure that we will not embarrass ourselves by choking, coughing, and turning red. If we already have mastered smoking a cigarette without a problem, we may be more likely to feel that we could successfully take a hit off of a joint without embarrassment. Likewise, if we have experience in maintaining appropriate behavior and not getting sick by using alcohol or lookalikes, we should feel more confident in our ability to handle the "harder" stuff. Youths without prior experience may lack use-related self-efficacy, which may increase the probability that they will remain abstinent, even in the face of peer pressure.

COMPREHENSIVE THEORIES

There have been several attempts to integrate this body of research and develop more comprehensive theories that cross discipline domains.

Problem Behavior Theory

Problem Behavior Theory, developed by R. Jessor & Jessor (1977), is unique in that, according to this model, substance abuse is viewed as one of several deviant adolescent behaviors. Thus, this theory is not limited to substance use but applies also to other deviant adolescent behavior such as crime, sex, and truancy.

According to this theory, many problem behaviors that teens engage in are behaviors that are acceptable for adults but not for teens. Examples of these would be smoking, drinking, sex, and discontinuation of academic endeavors. Each of these activities has either an explicit or an implicit age at which it becomes permissible. However, as long as one maintains "child" status, such behaviors are prohibited. One possibility, then, is that teens may engage in these behaviors as a way to assert their own maturity. Thus, we can think of some of these behaviors as similar to rites of passage: engaging in these behaviors is one way to claim one's adult status. Therefore, vulnerability to one of these behaviors is correlated with vulnerability to the others. This perspective is supported by data on the comorbidity of a variety of teenage problem behaviors. Silverman (1989) presented data from a number of different sources demonstrating that adolescent substance abuse is correlated with other problems such as suicide, homicide, school dropout, delinquency, mental illness, and unwanted pregnancy.

Rather than focusing on only one type of variable, in this model, the key to behavior is the interaction between the person and the environment. This theory integrates many of the variables that have been discussed separately in the theories described previously. For example, environmental factors would include the relative influence of friends versus family and immediate social models. Person factors would include one's level of commitment to conventional societal values, self-esteem, personal goals, attitudes, and expectations regarding possible outcomes of various behavioral options. Although acknowledging the role of many variables, this model significantly downplays the role of cognition and places a heavy emphasis on peers.

The Domain Model

Huba & Bentler's Domain model of substance abuse (Huba, Wingard, & Bentler, 1980) includes over 50 possible causes of substance use, divided into 4 domains. Vulnerability factors from the biological domain include genetic susceptibility to addiction, an individual's physiological reactions to substances, and general health. Factors from the intrapersonal domain include expectations regarding consequences of substance use; personal values (e.g., success, achievement, independence) and individual personality traits (e.g., depression, self-esteem, impulsivity, extraversion). The interpersonal domain includes factors such as the makeup and availability of one's social network, including the attitudes and characteristics that the individual perceives one's social network as espousing. Lastly, the sociocultural domain includes media images of alcohol and other drugs, market availability, social sanctions, and laws regarding substance use. This last domain represents an important factor in substance abuse vulnerability that is overlooked in most other theories.

CUTTING THROUGH THE SEMANTIC FOG: ARE WE COMPARING APPLES AND ORANGES?

Now that we have briefly examined about a dozen major theories of substance use, we may find ourselves feeling overwhelmed, not only by the number of ideas, but also by the urge to integrate them or to consider them as competing alternatives calling for a meaningful and useful arbitration. Of course the plethora of theories and factors studied may be due to the fact that researchers have not adequately defined their terms, and, thus, may be studying entirely different phenomena. Hawkins, Lishner, and Catalano (1985) caution that, before etiological research can be informative for prevention, we must first define what it is we are trying to prevent. Is our goal to prevent any and all use? Misuse? Use of particular substances? Several researchers have suggested (Hawkins *et al.,* 1991; McGue, 1994; Pickens & Svikis, 1991) that there may be different causal factors for different types of use, and that there may indeed be different types of alcoholism (Sher, 1994; Zucker, 1994). For example, it is reasonable to expect that one set of factors may lead to experimentation—factors such as attitudes, environment, and so forth. However, once the effects of the substances are experienced, other factors, perhaps more of the biogenetic variables, may be more important in maintaining use or in changing patterns to misuse and addiction. Similarly, although correlations have been found between drug abuse and other rebellious (Segal, Huba, & Singer, 1980) and deviant (R. Jessor & Jessor, 1978) behaviors, no such correlation with an antisocial character has been found with experimental drug use, with the exception of initiation of marijuana use by adolescent males (Kandel & Yamaguchi, 1985; Yamaguchi &

Kandel, 1984) As yet, no models have attempted to account for these possible distinctions in etiology. The answers to such questions, however, have important implications for prevention, particularly once prevention personnel can agree on what exactly it is that they are trying to prevent.

SUBSTITUTING COMPETING THEORETICAL POSITIONS WITH RESEARCH-BASED ASSESSMENTS

The current plethora of competing and, more or less, conflicting theoretical positions suggests that the pathogenic behavior of substance abuse has a broad multifactorial foundation. Attempts to find solutions based on a single general theoretical foundation appear to be impractical and misguided. The vast array of diverse psychological factors, environmental influences, situational conditions, and their many combinations present indeed an exceptional challenge for educators and prevention specialists. This challenge is truly unmanageable in the absence of information about what the key factors are that need to be addressed in dealing with a particular population.

In facing this challenge of countless factors of potential but unknown relevance, our strategy is to begin with a diagnostic assessment that identifies the factors that deserve primary attention regarding a particular student or adolescent population. Rather than searching for a solution for drug prevention based on the numerous theories of substance abuse, our approach follows a different rationale. We start with a diagnostic assessment and propose that program development follow the results of the assessment, targeting the variables found to be most influential in shaping drug-related decisions for the populations under consideration. We may characterize this approach as based on a theory of human behavior founded on the system of cognitive–semantic representations rather than on a specific theory of substance abuse.

The Latest Scientific Developments
Open a Window on Propensities

The window opened by the technology of comparative imaging and mapping reveals psychological dispositions and environmental influences previously beyond the reach of empirical assessment. This new knowledge fundamental to the present strategy of substance abuse prevention deserves special attention. It is based on the assessment of psychological dispositions as powerful contributors to people's decisions to use or not to use harmful substances. Furthermore, powerful as they are, because they work below people's conscious awareness, there is a natural tendency to ignore them. As the review of the literature discussed in the previous chapter indicates, they receive little attention in prevention. The latest developments in the cognitive sciences and neurosciences are used to place our findings on the power of psychological and social influences into timely perspective.

A WINDOW ON INVISIBLE FORCES

The single most central feature of our strategy pursued in prevention is the identification of hidden forces—perceptual and motivational dispositions that shape decisions related to the use of harmful substances. The success of our approach hinges on our capability to identify and measure psychological dispositions and environmental influences that shape people's choices without their conscious awareness. A new window has been opened by the technology of comparative imaging and mapping. What it reveals are psychological and environmental forces previously beyond the reach of assessment. Now these forces can not only be identified; they can also be quantitatively measured.

A systematic identification of these influences is naturally a special challenge, a task edging on the impossible and likely to be accompanied by sober skepticism. Although our views on substance abuse do not run counter to those widely held in alcohol and drug prevention (Chapter 17), our approach is fundamentally different. Its primary focus is on psychological dispositions working below people's conscious awareness. The more hidden the psychological and environmental influences promoting vulnerability are, the more they are beyond the reach of traditional methods of assessment, and naturally the stronger the inclination is to ignore them.

Our approach to substance abuse is based on the identification of internal dispositions that aggregate into propensities, such as vulnerability/resistance, and result in influences of which people are mostly unaware. These are also influences to which most of the behavioral science disciplines are not attuned.

Fortunately, recent developments in cognitive psychology and neurobiology show increasing awareness and sophistication in addressing the latent forces that shape behavior. Because these developments are so closely relevant to our method of identifying psychological dispositions, we next review some developments in related fields that inform on factors that shape behavior below awareness. We discuss how some of the latest advances in cognitive psychology and the cognitive sciences support our focus on implicit cognitions and cognitive–semantic representations.

In Chapter 3 we showed how neurobiology yields new knowledge of the working of neural images in correspondence with our findings on mental images. Next we discuss a few main conclusions of neurobiology about the working of the system of neural representations. These conclusions are of special relevance because they bear on our findings about the importance of large systemic influences that shape people's choices and decisions below their awareness.

Neurobiology is also of critical relevance in identifying variables that prevent cognitive psychology from using its full potential to address implicit cognitions and cognitive–semantic representations. It also offers an incisive analysis of the dispositional foundation of neural images and systems of neural representations as the foundation of choices shaping behavior. These insights help explain the success of recent Behavioral Decision Theory-based investigations using the mental imaging approach. We discuss next three main areas: the cognitive sciences, neurobiology, and research on decisions and behavior.

Cognitive Psychology and the Cognitive Sciences— The Effects of Implicit Cognitions

Cognitive psychology, one of the most dynamic fields of contemporary psychology, is rich in research that supports the hidden nature and power of cognitive–semantic representations. Recent work has addressed *implicit cognitions*—those thoughts and attitudes that operate without our conscious awareness. After a long history of predominantly philosophical debates about the myths and realities of thought processes, contemporary cognitive psychologists are producing intriguing empirical evidence in controlled laboratory experiments. They have found that there are memories and cognitions that affect choices and decisions beyond people's awareness. Reviews by Schachter (1987), Reber (1993), Stacy and associates (1996), and Berry and Dienes (1993) offer timely accounts of developments regarding the distinction between two main types of thought processes: explicit and implicit cognitions. The first involves our normal, meditative, reflective thinking, a process we are mostly aware of. *Implicit cognition* or *representation* is characterized as just the opposite: hidden below awareness and inherently inaccessible to introspection.

Two characteristics of implicit cognitions are of special relevance to our interest in substance abuse prevention. One has to do with the power and influence of implicit thought. The leading investigators in this field tend to agree about several important characteristics of implicit cognitions, including their ubiquity and their power to influence choices and decisions without people's awareness (Greenwald & Banaji, 1995; Jacoby, Lindsay, & Toth, 1992; Nelson *et al.*, 1992; Nisbett & Ross, 1980; Nisbett & Wilson, 1977; Reber, 1993; Roediger, 1990; Stacy *et al.*, 1996; Wilson & Schooler, 1991). There are differences in emphasis and in assumptions about whether and in what way the implicit and explicit modalities mix. Nonetheless, the evidence shows that implicit cognitions are important sources of influence, previously little recognized. Their impact on shaping behavior appears particularly powerful. Choices previously believed to be free are apparently open to influences by past experiences, subjective understanding of the world, and social environments. These findings have direct relevance to substance abuse.

A second important characteristic of implicit cognitions is that they are inaccessible to introspection. Banaji and Greenwald (1994), Greenwald (1990), Wilson, Hodges, and LaFleur (1995), and Wilson and Schooler (1991) have made the observation that attempts to reconstruct and report the content of implicit cognitions not only tend to fail, but also produce unreliable and misleading results. As Banaji observes, this is not a matter of lack of candor or willful deception, but rather a consequence of the fact that the respondent is unaware of his or her own implicit cognitions. Because implicit cognitions are unavailable to introspection, respondents tend to produce some plausible reasons for their behavior, while being unaware of their own deeper reasons. Consider, for instance, cases in which a respondent is asked what made him or her get drunk for the first time. Queries such as this address implicit cognitions, reasons beyond the reach of the respondents' introspection. Thus, the answer offered cannot be accepted simply at face value. Direct questions that ask the respondents to explain the reasons behind their own behavior are frequently rich sources of misinformation. As we have said, neurobiology has helped us recognize how subcortical, limbic centers contribute to behavior without conscious awareness.

Limited Use in Substance Abuse Research

The theoretical underpinnings of research in the cognitive sciences vary considerably. Hopfield and Tank (1986) and Masson (1995) use a biology-based approach that models neural networks. Roediger (1990) relies on transfer of memory performance from one situation to another. Graf and Schacter (1987) and Schacter (1987) build on neurological systems underlying implicit memory. Schacter (1987) views the neurological systems supporting implicit cognitions as distinctly different from those involved in explicit cognitions. As Stacy and his associates (1996) observe, the number of studies documenting the relevance of implicit cognitions is large and the importance of this phenomenon to practical human problems is obvious; however, only a few of the research findings have been put to work in health research. This includes Tiffany's (1990) study of how drug use may be motivated by automatic memory process. Goldman and associates examined how motivations to use alcohol may be accessed by a semantic network of associations in memory (Goldman, Brown, Christiansen, & Smith, 1991). Several studies by Stacy and his colleagues (1996) show that implicit measures of cognitions reflect patterns of activation in memory that are elicited by drug-related experiences.

Decisions and Behavior: Their Foundation in Implicit Cognitions

The noninvasive, nontransparent, multiple-response elicitation task used in comparative imaging and mapping was especially designed for reconstructing cognitions and systems of cognitive–semantic representations that shape behavior without people's conscious awareness (Szalay & Deese, 1978). Recent developments in cognitive psychology distinguish implicit and explicit thought processes and demonstrate the previously ignored importance of implicit thought processes in shaping decisions. Such developments help to place our imaging and mapping technology in proper perspective.

All of our findings showing differences in the perceptions and attitudes of the users and the nonusers have their foundation in implicit thought processes and in the systems of cognitive–semantic representations beyond people's conscious awareness. This explains why imaging and mapping offers insights into internal processes frequently beyond the reach of survey questions. It explains why our finding that users have limited awareness of consequences not only supports the longitudinal University of Michigan ISR surveys but also increases the understanding of psychological dispositions that differentiate users and nonusers. This linkage between our findings and implicit thought processes also explains why our imaging results can provide useful information to program planners for developing prevention programs to reduce vulnerability and build resistance.

We have referred several times throughout this volume to mapping in new perspectives. Like the ISR's "Monitoring the Future" surveys showing the link between perceived harm and substance use, our findings, based on large student samples, also show how perceived harm is most influential in shaping choices related to substance use: Heavy drinkers and drug users tend to ignore the risks whereas nonusers show concern about negative consequences—loss of control, addiction, debilitating effects. Users are unaware of their tendency to overlook risks and harmful consequences, just as they tend to deny dependency. The ISR research has been showing since the late 1970s that there is an inverse relationship between perceived harm and substance abuse. In the years when reported awareness of harm grows, substance abuse decreases, and vice versa. The AGA-based findings show a similarly close relationship between perceptual dispositions and substance use, backed by extensive details on the dispositions that make people vulnerable and the dispositions that make people resistant to the use of harmful substances. Naturally, users are just as unaware of their dispositions that make them vulnerable as nonusers are unaware of those that make them resistant. The following discussion of neurobiology offers important insights that explain, based on the functioning of the neural system, the success of implicit thought processes and of the systems of cognitive–semantic representation to inform on behavioral dispositions that shape behavior. Neurobiology offers some important clues as to why some of the contemporary approaches of cognitive psychology are not as successful as they could be in producing information of direct utility to health and drug research.

NEUROBIOLOGY: THE SYSTEM OF REPRESENTATION AND BEHAVIORAL ORGANIZATION

Neuroscience is another field in a state of explosive growth. Two main developments are especially relevant to our work: neuroimaging and neurobiology.

Neuroimaging offers revolutionary opportunities in diagnostics. Neuroimaging refers to developing advanced diagnostic tools such as the Magnetic Resonance Imaging (MRI) and Positron Emission Tomography (PET) scans. These new instruments offer images of internal processes and functioning of the human body, both normal and pathological. They are used to monitor physiological changes and neural activity that could not be observed through older technology, such as X-rays. The neuroimaging developed for medical diagnoses and our comparative mental imaging, which focuses on the perceptual and motivational foundation of behavior, have a similar foundation in neural activations. The comparative mental imaging technology promises to be a useful tool for connecting the neural activity revealed by neuroimaging with the cognitive–semantic correlates of this activity involved in behavior. This means that dominant perceptions and emotions involved in internal processes that were previously inaccessible may now find cognitive–semantic expression. To make effective use of this new information requires additional research and testing because the solution is likely to vary along the different technologies of neuroimaging. This is discussed later in the context of future applications.

In Chapter 3, we discussed images as units of the system of cognitive–semantic representations; there we showed mental images of the system as they emerged from our data, parallel to neural images identified by neurobiology (Damasio, 1994; A. Damasio & Damasio, 1993; Dennett, 1991; Kosslyn *et al.,* 1993; Shepard & Cooper, 1982). The correspondence found at the level of images is remarkable. Now, after we have progressed from the analysis of images to the analysis of the larger system and of the propensity for vulnerability or for resistance, it is time to take another look. How much correspondence do we find at the level of the system of neural representations? Or more precisely, we are eager to explore what insights neurobiology offers to explain our findings at the broad systemic level. Since Damasio's (1994) book provided a host of valuable insights, we focus our attention on three critical parameters that appear to be particularly relevant to our interest.

Awareness in New Perspectives

Probably the most fascinating insight from neurobiology is its recognition of behavior as a product of a single integrated system of neural representations, a system that exerts a myriad of influences on behavior all the time. This means that influences whose sources lie below the level of conscious awareness are not rare or exceptional but do occur continuously.

In light of the experiences of neurobiology, what cognitive psychologists have tried to isolate, by studying implicit cognitions as mental representations in their laboratories under controlled conditions, happen to occur naturally, constantly, and spontaneously. Based on the experiences of neurobiology, implicit thought processes, their origin, and their potential to shape behavior are readily explicable in several ways. Implicit thought processes are influences promoted naturally through the subsystems of chemical and hormonal regulations, through the input of the limbic centers, and through the highly integrated nature of this system of neural representations. As this follows from the working of the system, even the most rational choices and behavior are not beyond influences from the centers that work below conscious awareness. Because it is intrinsic to the system that its working depends on the integrated system as a whole rather than its isolated parts, decisions considered under the control of conscious awareness may be more the exception than the rule.

In chapter 3 we used the image of alcohol to illustrate how mental images of users and of nonusers are shaped by two contrasting propensities: the propensity to use harmful substances and the propensity not to use them. We labeled these propensities Vulnerability and Resistance. In the later chapters we have presented findings showing how Vulnerability/Resistance involves two contrasting systems of representations that result, with a high degree of predictability, in alternative behavioral organizations that promote different behavior: use versus no use of harmful substances.

The conclusions of neurobiology on the dispositional foundation of neural images are congruent with our findings on the role of perceptual and attitudinal dispositions shaping behavior. The conclusions of neurobiology on the integrated influences of the system of neural representations also find extensive support in our findings on the contrasting propensities of vulnerability and of resistance registered in the comparisons of users and nonusers. The details in part I of this volume illustrate simultaneously how these underlying behavioral dispositions work to a large extent without the person's awareness. For instance, users are genuinely unaware that they tend to ignore negative consequences, not only of alcohol and other drug use but in other domains of life as well. The Vulnerability/Resistance measure, which assesses propensities toward use of harmful substances, taps dispositions that have a broad systemic foundation and that are characteristically beyond the respondents' awareness.

The Reason–Emotion Dichotomy in New Perspectives

A central subject of Damasio's (1994) book is the evidence from patients and from experiments that the traditional contrast between cognitions and emotions is superficial and misleading. Decisions and behaviors based on thought processes of reasoning and logic have been touted as superior to the supposed "blind" and "dumb" behaviors guided by emotion. However, there is growing evidence that emotions provide the organism with input essential for its survival in the shortest and most practical ways. As Damasio demonstrated, cognitions and reasoning deprived of the capability to rely on the wisdom of lower centers of biological regulation can become blind and dysfunctional.

This new evidence is of special relevance to fields of the behavioral sciences that tend to address cognitions and emotions separately. Neurobiology shows that such a separation is artificial and alien to real-life settings. This is one reason that laboratory experiments conducted with a narrow cognitive focus have shown limited success in using their findings on implicit cognitions to address human problems outside of the laboratory. A second explanation suggested by neurobiology, as well as by our own research, follows from a research strategy to rely on newly built connections in laboratory experiments using meaningless, artificial language material such as nonsense syllables. This strategy systematically attempts to establish independence from the existing system of neural representations that is the foundation of thought processes and behavior. Thought processes are based on the accumulated perceptual and affective content of human experience. Attempts to work outside of the existing system eliminates for the sake of control the systemic foundation on which implicit cognitions draw their power and influence.

Our many examples from comparative imaging (e.g., Figure 3.2 on the image of ALCOHOL) show that practically all of the particular responses, as mosaic pieces of the users' and the nonusers' images, have their foundation in external reality but emerge in combination with emotional, attitudinal elements that have their foundation in the positive as well as in the negative experiences of the responding person. All of the characteristics supporting the inseparability of reason and emotion emerge also in combination with the highly predictable systemic influences of Vulnerability/Resistance.

Behavior in New Perspectives

Along our interest to identify etiological factors that promote the use of harmful substances, a third major question is how the system of neural representations shapes and organizesbehavior. This question is particularly intriguing from the neurobiological perspective of a highly integrated system of representation of the environment. As we have seen, neurobiology shows the system of neural representations working along two complementary roles or functions: The system is a natural source of thoughts and representations that informs on external realities and requires conscious awareness and the system includes emotions that result from past positive or negative experiences and that affect choices and decisions without the person's awareness.

This particularly revolutionary view of neurobiology contrasts most fundamentally with stimulus–response behaviorism that focuses on objective characteristics, which in the present case would mean a faithful reproduction of the stimulus in the system of neural representations. Damasio (1994) presented a convincing case that, in reality, what matters is not so much the stimulus but rather the system of neural representations that defines the response. Neurobiology shifts the focus of attention from the stimulus to the dispositions of the responding person, dispositions as shaped by past experiences and history and registered in his or her system of neural representations. This system has a composite nature constantly formed and updated by new experiences and new situations. Clearly, behavior emerges as a product of countless dispositional elements that are continuously online, ready to feed into new choices and behaviors.

The dispositional foundation built on aggregate propensities accumulated across the images of the neural system was illustrated by the prevalence profiles of users and of nonusers reconstructed from images in three domains of life (Figure 3.3). This ties in closely again with our findings on the contrasting propensities of vulnerability- and of resistance-based results reflecting close agreement with behaviors reported or observed.

Previously (Chapter 3) we discussed our findings on mental images compared with the observations and findings of neurobiology on neural images. We described the role of select images parallel to the conclusions of neurobiology. In this chapter we have examined how our findings on dominant behavioral dispositions and propensities of vulnerability and resistance relate to three revolutionary conclusions of neurobiology that bear on systemic influences operating below awareness, on the artificial contrast between the emotional and the rational, and on the role played by the system of neural representations as a source of continuous input shaping behavior.

Naturally, the related views of neurobiology about how behavior is formed and organized are based on extensive experience with the neural system and its functioning. Of special relevance to our interest is that the principles registered by neurobiology are in agreement with our findings on the perceptual and attitudinal foundation of behavior. The neurosciences offer valuable insights into the systemic neurological foundation of behavioral dispositions. They are also in good agreement with the latest results of investigations based the theory of decision research.

RESEARCH ON FACTORS AFFECTING DECISIONS AND BEHAVIOR

Expectancy and Decision Research on Factors Affecting Behavior

Along a third line of development, Expectancy Theory and Behavioral Decision Theory have stimulated investigations resulting in new findings and insights that bear on the etiology of behavior and its foundation on internal dispositions. These theories demonstrate the intrinsic relationship between perceptions and attitudes as behavioral dispositions and choices and decisions that shape behavior. Expectancy theory has built on the work of Tolman (1932), Lewin (1951), Rotter (1966, 1981) and later on the work pursued by Chritchlow (1986) and Marlat (1987). Particularly in its adaptation by Goldman, Brown, and Christiansen and Smith (1987), and Goldman *et al.* (1991), it has produced useful insights about alcohol abuse, showing that respondents' expectations influence their behavior regarding the use of alcohol.

Behavioral Decision Theory is traced back to Edwards' (1961) review of the psychological approaches to decision making. Early work reflected economic issues, utilitarian interest, how to reduce risks, how to promote decisions based on actual probabilities, and how to cope with uncertainties (Kahneman, Slovic, & Tversky, 1982; Slovic, Fischoff, & Lichenstein, 1979, 1984). Within decision theory, recognition of the difference between objective and subjective probabilities gained growing importance, with emphasis on the role of perceived risks (Slovic, 1987, 1993).

Expectancy theorists speak of perceived expectations as well. A difference between expectancy theories and decision theory relevant to our interest is that representatives of the behavioral decision theory have been using comparative imaging adapted from the AGA method to assess perceptions, perceived outcomes, and anticipated consequences.

Use of Mental Imaging in Decision Research

Since the late 1980s, research based on multiple-response association strategies have ranged across a wide variety of research topics: assessing public images of nuclear waste (Slovic, Layman, & Flynn, 1990); perceived risks and trust in politics (Slovic et al., 1991); perceptions and attitudes related to the Yucca Mountain, stigma, and economic impact associated with risks (Slovic, Layman, & Flynn, 1991); the psychometric paradigm in risk perception (Slovic, 1992); perceptions of environmental hazards (Slovic, 1992); adolescents health-threatening and health-enhancing behavior (Benthin et al., 1995), and others. After listing a variety of sources of biases in judgment of risks, Slovic (1993) observed that experts appear to be prone to the same biases as laypersons, particularly when experts go beyond the limits of available data and rely upon their intuitions (Henrion & Fischoff, 1986; Kahneman et al., 1982).

Regarding the research technology, Slovic (1995) concludes:

> The word association methodology provides a useful technique for exploring adolescents' cognitions and affective reactions with regard to health-related behaviors. The data provided by this method have implications for prevention and intervention programs, as well as for future research. (p. 143)

The Etiology of Health-Threatening Behaviors

Over the years researchers with interest in Decision Theory have adopted our multiple-response elicitation strategy of mental imaging. In earlier investigations they used this approach to reconstruct the dominant perceptual and motivational composition of images characteristic of particular populations. This reflected a recognition that continuous free associations offer useful information about how people's images shape their decisions and their behavior. More recently, applications of the multiple-response elicitation strategy have combined the reproduction of mental images with a focused etiological interest. These applications identify behavioral dispositions of people with contrasting behavior: people who drink compared with those who do not, people who engage in protected sex compared to those who do not. Although some of these applications by researchers from decision theory use categories of analysis (e.g., positive vs. negative outcomes and concept categories) that are broader than what we use in our analysis of dominant perceptions and attitudes, they do reflect the same rationale.

A comparison of the images of people who behave differently offers insights into their differences in perceptions and attitudes that are at the foundation of their differences in behavior. The strategy of analyzing the mental images of people whose behavior differs (drinkers vs. nondrinkers) to reconstruct the perceptual and attitudinal sources of their behavior is a strategy of etiological analysis that is closely analogous to our present investigations and to those, for instance, pursued in the recent study of health-threatening and health-enhancing behaviors by Benthin, Slovic, Moran, Severson, Mertz, and Gerard (1995).

LOOKING UNDER THE HOOD

In an age of progressive scientific specialization it is a rare experience that disciplines with a different focus of interest and with different approaches and diagnostic methods produce results with the close resemblance we have noted in this chapter. The correspondence of our specific findings with some of the main conclusions of neurobiology about the working of the system of neural representations, the engine at the foundation of behavior, is naturally a welcome discovery. It cannot be accidental. It supports the lesson we have learned over many years from our imaging and mapping technology, namely, that human behavior has a foundation in a system of behavioral dispositions with roots beyond what is visible to the naked eye.

Since the late 1960s, our research has used the method of mental imaging and cognitive mapping and it has produced rich evidence that subjective images and meanings are part of a vast system of cognitive–semantic representations (Szalay & Brent, 1967; Szalay & Bryson, 1974; Szalay & Deese, 1978). Our many multicultural and multidisciplinary investigations have treated images as the natural units of a system that is the foundation of the subjective worlds of different cultures (Diaz-Guerrero & Szalay, 1991; Szalay & Bryson, 1973; Szalay & Diaz-Guerrero, 1985; Szalay & Kelly, 1982; Szalay & Maday, 1983). An adapted use of the imaging and mapping technology has served as the basis for the more recent applications in the field of substance abuse dealing with the assessment of perceived harm (Szalay, Inn, et al., 1993), psychological correlates of substance abuse (Szalay, Vilov, & Strohl, 1992), and treatment effects (Szalay, Bovasso, Vilov, & Williams, 1992). As several dozen large-scale investigations have shown, subjective images and meanings are the natural units of a subjective world, supported by a cognitive–semantic organization that provides an enduring organization of behavior. They all support the conclusion that human choices and decisions are rooted in subjective images in the system of cognitive–semantic representations.

The correspondence between our findings on mental images in the system of cognitive–semantic representations and the contemporary conclusions of neurobiology on the working of neural images in their system of neural representations is remarkably close indeed. It contrasts vividly with the diversity of views among the various behavioral science disciplines. Our tentative explanation is that much of the contemporary differences come from high-level abstractions and speculation. They are likely to disappear gradually as disciplines seriously interested in behavior begin to follow the example set by neurobiology and take a closer look at the system that is the origin and foundation of behavior. The system that is central to the working of a car has to be understood as a system built on the integrated working of several subsystems of transmission, fuel, lubrication, electrical circuitry, and so forth. That is, much of the present confusion may disappear if the disciplines interested in behavior take a closer look at the system under the hood. This will lead to a paradigm shift, but it will naturally follow from lifting the hood.

Regarding substance abuse prevention, this implies that we use as a point of departure the assessment of behavioral dispositions at the foundation of vulnerabilities. We are then in a position to develop programs that are systematically targeted on the most dominant propensities identified. A brief summary of a comprehensive prevention strategy is offered in the following final chapter.

Comprehensive Prevention

Future Perspectives

The findings support a comprehensive strategy of prevention built on three interrelated tasks: Diagnostics: assessment of dominant psychological dispositions, measuring the Vulnerability/Resistance of particular populations; Program Development: developing and targeting programs on dominant perceptual and motivational dispositions affecting the propensities of Vulnerability/Resistance; and Feedback: evaluation of the psychological and environmental effects of the program. The success in the field of alcohol and drug prevention supports the feasibility of extending this research-based assessment and targeting strategy to other problem areas, from education to mental health and from violence to crime.

A SYSTEMATIC PREVENTION–INTERVENTION STRATEGY IN THREE STEPS

The culmination of our extensive investigations conducted with tens of thousands of student is a comprehensive strategy for alcohol and drug prevention. It includes three interconnected steps. Though each is useful on its own, they offer the most benefit when used combination.

1. Diagnostic Assessment

Comparative imaging and cognitive mapping offer a systematic research-based approach to identify dominant perceptual and motivational dispositions that are the hidden sources of psychological vulnerabilities, as well as being the foundation of resistance to use harmful substances. This comprehensive strategy supports systematic prevention by identifying dominant perceptual and motivational dispositions at the source of psychological vulnerabilities to substance abuse.

Supported by extensive research, internal dispositions previously beyond the reach of empirical assessment can now be identified as powerful sources that shape the students' decisions to use or not to use harmful substances. These new diagnostics, which offer up-to-date assessments of psychological dispositions leading to substance abuse, open a new chapter in prevention where programs generally lack factual knowledge about the psychological factors they are trying to impact.

There is conclusive evidence that the psychological dispositions affecting students' decisions to use harmful substances and impacting their overall vulnerability/resistance to substance abuse vary from group to group and from population to population, depending on their background, age, social environment, and so forth. This variability underscores the importance of etiologically focused diagnostics. To avoid shooting in the dark, systematic prevention must identify and address the dominant contributing and causative factors that are at the foundation of the vulnerabilities as well as those at the foundation of the resistance in any particular population.

A second main group of variables that affect drug use and that shape vulnerability/resistance involves socioenvironmental factors , frequently identified as social climate or drug climate. The influence of such environmental factors can be similarly powerful and similarly evasive to empirical assessment. Their power and influence on vulnerability/resistance, behavior, and lifestyle have also emerged from imaging and mapping.

A useful and reliable diagnostic assessment calls for testing medium-size samples (e.g., 200–400 students) in the representation of a particular school or college. The testing may include select word themes and/or pictures (16–32), depending on the focus of interest (drugs, alcohol, violence, academic motivation). Considering background questions and imaging and mapping, the data collection takes 20 to 40 minutes. For additional details, see chapter 12 and the appendix.

2. Program Development

Following diagnostic assessment, the development of successful prevention programs depends largely on the effective use of the information accumulated on the dominant psychological dispositions and environmental influences regarding the students sampled.

Imaging and mapping offer program developers up-to-date information on the dominant psychological propensities of the specific populations in which they are interested; that is, a mapping of the main directions of the propensities toward vulnerability or toward resistance. Comparative imaging provides details showing what these propensities involve in terms of dominant perceptions and attitudes characteristic of the particular samples and subsamples of students tested. As we have discussed in more detail in chapter 14, comparative imaging produces detailed information on the perceptual and attitudinal dispositions of the students. This information is useful first along diagnostic interests in showing what the sources of vulnerabilities are that require correction and what the sources of resistance are and then in building programs systematically designed to reduce vulnerability and to strengthen resistance.

From the angle of systematic and effective program planning, it is especially important to know how to take the students' perceptions and attitudes and their subjective world into careful consideration. The effectiveness of communications, program selection, and curriculum materials depends to a large extent on the appropriate selection of their content to be relevant to the students' frame of reference and to their own experiences and views regarding harmful substances, associated risks, and expectations. As we have discussed in the context of educational and training experiences (chapters 14,15), comparative imaging provides information on the students' images and meanings, which can provide a basis for extending their experiences in order to build their resistance to substance use and to social influences that pressure students to use alcohol and drugs.

Compared to the diagnostic assessment that offers information on the overall level of vulnerability or resistance of particular student populations to substance abuse, the detailed results of comparative imaging offer timely information for program development. This information can be used in targeting programs on the perceptual and attitudinal dispositions that offer optimal opportunities to reduce the students' vulnerabilities and to build their resistance by taking into systematic consideration their internal psychological dispositions and the external climatic conditions characteristic of their social environment.

Generally, the diagnostic assessment has been performed by our research organization (ICS—the Institute of Comparative Social and Cultural Studies, Inc.) in cooperation with the school or college interested in the assessment. The program development has been largely the task of the educational institution, drawing on the experiences of other schools and experts in program planning. Although the conditions and interests of the schools have varied a great deal in the past, the recent experiences we have summarized here and in other publications suggest that the schools are rising to the challenge of incorporating these psychological and environmental factors in developing and targeting their prevention programs.

3. Feedback and Evaluation of Program Effects

A major source of doubt and uncertainty about prevention stems from the difficulties associated with the evaluation of a prevention program's impact. The results of imaging and mapping, when used to trace changes in perceptions and attitudes and changes in vulnerability/resistance, offer noninvasive, indirect measures for use as sensitive tools in program evaluation. Compared to most contemporary measures based on asking participants what they liked or did not like about the program, the imaging and mapping technology provides feedback on how the program affected the participants' perceptions and attitudes and how it affected their vulnerability/resistance to substance abuse.

This capability to evaluate the psychological impact of a particular program focuses on the most central question: What did the program achieve, as gauged by changes along the key variables previously identified as informative on the respondents' overall propensities to use harmful substances? The evaluation tools work by tapping dominant perceptions and attitudes and their aggregate effects on vulnerability/resistance, a measure that has been extensively validated as informative regarding the respondents' propensity to use or not use harmful substances.

A particularly attractive feature of these new measures is that they tap the relevant changes without asking specific or direct questions. Questions concerning program evaluation can be of uncertain informational value; often they inform more on whether the respondent liked the program rather than on the extent to which it had any meaningful impact on the respondent's propensity to use or not to use harmful substances. As we have discussed in the previous chapter, our assessment measures psychological dispositions and their changes that affect the person's propensities to use harmful substances, propensities that work largely below the respondent's awareness. Over the recent years we have tested the analytic sensitivity and validity of these noninvasive measures, as discussed in chapter 6 and also in the context of various program evaluations (chapter 16).

The results support the general conclusion that using these analytic measures before and after the completion of a particular prevention program offers sensitive and valid indicators of the psychological impact of select programs. In the present situation characterized by demoralizing uncertainties and doubts about the effectiveness of drug prevention in general and the effectiveness of specific programs in particular, the solution offered by the pre and postadministration of the comparative imaging task and the calculation of the Vulnerability/Resistance measures offers a valuable solution for program evaluation. Repeated use of these feedback measures offers a continuous solution that supports progressive improvement through program revisions following each feedback loop, using the feedback to make changes designed and evaluated to enhance program effects. A postprogram administration of the measures can be performed on a reduced scale and the associated expenses are likely to be modest.

FUTURE VISTAS AND OPPORTUNITIES

Compared to a narrow focus on the substances abused, our findings support substance abuse prevention from the human perspective, people's dispositions, and their social and cultural environments. Such a strategy is especially compelling when we realize that a person's decision to experiment with harmful substances depends on his or her internal dispositions variously shaped by the environment. Our research conclusions are supported by the latest findings of cognitive psychology showing the influences of implicit cognitions, which are mental representations that shape choices without people's conscious awareness. They receive particularly strong support from the field of neurobiology, which has accumulated advanced knowledge on the functioning of the neural system as it shapes behavior. In light of the findings of neurobiology, any attempt to prevent substance abuse without considering its broad foundation on human dispositions and environmental influences is like trying to avert a tornado by plugging up a keyhole.

Progress in prevention requires overcoming the vestiges of stimulus–response behaviorism and recognizing that behavior is the product of a highly integrated system of mental and neural representations and organization. That amounts to a genuine paradigm shift, which is already in progress in several fields and dimensions. The solution offered by the AGA imaging and mapping approach to systematic drug prevention promises several practical applications.

The Combined Use of Neural Imaging and Mental Imaging

Much progress is being made in neuroimaging-based diagnostics. The results produced by the diverse neuroimaging technologies specific to particular sensory modalities do contribute to the broad systemic picture presented by Damasio's (1994) review. We believe that our approach to mental imaging is closely related to the diagnostic approaches of neuroimaging. At present we do not have the direct empirical evidence, but it will be relatively easy to develop combined applications. Neuroimaging and mental imaging technologies have their foundations on analogous capabilities to trace and to reproduce neural activation. The utility of the neuroimaging technologies speak for themselves. The utility of the mental imaging technology follows from its ability to identify dominant perceptual and motivational dispositions previously beyond empirical assessment. That is, it identifies psychological dispositions, perceptions, and attitudes linked to specific mental images. Their aggregate effects inform on propensities that shape behavior, or in the present context, vulnerability/resistance to substance abuse. In the context of particular neuroimaging technologies, the mental imaging approach promises new opportunities to communicate diagnostic results in simple language and in perceptual and attitudinal terms.

Complementing Epidemiological Data with Etiological Data

An effective use of available resources calls for combining surveys of reported use with cognitive mapping. The epidemiologically oriented surveys assess the level of use characteristic of particular schools, institutions, or jurisdictions. Surveys are fast, inexpensive, and effective in showing changes in the level of use. Cognitive mapping, which requires smaller samples and less frequent testing, offers insights into the students' dispositions and other psychological factors. Combined with survey data, mapping can provide a solid foundation for policy and planning decisions over several years. The complementary use of survey and cognitive mapping methods is a simple and viable solution, granted that it is done with well-coordinated planning. Most colleges have experience in developing sampling strategies and in administering surveys; adding a comparative imaging and mapping component can be done through cooperative arrangements with the Institute of Comparative Social and Cultural Studies in Chevy Chase, Maryland.

Extending Risk Assessment to Include Psychological Vulnerability

Information on psychoenvironmental risk factors adds an important dimension to risk assessment. Comprehensive risk assessment based on identification of dominant psychological dispositions and on the measurement of aggregate propensities for substance use opens the opportunity to address perceived risks. As leading representatives of decision theory recognize, choices and behavior have their deep foundation in perceived risk and harm.

The Vulnerability data can be used to aggregate propensities for use and the image data offer detailed insights for addressing these propensities in programs that recognize the subjective foundation of perceived harm and risk. The new Vulnerability measures are backed by image data that show in specific detail the main sources of the vulnerability. For instance, differing male–female perceptions and attitudes at the foundation of their vulnerability to alcohol and other drug abuse offer information that prevention practitioners can use to address the respondents' psychological dispositions that affect their choices and their behavior.

Extending Prevention to Building Resistance

It is customary to think of prevention as an intervention focused on reducing vulnerability to substance use. New findings suggest that a true type of prevention of use is now possible through supporting and building resistance. Building resistance requires strengthening psychological dispositions that are strongly characteristic of nonusers.

The simultaneous use of both strategies, reducing vulnerability and building resistance, may provide the smoothest transition to focusing on building resistance. This second strategy promises several advantages. Relying on positive solutions promoted proactively is generally more effective than addressing deficits.

Building resistance on a broad natural foundation of personal interests and perspectives also offers a stronger and more viable approach to cope with the dispositions toward hedonism and instant gratification characteristic of users.

Extending Prevention toward Intervention

It may have occurred to the reader that we have made very few references to intervention. This is neither accidental nor a reflection of lack of interest. Rather it is an attempt to maintain a focus on prevention itself. Intervention is of immense practical importance, and what has been said here has implications for intervention. How individual investigators demarcate the fields of prevention and intervention varies considerably. The broad variation may explain our reluctance to address the issue, but this should not detract from the fact that imaging and mapping can be used to gain insights into the relevant psychological dispositions of people at any stage of use. Application of this technology in intervention will probably require a stronger focus on the individual. In intervention it is increasingly important to consider the combined effects of psychological dispositions and the particular substances used. The combined effects of substance abuse and other psychological impairments requires attention. Nonetheless, our experiences in treatment evaluation support the assessment of psychological dispositions as a part of any effort directed at overcoming impairments resulting from substance abuse. Tracing changes in dispositions along program objectives also offers feedback for improving program effects.

Extending Prevention to Younger Populations

In the present volume we relied mostly on data that came from college students. A next logical step is to apply the methods and results to younger student populations. How can we start addressing the prevention of alcohol and other drug abuse with elementary or middle school students? Our experiences with younger populations are more limited yet sufficient to draw three main conclusions. Application to younger populations can be done with the same basic strategy or principles already discussed. It does require some changes in the instrument, depending on the age and composition of the samples considered; every 2 to 4 years of age difference may require adaptation in the themes (or pictures) used in the elicitation tasks. Similarly, the norms developed for scoring vulnerabilities may require age-specific adaptations as well; the procedures for such adaptations are available.

It is easier to cope with vulnerabilities at an early stage rather than later when they are supported by more entrenched habits and chemical influences. Shifting the focus of prevention from fighting vulnerability to building resistance is certainly not new as an idea. What is new is the capability to pursue it systematically by relying on a combination of effective diagnostics and feedback.

Extending Prevention to Other Social Problems

As the reader may have already anticipated, our strategy of identifying and coping with psychological dispositions as antecedents of problem behavior has wider applicability. There are other clusters of psychological dispositions that are contributing to a variety of social problems. Certain types of crime, violence, antisocial behavior, suicide, and some mental health and educational problems have been shown to have a strong psychological foundation. The more the problems are shaped and accentuated by social experiences, socialization, and cultural influences, the more likely it is that imaging and cognitive mapping methods can make some useful contributions. As in the case of substance abuse, mapping the systems of semantic–cognitive representations can open a window on hidden forces and processes that provide the foundation of behavior.

Opening similar windows on crime, violence, suicide, and on many other environmentally driven problems with psychological foundations could be particularly helpful if approached in terms of their natural relationship rather than as separate and independent problems. Such recognition appears to be desirable for developing effective methods of social prevention with a sound educational foundation.

One of the important implication of the present strategy is that by tracing the dispositional foundation that promotes various personally and socially harmful behaviors, practical insights are gained. By taking into account the dominant perceptions and attitudes that promote vulnerabilities parallel to those that build resistance, it is possible to develop research-based programs, prevention and intervention strategies, communications, and information material systematically designed to reach and impact particular populations.

Appendix

Comparative Imaging and Mapping by the Associative Group Analysis (AGA) Method

Associative Group Analysis (AGA) is a computer-assisted method of comparative imaging and cognitive mapping. It uses tens of thousands of free responses produced by various groups for comparison: drug users and nonusers, males and females, Chinese and Americans, and so forth. AGA opens windows on their inner worlds through the identification of dominant perceptual and motivational dispositions in their respective systems of cognitive–semantic representations. By opening the worlds of different social experiences and cultures, these hidden systems become accessible to observation, measurement, and systematic intervention.

BACKGROUND

Roots in Empirical Research on Meaning

The development of the AGA method of assessing images and meanings and of reconstructing systems of mental representation was inspired by two main developments in the field of psychology. The original inspiration came from psychologist Charles Osgood, the author of the Semantic Differential. He developed his instrument based on a recognition of subjective meanings as the critical variables shaping behavior. As Osgood, Suci, and Tannenbaum (1957) put it:

> Of all the imps that inhabit the nervous system, that little black box in psychological theorizing—the one we call meaning—is held by common consent to be the most elusive. Yet again by common consent of social scientists, this variable is one of the most important determinants of human behavior.

Osgood's interest is pursued presently by psychologists in the field of cross-cultural research led by Harry Triandis and his associates. As Triandis explains, psychologists generally tend to approach culture through subjective meanings that form the mosaic pieces of people's subjective world or of their "systems of mental representations." Triandis, Vassiliou, and Nassiakou (1968) observed that this system of cognition constitutes a map of the ways people conceive their environment, and these maps probably serve as the basis for different kinds of behavior exhibited by people from different cultures.

Use of the Free Response Strategy to Reconstruct Meanings and Systems of Mental Representation

The second major development has to do with verbal associations. In his book *Structure of associations in language and thought* (1965) Deese pioneered a revolutionary reorientation in conceptualization of associations. Deese called attention to the importance of the meaning-mediated mechanism over the verbal habit-based mechanisms in the elicitation process. As Deese said in his preface, "The importance about associations is not what follows what, but how sets of associations define structured patterns of relations among ideas." This position bears closely on the distinction of explicit and implicit cognitions, which is central in the contemporary field of cognitive psychology.

Lorand Szalay and his associates developed the AGA method from a broad range of cross-cultural comparisons of multiple free responses elicited along a strategy designed to assess the respondent's subjective meanings, dominant perceptions and motivations (Szalay & Brent, 1967; Szalay & Lysne, 1970; Szalay, Lysne, & Brent, 1970; Szalay & Windle, 1968). These cross-cultural comparisons supported the findings of Clyde Noble (1952) and James Deese (1965). Noble was one of the first to demonstrate, with his measure of "meaningfulness," that the number of free responses elicited by a particular theme or image offers a valid indicator of the subjective importance of that theme or image in the inner world of the respondent.

Szalay's monograph *Subjective meaning and culture: Assessment through word associations,* coauthored with Deese (1978), describes the AGA method, including its rationale for reconstructing subjective images and systems of meanings, for reproducing dominant perceptions and attitudes, and for mapping the respondent's subjective world from hundreds of free responses.

AGA works by reconstructing people's dominant perceptions and attitudes, mapping their subjective world from the computerized analysis of their free associations. Thousands of free associations are used to reconstruct subjective images and meanings from these mosaic pieces in their main perceptual and attitudinal components. Specialized software was developed to map the system of mental representation, that is, to reconstruct each group's subjective world from free associations elicited by strategically selected key stimulus themes.

Features of the AGA Method

- AGA uses an indirect, inferential approach. It does not ask direct questions about people's opinions but reconstructs their dominant perceptions, motivations, and beliefs from the distribution of free associations to selected themes.
- AGA is a nontransparent method of assessment. Presented as a simple paper and pencil word-association task, it can assess dominant perceptual and attitudinal dispositions that lie below people's conscious awareness.
- There are no right or wrong answers. People respond spontaneously during the time-limited free-association tasks.
- Because it is nontransparent, it is relatively free of biases of acquiescence and social desirability.
- The continued, multiple-response free-association task is simple and easy to administer, particularly in a classroom environment or other group settings.
- AGA-based results on psychological dispositions show a close relationship to behavior; validation studies have identified drug users and nonusers with high accuracy.
- AGA is a sensitive tool for assessing program effects along perceptual and motivational dimensions that are beyond the reach of direct methods of assessment.

The AGA method offers empirically based insights into the perceptions, attitudes, and other hidden psychological dispositions that shape behavior. These dispositions operate mostly below the level of people's conscious awareness, and therefore beyond the reach of direct survey questions. Respondents have no idea of the selectivity of their perceptions and attitudes. Dispositions in combination reinforce each other and shape a person's propensity to act in certain ways (e.g., experiment with drugs). Findings based on thousands of students demonstrate the power of the AGA comparative imaging and mapping technology to trace and reconstruct these dispositions. The assessment relies on a sophisticated software system to analyze the spontaneous distributions of tens of thousands of free responses.

The AGA method has been in use since the late 1960s. The nondirective, open-ended nature of the method provides an opportunity to assess perceptual and motivational dispositions characteristic of individuals or of groups, and to map the dominant parameters of their systems of behavioral organization or of mental representation. The primary units of analysis are subjective images and meanings, these being the main elements of cognition—of systems of mental representation. Various schools of thought, from cognitive psychology to clinical psychology, ethnoscience, semantics, linguistics, and philosophy are converging in their views that differences in human behavior come, to a large extent, from differences in people's understanding or subjective view of their environment. This reasoning has led to a growing interest in people's inner worlds as a key to understanding and guiding behavior.

The AGA approach has its roots in two main lines of development in the field of psychology. The first is earmarked by Charles Osgood (Osgood, Suci, & Tannenbaum, 1957) and Harry Triandis (Triandis, Vassiliou, & Nassiakov, 1968, 1972, 1990) who performed groundbreaking work in approaching subjective culture through the empirical study of subjective meanings. The second line was started by the work of Clyde Noble (1952) and James Deese (1962), who initiated a reorientation in the field of free associations by recognizing the role of subjective meaning.

The AGA model has similarities to such other systems of cognitive organization as "meaning systems" (Osgood, Suci, & Tannenbaum, 1957), "cognitive map" (Tolman, 1948), "thought world" (Whorf, 1956), "world view" (Black, 1973), "system of perceptual/semantic representation" (Szalay et al., 1984), "mental representations" (Piavio, 1986), and "social construction of reality" (Gergen, 1985).

Briefly, AGA is a free association-based, noninvasive technology. It relies on the computer-assisted analysis of thousands of spontaneous reactions elicited in continued multiple-response tasks to strategically selected words (or pictures; Szalay & Deese, 1978). It works by tracing the organization of behavior, by mapping its foundation on implicit cognitions, on systems of cognitive–semantic representations.

DATA COLLECTION AND ORGANIZATION

Administering the Test

The standard AGA testing conditions of group testing, written responses, and working with little time pressure help promote spontaneous meaning-mediated responses. Individual respondents remain anonymous (demographic data are obtained using a brief questionnaire that carries the same code number as the respondent's test slips). Assurance of anonymity helps to reduce the likelihood of bias in the form of acquiescence or social desirability; it opens up a variety of emotion-laden issues to objective inquiry. The respondents are instructed to write free responses to each of the stimulus themes presented on randomly sequenced cards.

AGA Test Instructions
This experiment is part of a study in verbal behavior, and this particular task involves word associations. They are group experiments, and your responses will not be evaluated individually but collectively for your group. Your responses are completely anonymous, and you are free to give your associations concerning any subject. There

are no bad or wrong answers, so do not select your responses but put them down spontaneously in the order that they occur to you.

The task is easy and simple. You will find a word printed on each slip of paper. Reading this stimulus word will make you think of other associated words (objects, ideas, issues, etc.). You are asked to write as many separate responses as you can think of in the time allotted. Try to think of one-word responses and avoid long phrases or sentences.

It is important that in giving your responses you always take the given stimulus word into consideration. For example, if the stimulus is TABLE, and your answer is *writing*, in giving the subsequent responses you must refer back to TABLE and avoid "chain" responses (i.e., *writing pen, ink, blue, ocean, sail.* . . .). Please work without hurrying, but do your best to give us as many answers as possible. One minute will be given for each word. At the end of each minute I will ask you to go on to the next word. Do not work longer than one minute on any word and do not read ahead or return to others later.

Scoring the Responses

A logical assumption is that earlier responses are more meaningful than later ones and that the first response has more salience to the respondent than the last. This assumption is supported by empirical evidence. The stability of responses obtained at different rank places was studied by comparing the responses obtained from the same group in two separate sessions one month apart (Szalay & Brent, 1967). The responses obtained at higher rank places in the first test showed higher stability in the second test than did the responses first obtained at lower rank places. The coefficients of stability obtained in the comparative study provide the weights for the various rank places. The weights, beginning with the first response, are 6, 5, 4, 3, 3, 3, 3, 2, 2, 1, 1, 1. Respondents generally give six to eight different associations to each theme.

The cards are organized by stimulus words, and the individual responses from all of the respondents are tallied into group response lists (see Figure 1). Certain responses (e.g., *drug* to MARIJUANA) will occur to many members of the group; other responses may be given by only one or two members. In order to focus on the shared meaning for a particular group, the responses given by only one person are excluded from analysis. Dropping the idiosyncratic responses helps us to concentrate on the more stable, shared responses and simplifies the data processing and analysis.

If we look at responses produced by members of our own social group, they appear to be just plain common sense. We tend to feel that everybody would produce similar responses and that the responses do not tell us anything new. This impression is probably the major reason that the potential information value of associative response distributions had not been clearly recognized in the past. The systematic exploitation of associations as an important information source is the central objective of the AGA method.

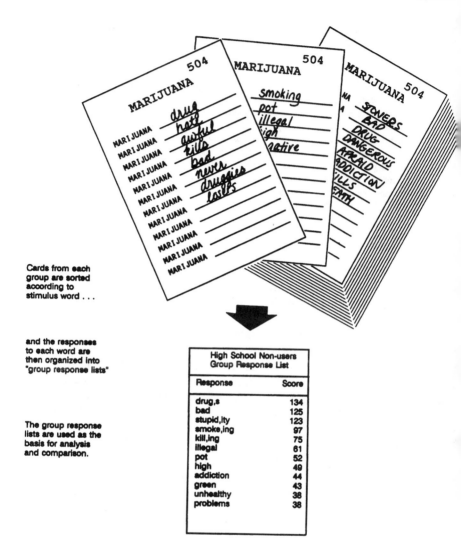

Cards from each group are sorted according to stimulus word . . .

and the responses to each word are then organized into "group response lists"

The group response lists are used as the basis for analysis and comparison.

High School Non-users Group Response List	
Response	Score
drug,s	134
bad	125
stupid,ity	123
smoke,ing	97
kill,ing	75
illegal	61
pot	52
high	49
addiction	44
green	43
unhealthy	38
problems	38

FIGURE A1. Formation of group response lists.

Based on the distribution of hundreds of spontaneous responses, the group response lists offer the main mosaic pieces of the respondent's subjective perceptions and evaluations. Each response has a score value. These values reveal how salient a particular idea or attribute is as a mosaic element of the group's perception of the stimulus word. A comparison of group response lists suggest some characteristic differences in the high school drug users' and nonusers' views. For instance, an in-depth analysis of how these groups view marijuana can be used to trace the effects of perceived harm and risk as factors affecting drug use. As other examples demonstrate, AGA can be used to assess the subjective culture of different social groups by reconstructing their priorities, measuring distances in views, or mapping their cognitive organization.

Comparability of Response Lists

Systematic examination of response lists has shown that every response contains a piece of valid information about the group's characteristic image and understanding of the stimulus theme. Responses with a sizable score value (10 to 15) are rarely accidental. Using conservative estimates, score differences of 18 can be considered significant at the .05 level and score differences of 24 can be considered significant at the .01 level. The wealth of information provided by the group response list is impressive, because even small score differences can have significant implications for communication and behavior (Szalay, Lysne, & Bryson, 1972).

The treatment of the responses is consistent with the conceptualization of subjective meaning or image as a composite of perceptual and evaluative components. The aim is to reconstruct this composite image or meaning in its main components and in their actual salience. In the framework of our analysis, the subjective salience of specific perceptual elements is inferred from the response scores. The more people give a particular response like *harmful,* the greater is the salience of this mosaic element, for instance, in the subjective image of MARIJUANA. To bring together responses that have the same linguistic root but are artificially separated because of different suffixes or prefixes, the response distributions are processed through by a custom-designed editing program. In our effort to achieve a faithful proportionate reconstruction of the group's subjective images or meanings, we rely on all of the shared responses given by the members of a group to a particular issue or theme. The salience of each mosaic element revealed by a particular shared response is revealed by the response score, which is a function of how many people gave this response and with what subjective weight. Along this rationale of proportionate representation, the relative salience of a specific response or of a particular response cluster is not only a function of the absolute score value but depends also on the relationship of the responses to the total score accumulated by all shared responses given to that particular stimulus theme. The same score value shows less salience in the context of a group that produces many responses than in the context of another group that produces fewer responses.

Main Analytic Measures and Procedures

Comparative Imaging

Comparative imaging reveals two or more group's characteristic image or understanding of the stimulus theme, including perceptual and affective details that are frequently unverbalizable and below their level of awareness. A comparison of drug users and nonusers' responses to the stimulus MARIJUANA, for instance, shows that most of the nonuser's high-ranking responses (e.g., *bad, stupid, killing, addiction*) do not even appear on the list of most frequent responses for the drug users (see Figure 2). Similarly, most of the high-ranking responses made by the user group do not immediately occur to the nonusers (e.g., *joint, bong, stoned, fun, friends, laughter*). These lists contain numerous responses that have high scores or salience for one group and low or no salience at all for the other group. A quick glance at the most frequent responses readily reveals that they are not accidental, but deeply rooted in the contemporary experiences of the respective groups.

The group response lists contain a rich variety of responses, each reflecting a different mosaic element of the total image or psychological meaning. Similar responses are grouped together, which helps to identify the main components and

USERS			NONUSERS	
Response	Score		Response	Score
high	141		drug,s	134
smoke,ing	140		bad	125
pot	125		stupid,ity	123
joint,s	86		smoke,ing	97
drug,s	81		kill,ing	75
fun	76		illegal	61
bong,s	59		pot	52
green	58		high	49
weed,s	56		addiction	44
illegal	40		green	43
friend,s	36		unhealthy	38
stone,d	36		problem,s	38
grass	34		danger,ous	37
bowl,s	32		never	31
laugh,ter	32		plant,s	31

Figure A2. 15 top-ranking responses to MARIJUANA by high school drug users and nonusers.

their relative salience. Each category has a score and a label. The category score is the sum of the scores of each subsumed response and expresses the importance of the category for a particular group. If a category yields a high score for a group, it is considered to be an important component of that image or theme for that group. The categories and category scores present a logical set of data from which the

MAIN COMPONENTS AND RESPONSES

	User	Non		User	Non
BAD, STUPID	96	498	ADDICTION, HARMFUL	42	381
bad	30	125	addiction	–	44
stupid,ity	20	123	harm,ful	7	22
dumb	–	18	danger,ous	19	37
never	–	31	unhealthy	–	38
waste,ful	–	12	dead,ly	7	30
not good	–	9	death	–	15
loser,s	–	11	kill,ing	4	75
sad,ness	–	11	sick,ness	5	–
gross	–	30	damage,ing	–	10
scare,d	7	14	hurt,ing	–	10
crazy	11	6	problem,s	–	38
hate,ful	7	22	brain cells	–	6
useless,ness	–	18	pain,ful	–	5
awful	–	10	ruin,ed	–	9
suck,s	–	24	cancer	–	19
trouble	5	9	kills brain	–	14
wrong	6	6	die, dying	–	9
terrible	–	14			
lame	10	–	FUN, GOOD	196	17
don't need	–	5	fun	76	17
			laugh,ter	32	–
SMOKING, JOINT	373	126	good,ness	27	–
smoke,ing	140	97	happy,ness	6	–
joint,s	86	23	enjoy,ment	9	–
toke,ing	9	–	great,est	15	–
reefer	4	–	wild	5	–
bong,s	59	–	help,ing,ed	13	–
pipe,s	29	–	like	13	–
bowl,s	32	–			
taste,ing	6	–			
paper,s	–	6			
light	8	–			

FIGURE A3. MARIJUANA: Selected clusters of responses.

central meaning of the stimulus may be deduced, either directly or through advisors or background literature on the culture of the group.

Using this procedure to analyze the stimulus MARIJUANA, for example, we find that the nonusers' negative references reflect strong disapproval and criticism of marijuana, as well as recognition of the harmful social and health consequences (see Figure 3). These categories barely even occur to the user group. On the other hand, the users' extensive references to different methods of use and types of paraphernalia reflect direct personal experience, whereas the nonusers show only modest familiarity with these aspects. The cluster of positive evaluations reveals that this component is an important part of the users' image of marijuana, but not of the nonusers'. The scores the various components accumulated in this process reflect the subjective salience of each component for the cultural groups compared.

In the case of the responses to MARIJUANA the analysts used 13 categories to identify the salient components of each groups' image of marijuana. Because there is usually a difference between the two groups in their level of responding, the category scores are converted to percentages of the respective total scores in order to make them directly comparable (see Table 1). The main content categories obtained by this analysis describe the total subjective meaning of the theme in terms of the main components characteristic of each group's understanding.

Further examination of Table 1 reveals additional perceptual and motivational trends. For example, the users express considerable awareness of the psychoactive effects of marijuana use such as high, stoned, relaxation, hunger, and so forth.

TABLE 1. Image of MARIJUANA: Main Components of Perceptions and Evaluations Among High School Users and Nonusers

Main components	Percentage of total score	
	Users	Nonusers
POT, PLANT	21	11
SMOKING, JOINT	21	7
EFFECTS: HIGH, STONED	16	6
FUN, GOOD	11	1
PARTY, CONCERT	1	3
ADDICTION, HARMFUL, DEATH	2	21
BAD, STUPID	5	28
SMELL, STINK	1	4
ILLEGAL, POLICE	3	5
DRUGS, ALCOHOL	7	7
MONEY, SELLING	5	2
FRIENDS, DRUGGIES	3	3
MISCELLANEOUS	3	1
Total Scores	1753	1794

They also demonstrate knowledge of the terminology used in buying and selling drugs. In contrast to the users, who show almost no concern with the harmful effects of smoking marijuana, the nonusers are extremely concerned that marijuana can lead to brain damage or even death. The nonusers are more aware of the illegality of marijuana and the legal consequences that can result from its use. The nonusers place slightly more emphasis on the use of marijuana among friends at social gatherings such as parties and concerts.

Another way to present these results of comparative imaging is the semantograph (Figure 4). It shows the main components of the image by using radially arranged bars: the solid dark bars represent the main components of the high school nonusers' image, and the outlined bars show the main components of the users' image. The bars on the left are especially strong (salient) for the users and those on the right are especially strong for the nonusers. This form of presentation helps to recognize components that most distinguish the two groups.

The reliability of this analytic method of comparative imaging was tested by comparing the performance of five judges working independently from each other. The interjudge reliability measured by product-moment correlation across 76 categories was .70. The validity of such inferences on particular single meaning components cannot be directly assessed because simple criterion measures are not available. There are, however, findings that show that the salience of these meaning components provides valid predictions on the meaningfulness of messages in intercultural communications. Communication material that capitalized on salient components of cultural meanings was judged by members of this culture as more meaningful than comparable communication material produced by cultural experts (Szalay et al., 1972).

The analysis of several related concepts within a particular domain (e.g., marijuana, drugs, and alcohol) informs on dominant trends of perceptions and evaluations that set drug users and nonusers clearly apart. The data reflect general trends of perceptions and motivations that reveal psychological factors and dispositions related to substance abuse. The consistency of such trends indicates that the differences observed are not confined to specific isolated images but reflect broader trends characteristic of the frame of reference and cognitive organization of the groups compared. Further analyses can inform on perceptual trends across several domains (i.e., self, family, social values) and reveal important parameters of people's systems of mental representations.

Dominance Measures of Subjective Priorities

In a person's subjective representation of the world some subjects, issues, and ideas play more important roles than others. Drugs may be dominant in the lives of drug users but not in the lives of nonusers. A valuable feature of the AGA method is that

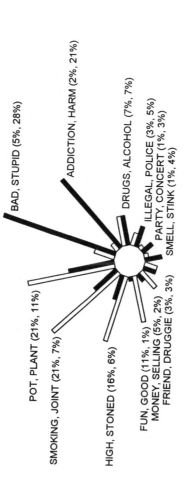

MARIJUANA
Perceptions and Attitudes by High School Drug Users and Nonusers

BAD, STUPID (5%, 28%)

ADDICTION, HARM (2%, 21%)

DRUGS, ALCOHOL (7%, 7%)

ILLEGAL, POLICE (3%, 5%)

PARTY, CONCERT (1%, 3%)

SMELL, STINK (1%, 4%)

POT, PLANT (21%, 11%)

SMOKING, JOINT (21%, 7%)

HIGH, STONED (16%, 6%)

FUN, GOOD (11%, 1%)

MONEY, SELLING (5%, 2%)

FRIEND, DRUGGIE (3%, 3%)

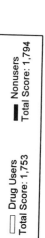

Drug Users
Total Score: 1,753

Nonusers
Total Score: 1,794

FIGURE A4. Image of MARIJUANA presented in semantograph form.

respondents are not *asked* to judge what is important to them. They reveal what is important or dominant to them without being aware that they are doing so by giving many or few responses to a given stimulus theme. We have several individual and group measures of dominance. Through comparisons of Dominance scores of each theme we can determine their ranking of priority within the system of a particular person or group, as well as the differences in priorities between two systems.

The Dominance scores calculated both on an individual and on a group basis are analogous to Noble's (1952) widely tested measure of meaningfulness. (Noble first demonstrated that the number of associations given by a person in a continued association task of one minute provides a measure of "meaningfulness" that is highly correlated with the person's familiarity with the word and its meaning.) Dominance scores have been used to measure differences between groups in their subjective priorities, as well as to trace changes in priorities over time. The group Dominance score is the sum of the scores of all responses elicited by a particular theme or domain by all members of a group. The reliability of the group Dominance score ($r = .93$) was measured by test-retest comparison (Szalay & Bryson, 1973). Individual Dominance scores are computed as the number of responses given to each stimulus theme, which results in a score ranging from 0 to 12. A Dominance Similarity score, calculated on the basis of discriminant function coefficients for the individual Dominance scores, can show whether a person belongs more to a user group or to a nonuser group, or to a pretreatment or posttreatment group. Discriminant function analysis of this measure correctly identified 64% of the respondents in one study as frequent users or nonusers (can. corr. = .33, $x^2 = 45.69$, $p < .005$), and in another study correctly identified 75% of the respondents as pretreatment addicts or posttreatment addicts (can. corr. = .56, $x^2 = 140.36$, p < .001; Szalay, 1990, 1994).

Different social or cultural groups can be compared by looking at their Dominance scores on the same concepts. Dominance scores reveal the subjective importance not only for single issues but also for larger domains of life. Table 2 compares the relative importance of selected themes in four domains of life for three student groups (high school, junior high, and elementary school). The results indicate that the meaningfulness of certain themes grows with age (see Work and Goals domains) whereas other themes show little change in meaningfulness with increased age (see Family domain). Although the subjective importance of school and teacher remains relatively constant, the meaningfulness of authority and discipline in particular grow considerably with age.

Evaluative Dominance: Inferences on Attitudes

Our perception of the environment is loaded with positive and negative evaluations and affects. We see certain elements as desirable and attractive and others as aversive and harmful. Evaluations and affect loading are terms closely synonymous

Table 2. Dominance Scores of High School, Junior High, and Elementary Students

Domain/theme	High school	Junior high	Elemen.	Domain/theme	High school	Junior high	Elemen.
WORK				FAMILY			
work	165	168	141	family	187	160	205
money	185	183	157	mother	165	126	161
help	146	148	101	father	150	158	153
responsibility	159	142	89	respect	150	149	130
Overall mean	164	160	122	Overall mean	163	169	162
GOALS				SCHOOL			
goals	158	136	102	school	191	204	182
happiness	158	152	131	teacher	166	164	169
health	165	156	113	authority	149	145	127
values	152	138	107	discipline	146	131	94
Overall mean	158	146	113	Overall mean	163	161	143

with attitudes, the most widely researched subject area of psychology. As extensive attitude research has demonstrated, affects, positive vs. negative evaluations, are important psychological variables. In our research we use several individual and group based measures of attitudes.

A simple and direct method of assessing connotations or attitudes is to ask the respondents to give a general evaluation of each stimulus word after performing the free association task. To express whether the words mean something positive, negative, or neutral, the respondents use the following scale:

- +3–strongly positive, favorable connotation
- +2–quite positive, favorable connotation
- +1–slightly positive connotation
- 0–neutral (neither positive nor negative conn.)
- −1–slightly negative connotation
- −2–quite negative connotation
- −3–strongly negative connotation

A mean group attitude score is obtained for each stimulus. The attitude scores ranked by greatest difference between high school students in our reference groups of users and nonusers are presented in Table 3. As expected, the nonusers express strongly negative attitudes toward alcohol and other drugs, reflecting the greatest differences between users and nonusers. Another clear distinction is that nonusers are more positive toward themselves as well as toward authority.

How people evaluate images, ideas, and events can be assessed without asking them directly. Attitudinal inferences are derived from the distribution of associative responses with positive, negative, and neutral connotation. Based on empirical evidence that the evaluative content of associative responses is a valid

TABLE 3. Connotation Scores Ranked by Greatest Difference Between High School Users and Nonusers

	Average connotation score		
Theme	Users	Nonusers	Difference
Marijuana	.0	−2.6	2.6
Drugs	−.2	−2.	2.2
Alcohol	.7	−1.1	1.8
Smoking	−.8	−2.2	1.4
School	−.3	1.1	.8
Party	2.2	1.4	.8
Me	1.3	2.0	.8
Authority	−.0	.7	.7
Mother	2.0	2.6	.6
I Am	1.1	1.7	.6
Religion	.7	1.3	.6
Sex	2.3	1.7	.6
Fear	−.8	−1.4	.6
Happiness	2.2	2.7	.5
Discipline	.4	.9	.5

indicator of the evaluative content of the stimulus word (A. Staats & Staats, 1959), we developed an Evaluative Dominance Index (EDI) to express the relative dominance of responses with positive or negative connotations (Szalay, Windle, & Lysne, 1970). (In previous experiments this grouping task was performed with an interjudge agreement of .93 measured by product-moment correlation across categories.) Next, using the total response score for each grouping, an Index of Evaluative Dominance is calculated by the following formula:

$$EDI = \frac{\text{scores of positive responses} - \text{scores of negative responses}}{\text{scores of all responses}} \times 100$$

Based on this formula, group indices are obtained on each stimulus for each group. The distance between groups in their evaluations is measured by comparing EDI scores using Pearson's r. A higher index implies more intense group evaluation, in either a positive or negative direction. The Evaluative Indices produce very high positive correlations of .88 to .91 with independent attitude measures (e.g., semantic differential; Szalay, Windle, & Lysne, 1970).

Another more automated measure of Evaluative Dominance has been developed using reference norms of preassigned positive or negative evaluative scores for each response in the current database. Each response a person gives to a particular theme is assigned an evaluative score (ranging from 1 to 7). The mean evaluative score indicates the degree of positive or negative dominance of a theme (image). This inferential evaluative measure has a score range comparable to the direct connotation measure.

Evaluative scores can also be calculated on an individual basis. Discriminant function analysis of this measure has correctly identified 69% of the respondents in one study as frequent drug users or nonusers (can. corr. = .456, x = 90.94, p < .001) and in another study 77% of the respondents as pretreatment addicts or post-treatment addicts (can. corr. = .62, x = 187.56, p < .001; Szalay, 1990, 1994). An Evaluative Similarity score, calculated on the basis of discriminant function coefficients for the Individual Evaluative Scores, can show whether a person belongs more to a user group or to a nonuser group, or to a pretreatment group or to a post-treatment group on the basis of their attitudes and evaluations.

The Affinity Measure of Relatedness

With the AGA method we have developed several measures of affinity to reconstruct how images are related for one group compared to another. They provide a means for assessing how particular groups organize and interrelate elements of their environment. The Affinity measures indicate which images and themes are related by a group to which other themes and to what extent. The degree of relationship among these elements of a group's subjective world is an important dimension of their cognitive organization.

Similar concepts based on various theoretical positions are: overlap coefficient (Deese, 1962); verbal relatedness (Garskof & Houston, 1963); mutual frequency (Cofer, 1957); co-occurrence measure (J. Flavell & Flavell, 1959); and measure of stimulus equivalence (Bousfield, Whitmarsh, & Danick, 1958). These concepts, however, use single-word associative responses rather than continued associations. One of our measures, the Index of Interword Affinity, is a modified relatedness measure similar to those reviewed by Marshall and Cofer (1963), and it was developed for use with continued associations.

The Index of Interword Affinity (IIA) is defined as the shared associative meaning of stimulus themes as measured by the number of associations produced in common to these words (Szalay & Brent, 1965; Szalay & Bryson, 1974). It measures the relationship of one theme (A) to another (B) for a particular group based on the responses in common to the two themes. The formula for the affinity of theme A to theme B is as follows:

$$\frac{\text{aggregate score for responses in common}}{\text{total score }(A+B)/2} \times 100 = \text{Index of Interword Associative Affinity}$$

Indexes on single word pairs provide empirical data on single relationships; index averages calculated on the affinity of one word with a set of words representing a particular domain have more generality. Indexes calculated between domains may be expected to gauge cognitive organization at an even higher level of generality by revealing how closely interrelated are such areas for a particular group. Advanced statistical methods like factor analysis or multidimensional scaling are used to reconstruct the organization of systems of mental representation.

The reliability of IIA in split-half comparisons was in the range of .90 (Szalay & Windle, 1968). The validity of this measure was estimated in a comparative study based on correlations of this measure with other independent measures: for similarity judgment, $r = .73$; for judgment of relationship, $r = .77$; and for grouping task, $r = .84$ (calculations based on 66 index pairs; Szalay & Bryson, 1972).

Table 4 shows the interrelatedness of two domains of life in the systems of mental representation of users and of nonusers (based on reference groups of 400 college students). For users the domains of Alcohol/Drugs and Entertainment are very closely related, suggesting that among users there is a strong expectation that alcohol and/or drugs will be present in their social life with friends and at parties. The results for nonusers show a very different relationship between these two domains. They see very little relationship between friends and alcohol or other drugs, and getting high is not a part of their idea of having fun. Getting high is strictly a drug concept and does not overlap with their views of friends or entertainment as it does for the users. Following this procedure of calculating the affinity of key concepts representing the various domains of life, it is possible to get a clearer overall picture of the organizational structure within the minds of users and those of nonusers.

TABLE 4. Affinity (Relatedness) of Alcohol/Drugs and Entertainment Domains for College Users and for Nonusers

DOMAINS

	Alcohol		Drunk		Drugs		Mariju.		Friends		Fun		Party		Getting high	
	user	non	user	non	user	non	user	non	usee	non	user	non	user	non	user	non
Alcohol/drugs																
Alcohol			48	44	18	33	20	32	19	5	24	8	35	17	26	31
Drunk					20	29	16	22	21	5	24	10	38	17	26	35
Drugs							35	41	11	3	8	3	16	9	39	42
Marijuana									12	1	11	2	18	6	50	44
Entertainment																
Friends											24	21	26	22	24	5
Fun													40	32	21	7
Party															34	13
Getting high																

A simpler way to measure the interrelatedness of these images as building blocks of the cognitive–semantic representation system is a correlation of the response distribution generated by one group or by another. These *within*-group correlations reveal the internal structure of a system. Correlational measures are also used as a means of measuring of measuring the similarity or distance *between* groups, as discussed next.

Similarity, Distance, and Homogeneity

All of the measures discussed so far were developed for measuring parameters *within* the system of one group or another. We have also developed measures for comparing the similarity or distance of one system to another. Without considering the actual nature of differences one may ask generally to what extent two groups differ in their understanding of a particular image or theme. Free associations offer an empirical answer to this question based on the principle that the closer the agreement between the associations of two groups on a particular theme, the more similar their images and perceptions are; the less agreement, the greater the psychological distance between them.

The Coefficient of Similarity is a measure of the extent to which two groups agree in their perception and understanding of a particular theme, idea, or issue. Similarity in subjective meaning is inferred from the similarity of response distributions measured by Pearson's product-moment correlation. Close similarity (high coefficient) means that the high-frequency responses produced by one group are also high-frequency responses for the other group; similarly, the low-frequency responses produced by one group will generally be the same as those produced by the other group. The scores for the same responses from two groups represent the pairs of observations (x, y) used in this calculation. N represents the number of pairs of observations, that is, the number of word responses used in the calculation of a particular coefficient. The reliability of this group measure based on split-half comparison over 40 themes was .82 (Szalay & Bryson, 1973). The coefficients provide a global measure of the level of similarities and differences without elaborating on the semantic components on which they are based.

Table 5 shows correlations from selected domains based on the responses of students in high school, junior high, and elementary school. In all instances, the least similarity is shown between high school and elementary students, whereas the closest similarity is between high school and junior high students. The junior high and elementary school students show slightly less similarity than the junior high and high school students, reflecting the intermediary position of the junior high group. The least agreement is on concepts such as goals, responsibility, and discipline, themes that also varied considerably in their meaningfulness or dominance for these three groups of students. Although dominance scores in the Family domain were comparable, there appear to be sizable differences in the groups'

TABLE 5. Psychological Similarity between High School, Junior High, and Elementary Students

Domain and theme	H.S. & Jr.High	Jr.High & Elem.	H.S. & Elem.	Domain and theme	H.S. & Jr.High	Jr.High & Elem.	H.S. & Elem.
WORK	r	r	r	FAMILY	r	r	r
work	.92	.86	.75	family	.85	.89	.67
money	.72	.54	.43	mother	.85	.78	.52
help	.84	.75	.63	father	.73	.78	.46
responsibility	.78	.64	.40	respect	.86	.81	.63
Overall mean	.83	.72	.57	Overall mean	.83	.82	.58
GOALS				SCHOOL			
goals	.67	.35	.11	school	.86	.75	.64
happiness	.94	.74	.69	teacher	.74	.69	.53
health	.85	.82	.75	authority	.90	.84	.74
values	.66	.76	.40	discipline	.63	.56	.23
Overall mean	.82	.70	.53	Overall mean	.80	.72	.56

perception of family, particularly between the elementary and the high school students. These findings underscore the differences between the age groups and reflect changes in meaning over time.

The Distance score measures express, by a single numerical value, how far apart individuals or groups are in the images reconstructed by the comparative imaging process. A single measure of distance is the similarity correlation subtracted from 1.00. Another measure of distance is found by calculating the degree of overlap of the response sets from the two groups (i.e., their similarity) and subtracting that number from 100% (perfect) overlap. The larger the Distance score, the more the two groups are different with respect to their subjective reaction to the various stimulus concepts. The Distance measure is inversely related to the degree of similarity of the user and the nonuser responses to the same stimulus concept; the more alike the two groups are, the smaller the distance between them.

The reliability of the Coefficient of Similarity measure was tested by comparing two groups obtained by splitting a larger group randomly into two halves. A comparison resulted in an r of .82, calculated over 40 themes (Szalay & Bryson, 1973).

Behavioral Propensities: Measuring Vulnerability/Resistance to Substance Abuse

Response distributions elicited by themes like ALCOHOL or GETTING HIGH provide the empirical database for reconstructing the respondents' subjective propensities to use or not to use alcohol and other drugs. These propensities vary in their intensity and fall into two major categories: vulnerable to or resistant to substance abuse.

The Vulnerability/Resistance measure provides an innovative assessment of the predominant psychological dispositions for an individual or for a group. This measure is inferential and nontransparent. Rather than asking students directly about their involvement with alcohol and with other harmful substances, this measure is based on an assessment of their psychological dispositions. It relies on the computer-assisted analysis of the hundreds of spontaneous responses elicited from each student to 24 systematically selected themes, from alcohol to party, and from society to discipline. The Vulnerability/Resistance score is derived by giving the student a +1 for every response that is given predominantly by frequent users and −1 for every response that is given predominantly by nonusers; the sum is the final Vulnerability/Resistance score indicating the degree to which the student is more like a user or a nonuser in his or her perceptual dispositions. The Vulnerability/Resistance scores can range from about +50 to −50. The higher the score the higher the student's vulnerability. Conversely, the lower the score the stronger their resistance. Students with scores above zero (positive scores) are identified as vulnerable, having user-type psychological dispositions and students with scores of zero and below (negative scores) are identified as resistant, that is, having nonuser-type dispositions.

The underlying assumption of this measurement is that students with high scores are at greater risk because they are thinking and feeling in ways that are more similar to frequent users than to nonusers. Students with low scores show stronger resistance because they are more like nonusers in their frames of reference.

Validation poses different tasks, depending on the behavior that can serve as the criterion. In our substance abuse prevention research we have used frequency of alcohol and other drug use as the criterion behavior. A simple dichotomous measure based on the Vulnerability/Resistance scores is used as an indicator of the proportion of students having psychological dispositions that are more characteristic of users (respondents with scores above zero) or of nonusers (respondents with Vulnerability/Resistance scores of zero and below).

The 24-theme Vulnerability/Resistance measure based on a student's perceptual similarity to frequent drug and alcohol users or to nonusers consistently shows a strong relationship to behavior (self-reported use). Of the 29,350 students tested to date, we have correctly identified approximately 80% of the abstainers and heavy alcohol and drug users based solely on their perceptual dispositions. Correlation of reported drug use behavior with the Vulnerability/Resistance measure was .50 (with the dichotomous Vulnerability/Resistance measure of user–nonuser type, it was .42, $p < .001$). These findings are of particular importance because they demonstrate that underlying perceptions and attitudes are at the core of people's decisions regarding drug use. They also suggests that a deeper understanding of people's psychological dispositions could be the key to successful proactive prevention. More information on validation can be found in chapters 4, 5, and 6 of this volume.

A Model of Cognitive–Semantic Representations

The analyses performed in these investigations based on many millions of spontaneous reactions are of two main types. They have been discussed under the label of *imaging* (chapters 1–2) and *mapping* (chapters 3–9). The Model of Cognitive–Semantic Representations (Figure 5) is used to illustrate and explain the relationship of these related but independent analytic approaches. The mapping relies predominantly on analyses performed along the vertical dimension of this system. Comparative imaging, which is supportive of program development, has a predominant interest in images, their relationship, and the dispositions they reveal across units of cognitive–semantic representation, characterized primarily by horizontal ties.

Imaging aims to reconstruct selected images of the respondents by their salient perceptions and attitudes. The comparative reconstruction of images held by users and by nonusers is used to identify psychological dispositions that are most instrumental in promoting the observed differences in behavior. The identification of these dispositions is important both in tracing the relevant internal differences and in using them in programs designed to prevent risky, harmful behavior.

Mapping aims to reconstruct the organization of the behavior along select parameters. The analysis can be focused on a number of variables—vulnerability/ resistance, priorities, attitudes/evaluations—depending on the focus of research

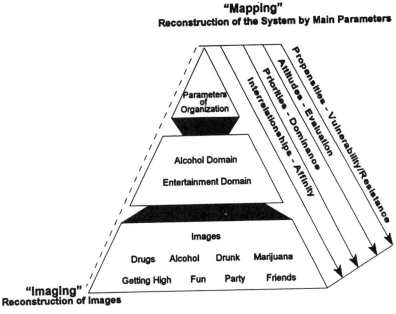

FIGURE A5. Model of cognitive–semantic representations: Sphere of "alcohol, entertainment."

interest. The main parameters used in applications of the AGA method have already been described here.

. Reconstruction of the system involves a systematic use of several analytic procedures and measures depending on the focus and depth of interest. These may range from predominantly diagnostic tasks of assessing vulnerability/resistance and their changes along policy interests, using predominantly the Vulnerability/ Resistance measures. Or they may involve program development taking into consideration the relevant details provided by comparative imaging. In most instances these two interests combine and can be effectively served in a variety of related applications.

Based on our experience with college-level applications in the field of prevention, the above multilevel, multiparameter imaging and mapping strategy offers opportunities to address the specialized interests of planners and educators. In the past we have offered several alternative options to each college (campus-level assessment or assessments focused on select student subpopulations, assessments focused on college climate or on the evaluation of selected activities, etc.). Although in all past applications both imaging- and mapping-based approaches have been used, the focus of interest has shown considerable variation. In a situation where the number of variables affecting substance use is extremely large, systematic identification and targeting of the most influential variables offers many important advantages for making decisions in where to focus attention in the planning of specific prevention programs.

MULTIDISCIPLINARY APPLICATIONS

Since the early 1970s, AGA has proven to be useful research tool in a broad variety of multidisciplinary and multicultural applications. These earlier applications served as the foundation of such instruments as the Environmental Assessment Instrument (EAI) and the Activities Assessment Instrument (AAI) developed for specific applications in substance abuse prevention. Over the years the terminology used in the related disciplines that use free associations have varied and undergone changes as well. Nonetheless our objectives and approach remain the same: to identify dominant perceptual and motivational dispositions that are key to human problems and behavior by reconstructing people's images and by mapping their inner world as the foundation of their behavior. In the following sections we address a few areas of applications that are the most relevant to substance abuse prevention.

Applications Relevant to Cultural Training and Language Instruction

Supported mostly by the U.S. Department of Education, we have produced over a dozen monographs focused on the identification of differences in meanings and cultural frames of reference. These volumes were designed to help overcome cultural differences, the most common causes of poor communication and misunderstandings. Szalay and his associates used the AGA method to create a series of Communication and Culture Guides (Russian, Chinese, Mexican, Middle-Eastern, Korean). Many of these are available through the ERIC system and commercial publications (e.g., Plenum), or in abbreviated form in professional journals dealing with culture and language. These include:

- *Russian-American communication and cultural guide for mutual understanding and cooperation* (1993)
- *American and Chinese public perceptions and belief systems* (1986, 1993)
- *Understanding Mexicans and Americans: Cultural perspectives in conflict* (1991)
- *A Colombian–U.S. communication lexicon of images, meanings, cultural frames of reference* (1982)
- *American, Jordanian, and Other Middle Eastern national perceptions* (1981)
- *Iranian and American perceptions and cultural frames of reference* (1979)
- *Hispanic American cultural frame of reference: A communication guide for use in mental health, education, and training* (1978)
- *Communication lexicon on three South Korea audiences,* 3 volumes (1971–1973)

These crosscultural comparisons were performed by a multidisciplinary group of behavioral scientists who believed that behavior is organized and guided by subjective images and maps—by different representations of reality. Triandis, Vassiliou, and Nassiakov (1968) spoke of a system of cognition that constitutes a map of the ways people conceive their environment. Tolman (1948) describes the maps as guidance or control systems that exert continuous influences on choices and behavior. Models of mental representation include such diverse notions as the cognitive map (Tolman, 1948), cognitive representation (Downs & Stea, 1973), internal representation (Posner & Keele, 1968; Osgood, Suci, & Tannenbaum, 1957), and thought world (Whorf, 1956).

Research Bridging Social, Educational, and Mental Health Problems

The AGA method has been used to promote a better understanding of psychological and cultural differences in a variety of primarily domestic applications as well, including the following work:

- Educational material on African-Americans and Hispanic-Americans to bridge differences in the training of minority populations (National Institute of Mental Health).
- Acculturation of U.S. Naval personnel of Filipino background relevant to job satisfaction and performance (Office of Naval Research).
- U.S.–Korean similarities and differences in population dispositions, community relations for U.S. forces stationed in Korea (ARPA).

- Cultural dispositions of Central American AID trainees (Agency for International Development).
- Population dispositions affecting the delivery of mental health services to Hispanic-American populations: Mexican-Americans, Cubans, and Puerto Ricans (National Institute of Mental Health, National Institute on Drug Abuse).
- Population characteristics and cultural change among Puerto Rican immigrants in the United States (National Institute on Drug Abuse, Department of Justice).
- Training Americans for communications with foreign populations (Department of State, Foreign Service Institute).

These applications are in agreement with the leading contemporary theories of social behavior and social influence. The approaches developed in these contexts represent integrated solutions developed on the basis of our representational theory of behavioral organization integrated with a key tenets of a leading theoretical positions in the field of social behavior. To mention just a few most influential and congenial: the cognitive social learning theory (Bandura, 1977, 1986; Botvin, 1983), the "theory of reasoned action" (Ajzen & Fishbein, 1980), and the "theory of acquired psychological dispositions" (Campbell, 1963).

Substance Abuse, Treatment Research, Prevention Research, and Program Planning and Evaluation

Of special relevance to this present volume are our investigations supported by the National Institute on Drug Abuse, (NIDA) the National Institute on Mental Health, (NIMH) the U.S. Department of Education, and the U.S. Department of Justice. In these projects we used the AGA method to address program planning and evaluation through the development of specific instruments (e.g., the EAI and AAI) adapted to particular tasks and populations. We have already discussed some of them. The publications most relevant to substance abuse include:

Kelly, R. M. (1985). The associative group analysis method and evaluation research. *Evaluation Review, 9,* 35–50.
Szalay, L. B., & Vilov, S. K. (1989). *Charting hidden psychological dispositions: In-depth assessment of perceptions, attitudes, belief systems.* Chevy Chase, MD: Institute of Comparative Social and Cultural Studies.
Szalay, L. B., Strohl, J. B., & Wilson, L. C. (1991). *Adolescent socialization: Changing views related to drug use: Comparison of elementary, junior high, and high school students.* Chevy Chase, MD: RAPPORT, Inc.
Szalay, L. B., Bovasso, G., Vilov, S. K., & Williams, R. (1992). Assessing treatment effects through changes in perceptions and cognitive organization. *American Journal of Drug and Alcohol Abuse, 18,* 407–428.

Szalay, L. B., Vilov, S. K., & Strohl, J. B. (1992). Charting the psychological correlates of drug abuse. In R.R. Watson (Ed.) *Alcohol and drug abuse reviews, Vol 4: Drug abuse treatment.* Totowa, NJ: Humana.

L. B. Szalay, & Vilov, S. K. (1992 to present). *Environmental assessment: The social climate on your campus relevant to substance abuse.* Series of reports, Chevy Chase, MD: Institute of Comparative Social and Cultural Studies.

Szalay, L. B., Canino, G., & Vilov, S. K. (1993). Vulnerabilities and culture change: Drug use among Puerto Rican adolescents in the United States. *The International Journal of the Addictions, 28,* 327–354.

L. B. Szalay, Carroll, J. F. X., & Tims, F. (1993). Rediscovering Free Associations for Use in Psychotherapy. *Psychotherapy, 30* (2), 344–356.

Szalay, L. B., Inn, A., Strohl, J., & Wilson, L. (1993). Perceived harm, age and drug use: Perceptual and motivational dispositions affecting drug use. *Journal of Drug Education, 23* (4), 333–356.

Szalay, L. B. (1996). Socialization into the t.c. culture. In G. DeLeon and F. Tims (Eds.), *Therapeutic Community Research*) National Institute on Drug Abuse Monograph).

Szalay, L. B., Inn, A., & Doherty, K. (1996). Social influences, their role in promoting substance abuse: The effects of the social environment, *Substance Use and Misuse, 31,* 343–373.

Doherty, K., & Szalay, L. B. (1996). Statistical risk versus psychological vulnerability: Why are men at greater risk for substance abuse than women? *Journal of Alcohol and Drug Education, 42,* 57–77.

Work in this field is based on the representational theory of behavioral organization and control. The findings consistently support the central assumption that substance abuse is controlled by the dominant perceptual and motivational dispositions that reflect a person's inner world. Dispositions combine into propensities to use or not to use harmful substances, that is, into a vulnerability or resistance to substance abuse. Identifying the differential propensities and targeting them in systematically designed programs offers a promising approach to substance abuse prevention.

Our research experience of the last decade suggests that, despite some differences, our approach fits well with many of the leading theoretical and practical positions in the substance abuse field. Among the theoretical positions, the most related are Social Problem Theory (R. Jessor & Jessor, 1980), Theory of Drug Subcultures (Johnson, 1980), Theory of Psychogenic and Sociogenic Factors (van Dijk, 1980), and Social Development (Hawkins, Lishner, & Cantalano, 1985), just to mention a few.

In placing social influences in relation to substance use and misuse, the most common topic is peer influence (Flay *et al.,* 1987; Huba & Bentler, 1980; Jessor & Jessor, 1977; Kandel & Andrews, 1987; Novacek, Raskin, & Hogan, 1991). Other social influence studies focus more broadly on the effects of the broad social environments, such as school culture (Berkowitz & Perkins, 1987; Boker, 1974; Burrell, 1990; Perkins & Berkowitz, 1986).

Our approach is in general agreement with the previously discussed positions in recognizing psychological and socioenvironmental factors. However, it differs in two major ways. Conceptually, our approach is guided by a theory of behavioral organization that assumes that in the organization and control of behavior the perceptual and attitudinal dispositions shaped by the respondent's subjective world play a more central and more influential role than is generally recognized. Methodologically, this leads us to place special emphasis on the reconstruction of dominant perceptions and motivations, which can vary from person to person as well as from group to group. Compared to mainstream social psychology, the difference lies in the distinction between perceptions and motivations of which people are aware and those that are below their conscious awareness. This distinction emerges from the field of cognitive psychology.

References

Adolphs, R. (1993). Bilateral inhibition generates neuronal responses tuned to interaural level differences in the auditory brainstem of the barn owl. *The Journal of Neuroscience, 13,* 3647–3668.

Aguilar, E., Narvaez, A., & Samaniego, N. (1990). *La farmaco-dependica en el Ecuador.* Ministerio de Salud Pública. UNFDAC.

Ajzen, I., & Fishbein, M. (1980). *Understanding attitudes and predicting social behavior.* Englewood Cliffs, NJ: Prentice-Hall.

Almeida-Filho, N., Sousa Santana, V., Matos Pinto, L., & Carvalho-Neto., J. A. (1991). Is there an epidemic of drug misuse in Brazil? A review of the epidemiologic evidence (1977–1988). *International Journal of Addictions, 26(3),* 355–369.

Alvy, K. T. (1987). *Black parenting: Strategies for training.* New York: Irving Publishers, Inc.

Alvy, K. T. (1994). *Parent training today: A social necessity.* Studio City, CA: Center for the Improvement of Child Caring.

Anthony, J. C., & Helzer, J. E. (1991). Syndromes of drug abuse and dependence. In L. Robins & D. Regier. (Eds.), *Psychiatric disorders in America* (pp. 116–154). New York: The Free Press.

Bachman, J. G., Johnston, L. D., & O'Malley, P. M. (1991). How changes in drug use are linked to perceived risks and disapproval: Evidence from national studies that youth and young adults respond to information about the consequences of drug use. In L. Donehew, H. E. Sypher, & W. J. Bukoski (Eds.), *Persuasive communication and drug abuse prevention* (pp. 133–155). Hillsdale, NJ: Lawrence Erlbaum Associates.

Bachman, J. G., Johnston, L. D., O'Malley, P. M., & Humphrey, R. H. (1988). Explaining the recent decline in marijuana use: Differentiating the effects of perceived risks, disapproval, and general lifestyle factors. *Journal of Health and Social Behavior, 29,* 92–112.

Bachman, J. G., O'Malley, P. M., & Johnston, L. D. (1984). Drug use among young adults: The impacts of role status and social environments. *Journal of Personality and Social Psychology, 47,* 629–645.

Bahr, S. J., Marcos, A. C., & Maughan, S. L. (1995). Family, educational and peer influences on the alcohol use of female and male adolescents. *Journal of Studies on Alcohol, 56,* 457–469.

Banaji, M. R., & Greenwald, A. G. (1994). Implicit stereotyping and unconscious prejudice. In M. P. Zanna & J. M. Olson (Eds.), *The psychology of prejudice, the Ontario symposium* (vol. 7, pp. 55–76). Hillsdale, NJ: Erlbaum.

Bandura, A. (1973). *Aggression: A social learning analysis.* Englewood Cliffs, NJ: Prentice-Hall.

Bandura, A. (1917). *Social learning theory.* Englewood Cliffs, NJ: Prentice-Hall.

Bandura, A. (1986). *Social foundations of thought and action: A social cognitive theory.* Englewood Cliffs, NJ: Prentice-Hall.

Bandura, A. (1992). Social cognitive theory of social referencing. In S. Feinman (Ed.), *Social referencing and the social construction of reality in infancy* (pp. 175–208). New York: Plenum Press.

Bandura, A., Ross, D., & Ross, S. (1961). Transmission of aggression through imitation of aggressive models. *Journal of Abnormal and Social Psychology, 63,* 575–582.

Barnes, G. M., Farrell, M. P., & Banerjee, S. (1994). Family influences on alcohol abuse and other problem behaviors among black and white adolescents in a general population sample. Special issue: Preventing alcohol abuse among adolescents: Preintervention and intervention research. *Journal of Research on Adolescence, 4,* 183–201.

Benedict, R. (1935). *Patterns of culture.* London: Routledge.

Benthin, A., Slovic, P., Moran, P., Severson, H., Mertz, C. K., & Gerrard, M. (1995). Adolescent health-threatening and health enhancing behaviors: A study of word association and imagery. *Journal of Adolescent Health, 17,* 143–152.

Berkowitz, A. D., & Perkins, H. W. (1987). Recent research on gender differences in collegiate alcohol use. *Journal of American College Health, 36,* 123–129.

Berry, D. C., & Dienes, Z. (1993). *Implicit learning: Theoretical and empirical issues.* Hove, England: Erlbaum.

Berry, J., Trimble, J. E., & Olmedo, E. (1986). Assessment of acculturation. In W. J. Lonner and J. W. Berry (Eds.), *Field methods in cross-cultural research* (pp. 291–324). Newbury Park, CA: Sage.

Bettes, B. A., Dusenbury, L., Kerner, J., James-Ortiz, S., & Botvin, G. J. (1990). Ethnicity and psychosocial factors in alcohol and tobacco use in adolescence. *Child Development, 61,* 557–565.

Black, M. (1973). Belief systems. In J. J. Honigmann (Ed.), *Handbook of social and cultural anthropology.* Chicago: Rand McNally.

Black, G. S. (1991). Changing attitudes toward drug use: The effects of advertising. In L. Donehew, H. E. Sypher, & W. J. Bukoski (Eds.), *Persuasive communication and drug abuse prevention* (pp. 157–191). Hillsdale, NJ: Lawrence Erlbaum Associates.

Boker, L. H. (1974). Student drug use and the perceived peer drug environment. *International Journal of Addictions, 9,* 851–861.

Booth, M. W., Castro, F. G., & Anglin, M. D. (1990). What do we know about Hispanic substance abuse? A review of the literature. In, R. Glick and J. Moore (Eds.), *Drugs in Hispanic communities.* New Brunswick, N.J.: Rutgers University Press.

Botvin, G. J. (1983). Prevention of adolescent substance abuse through the development of personal and social competence. In T. J. Glynn, C. G. Leukefeld, & J. P. Ludford (Eds.), *Preventing adolescent drug abuse: Intervention strategies* (Research Monograph 47) (pp. 115–140). Rockville, MD: National Institute on Drug Abuse.

Bousfield, W. A., Whitmarsh, G. A., & Danick, J. J. (1958). Partial response identities in verbal generalization. *Psychological Reports, 4,* 703–713.

Brook, J. S., Cohen, P., Whiteman, M., & Gordon, A. S. (1992). Psychosocial risk factors in the transition from moderate to heavy use or abuse of drugs. In M. D. Glantz & R. Pickens (Eds.), *Vulnerability to drug abuse* (pp. 359–388). Washington, DC: American Psychological Association.

Braucht, G. N., Brakarsh, D., Follingstad, D., & Berry, K. L. (1973). Deviant drug use in adolescence: A review of psychosocial correlates. *Psychological Bulletin, 79,* 92–109.

Brunswick, A. F., Messeri, P. A., & Titus, S. P. (1992). Predictive factors in adult substance abuse: A prospective study of African American adolescents. In, M. D. Glantz and R. Pickens (Eds.), *Vulnerability to drug abuse* (pp. 419–472). Washington, DC: American Psychological Association.

Buckhalt, J. A., Halpin, G., Noel, R., & Meadows, M. E. (1992). Relationship of drug use to involvement in school, home and community activities: Results of a large survey of adolescents. *Psychological Reports, 70,* 139–146.

Burnam, A. (1989). Prevalence of alcohol abuse and dependence among Mexican-Americans and Non-Hispanic Whites in the community. In D. L. Spilgler, D. A. Tate, S. S. Aitken, & C. M. Christian (Eds.), *Alcohol use among U. S. ethnic minorities* (NIAAA Research Monograph 18; DHHS Publication ADM 88–1435). Washington, DC: U. S. Government Printing Office.

Burrell, L. F. (1990). College students' recommendations to combat abusive drinking habits. *Journal of College Student Development, 31,* 562–563.

Caetano, R. (1984). Self-reported intoxication among Hispanics in northern California. *Journal of Studies on Alcohol, 45,* 349–354.

Campbell, D. (1963). Social attitudes and other acquired behavioral dispositions. In S. Koch (Ed.), *Psychology: A study of a science,* (vol. 6). New York: McGraw-Hill.

Canino, G., Anthony, J. C., Freeman, D., Shrout, P., & Rubio-Stipec, M., (1993). Drug abuse and illicit drug use in Puerto Rico. *Am I Public Health, 83*(2), 194–200.

Canino, G., Burnam, A., & Caetano, T. (1992). The prevalence of alcohol abuse and/or dependence in two Hispanic communities. In J. Helzer & G. Canino (Eds.), *Alcoholism-North America, Europe, and Asia: A coordinated analyses of population from ten regions* (131–158). New York: Oxford University Press.

Carlini-Cotrim, B., & Aparecida de Carvalho, V. (1993). Extracurricular activities: Are they an effective strategy against drug consumption? *Journal of Drug Education, 23,* 97–104.

Cervantes, R. C., Padilla, A. M., & Salgado de Snyder, V. N. (1990). Reliability and validity of the Hispanic Stress Inventory. *Hispanic Journal of Behavioral Sciences, 12,* 76–82.

Cochran, J. K. (1993). The variable effects of religiosity and denomination on adolescent self-reported alcohol use by beverage type. *Journal of Drug Issues, 23,* 479–491.

Cofer, C. N. (1957). Associative commonality and ranked similarity of certain words from Haagen's list. *Psychological Reports, 3,* 603–606.

Constantino, G., Malgady, R. G., & Rogler, L. H. (1988). *TEMAS* (Tel-Me-A-Story). Los Angeles: Western Psychological Services.

Coombs, R. H., Paulson, M. J., & Richardson, M. A. (1991). Peer vs. parental influence in substance use among Hispanic and Anglo children and adolescents. *Journal of Youth and Adolescence, 20,* 73–88.

Cooper, L., Russell, M., Skinner, J. B., Frone, M. R., & Mudar, P. (1992). Stress and alcohol use: The moderating effects of gender, coping, and alcohol expectancies. *Journal of Abnormal Psychology, 101,* 139–154.

Critchlow, B. (1986). Beliefs about the effects of alcohol on social behavior. *American Psychology, 41,* 751–764.

Cuellar, I., Harris, L. C., & Jasso, R. (1980). An acculturation scale for Mexican American normal and clinical populations. *Hispanic Journal of Behavioral Sciences, 2,* 199–217.

Damasio, A. R. (1994). *Descartes' error: Emotion, reason, and the human brain.* New York: Avon Books.

Damasio, A. R., & Damasio, H. (1993). Cortical systems underlying knowledge retrieval: Evidence from human lesion studies. In *Exploring brain functions: Models in neuroscience* (pp. 233–248). New York: Wiley and Sons.

Deese, J. (1962). Form-class and the determinants of association. *Journal of Verbal Learning and Verbal Behavior, 1,* 79–84.

Deese, J. (1965). *The structure of associations in language and thought.* Baltimore, MD: John Hopkins Press.

Dennett, D. (1991). *Consciousness explained.* Boston: Little, Brown.

Deykin, E. Y., Levy, J. C., & Wells, V. (1987). Adolescent depression, alcohol and drug abuse. *American Journal of Public Health, 77,* 178–182.

Diaz-Guerrero, R., & Szalay, L. B. (1991). *Understanding Mexicans and Americans: Cultural perspectives in conflict.* New York: Plenum Press.

Diem, E., McKay, L. C., & Jamieson, J. L. (1994). Female adolescent alcohol, cigarette, and marijuana use: Similarities and differences in patterns of use. *International Journal of the Addictions, 29,* 987–997.

Doherty, K., & Szalay, L. B. (1996). Statistical risk versus psychological vulnerability: Why are men at greater risk for substance abuse than women? *Journal of Alcohol and Drug Education, 42,* 57–77.

Downs, R. M., & Stea, D. (1973). *Image and environment: Cognitive mapping and spacial behavior.* Chicago, IL: Aldine.

Duncan, S. C., & Duncan, T. E. (1994). Modeling incomplete longitudinal substance use data using latent variable growth curve methodology. *Multivariate Behavioral Research, 29,* 313–338.

Eagly, A. H. (1987). *Sex differences in social behavior: A social-role interpretation.* Hillsdale, NJ: Lawrence Erlbaum Associates.

Eagly, A. H., & Johnson, B. T. (1990). Gender and leadership style: A meta-analysis. *Psychological Bulletin, 108,* 233–256.

Eagly, A. H., & Steffen, V. J. (1986). Gender and aggressive behavior: A meta-analytic review of the social psychological literature. *Psychological Bulletin, 100,* 309–330.

Edwards, W. (1961). Behavioral decision theory. *Annual Review of Psychology, 12,* 473–498.

Elliott, D. S., Huizinga, D., & Menard, S. (1989). *Multiple problem youth: Delinquency, substance use, and mental health problems.* New York: Springer-Verlag.

Engs, R. C., & Hanson, D. J. (1985). The drinking patterns and problems of college students: 1983. *Journal of Alcohol and Drug Education, 31,* 65–83.

Epstein, J. S., Botvin, G. J., Diaz, T., & Schinke, S. P. (1995). The role of social factors and individual characteristics in promoting alcohol use among inner-city minority youths. *Journal of Studies on Alcohol. 56,* 39–46.

Feigelman, W., & Lee, J. A. (1995). Patterns of cigarette use among black and white adolescents. *American Journal on Addictions, 4,* 215–225.

Flavell, J. H. & Flavell, E. R. (1959). One determinant of judged semantic and associative connection between words. *Journal of Experimental Psychology, 63,* 159–165.

Flay, B. R., Hansen, W. B., Johnson, C. A., Collins, L. M., Dent, C. W., Dwyer, K. M., Hocksteth, G., Grossman, L., Rauch, J., Sobal, D. F., Sussman, S. Y., & Ulene, A. (1987). Implementation effectiveness trial of a social influences smoking prevention program using schools and television. *Health Education Research 2,* 385–400.

Forman, S. G., & Linney, J. A. (1991). School-based social and personal coping skills training. In L. Donehew, H. E. Sypher, & W. J. Bukoski (Eds.), *Persuasive communication and drug abuse prevention* (pp. 263–282). Hillsdale, NJ: Lawrence Erlbaum Associates.

Frank, B., Schmeidler, J., Marel, R., & Maranda, M. (1988). Illicit substance use among Hispanic adults in New York State. In New York Statewide Household Survey of Substance Abuse, 1986.

Franzoi, S. L. (1996). *Social psychology.* Dubuque, IA: Brown & Benchmark.

Free, M. D. (1994). Religiosity, religious conservatism, bonds to school, and juvenile delinquency among three categories of drug users. *Deviant Behavior, 15,* 151–170.

Fritner, M. P., & Rubinson, L. (1993). Acquaintance rape: The influence of alcohol, fraternity membership, and sports team membership. *Journal of Sex Education and Therapy, 19,* 272–284.

Garskof, B. E. & Houston, J. P. (1963). Measurement of verbal relatedness: An idiographic approach. *Psychological Review, 70,* 277–288.

Gergen, K. J. (1985). The social constructionist movement in modern psychology, *American Psychologist, 40(3),* 266–275.

Gfroerer, J., & de la Rosa, M. (1993). Protective and risk factors associated with drug use among Hispanic youth. *Journal of Addictive Diseases, 12,* 87–107.

Glantz, M. D., & Pickens, R. (1992). *Vulnerability to drug abuse.* Washington, DC: American Psychological Association.

Goldman, M. S., Brown, S. A., & Christiansen, B. A. (1987). Expectancy theory: Thinking about drinking. In H. T. Blane & K. E. Leonard (Eds.), *Psychological theories of drinking and alcoholism* (pp. 181–226). New York: Guilford Press.

Goldman, M. S., Brown, S. A., Christiansen, B. A., & Smith, G. T. (1991). Alcoholism and memory broadening the scope of alcohol-expectancy research. *Psychological Bulletin, 110,* 137–146.

Goodwin, L. (1990). Social psychological bases for college alcohol consumption. *Journal of Alcohol and Drug Education, 36,* 83–95.

Goree, C. T., & Szalay, L. B. (1996). *Rethinking the campus environment: A guide for substance abuse prevention.* Newton, MA: Higher Education Center for Alcohol and Other Drug Prevention.

Graf, P., & Schacter, D. L. (1987). Selective effects of interference on implicit and explicit memory for new associations. *Journal of Experimental Psychology: Learning, Memory, and Cognition, 13,* 45–53.

Greenwald, A. G. (1990). What cognitive representations underlie social attitudes? *Bulletin of the Psychonomic Society, 35,* 603–618.

Greenwald, A. G., & Banaji, M. R. (1995). Implicit social cognition: Attitudes, self-esteem, and stereotypes. *Psychological Review, 102,* 4–27.

Hagan, J. (1989) *Structural criminology.* New Brunswick, NJ: Rutgers University Press.

Hall, E. T. (1959). *The silent language.* Garden City, NY: Doubleday and Co.

Hall, E. T. (1966). *The hidden dimension.* Garden City, N.Y.: Doubleday and Co.

Hardert, R. A., & Dowd, T. J. (1994). Alcohol and marijuana use among high school and college students in Phoenix, Arizona: A test of Kandel's socialization theory. *International Journal of the Addictions, 29,* 887–912.

Hawkins, J. D., Abbott, R., Catalano, R. F., & Gillimore, M. R. (1991). Assessing effectiveness of drug abuse prevention: Implementation issues relevant to long-term effects and replication. In C. G. Leukefeld & W. J. Bukoski (Eds.), *Drug abuse prevention intervention research: Methodological issues* (Research Monograh 107) (pp. 195–212). Rockville, MD: National Institute on Drug Abuse.

Hawkins, J. D., Lishner, D. M., & Catalano, R. F. Jr. (1985). Childhood predictors and the prevention of adolescent substance abuse. In C. L. Jones & R. J. Battjes (Eds.), *Etiology of drug abuse: Implications for prevention* (Research Monograph 56) (pp. 75–126). Rockville, MD: National Institute on Drug Abuse.

Hawkins, J. D., & Weis, J. G. (1985). The social development model: An integrated approach to delinquency prevention. *Journal of Primary Prevention, 6,* 73–97.

Helzer, J. & Canino, G. (1992). Comparative analysis of alcoholism in ten cultural regions. In J. Helzer & G. Canino (Eds.), *Alcoholism in North America, Europe and Asia* (pp. 289–308). New York: Oxford University Press.

Helzer, J. E., & Pryzbeck, T. R. (1988). The co-occurrence of alcoholism with other psychiatric disorders in the general population and its impact on treatment. *Journal of Studies on Alcohol, 43,* 497–516.

Henrion, M., & Fischoff, B. (1986). Uncertainty assessment in the estimation of physical constants. *American Journal of Physics, 54,* 791–798.

Hirschi, T. (1969). *Criminology of delinquency.* Berkeley, CA: University of California Press.

Hofstede, G. (1980). *Culture's consequences: International differences in work-related values.* Beverly Hills, CA: Sage.

Hofstede, G. (1990). *Culture's consequences.* Beverly Hills, CA: Sage Publications.

Hopfield, J. J. & Tank, D. W. (1986). Computing with neural circuits: A model. *Science, 233,* 625–633.

Hsu, F. L. K. (1961). *Psychological anthropology.* Homewood, Illinois: Dorsey.

Hsu, F. L. K. (1981). *Americans and Chinese: Passage to differences.* Honolulu: University of Hawaii Press.

Huba, G., & Bentler, P. M. (1980). The role of peer and adult models for drug taking at different stages in adolescence. *Journal of Youth Adolescence, 9,* 449–465.

Huba, G. J., Wingard, J. A., & Bentler, P. M. (1980). Longitudinal analysis of the role of peer support, adult models, and peer subcultures in beginning adolescent substance use: An application of setwise canonical correlation methods. *Multivariate Behavioral Research, 15,* 259–279.

Hyde, J. S., (1984). How large are gender differences in aggression? A developmental meta-analysis. *Developmental Psychology, 20,* 722–736.

Jacob, T., & Leonard, K. (1994). Family and peer influences in the development of adolescent alcohol abuse. In R. Zucker, G. Boyd, & J. Howard (Eds.), *The development of alcohol problems: Exploring the biopsychosocial matrix of risk.* (Research Monograph 26) (pp. 123–155). Rockville, MD: National Institute on Alcohol Abuse and Alcoholism.

Jacoby, L. L., Lindsay, D. S., & Toth, J. P. (1992). Unconscious influences revealed: Attention, awareness, and control. *American Psychologist, 47,* 802–809.

Jessor, R., & Jessor, S. L. (1973). Adolescent development and the onset of drinking: A longitudinal study. *Journal of Studies in Alcohol, 36,* 27–51.

Jessor, R., & Jessor, S. L. (1977). *Problem behavior and psychosocial development: A longitudinal study of youth.* New York: Academic Press.

Jessor, R., & Jessor, S. L. (1978). Theory testing in longitudinal research on marijuana use. In D. Kandel (Ed.), *Longitudinal research on drug use.* Washington, D.C.: Hemisphere Publishing Corporation.

Jessor, R., & Jessor, S. L. (1979). Marijuana: A review of recent psychosocial research. In R. L. Dupont, A. Goldstein, & J. O'Donnell (Eds.), *Handbook on drug use.* Rockville, MD: NIDA.

Jessor, R., & Jessor, S. (1980). A social–psychological framework for studying drug use. In D. Lettieri, M. Sayers, and H. W. Pearson (Eds.), *Theories on drug abuse: Selected contemporary perspectives* (vol. 30, pp. 102–119). NIDA Research Monograph.

Johnson, B. D. (1980). Toward a theory of drug subcultures. In D. Lettieri, M. Sayers, and H. W. Pearson (Eds.), *Theories on drug abuse: Selected contemporary perspectives* (vol. 30, pp. 110–119). NIDA Research Monograph.

Johnston, L., Bachman, J., & O'Malley, P. (1989). Drug Use, Drinking, and Smoking: National Survey Results from High School, College, and Young Adult Populations 1975–1988. Washington, DC: Government Printing Office.

Johnston, L., O'Malley, P., & Bachman, J. (1996). *National survey results on drug use from the Monitoring the Future Study,* 1975–1995. Volume I: Secondary school students (NIH Pub. No. 974139). Rockville, MD: National Institute on Drug Abuse.

Jones, E. G., & Powell, T. P. S. (1970). An anatomical study of converging sensory pathways within the cerebral cortex of the monkey, *Brain, 93,* 793–820.

Kahneman, D., Slovic, P., & Tversky, A. (Eds.; 1982). *Judgement under uncertainty: Heuristics and biases.* New York: Cambridge University Press.

Kandel, D. B. (1980). Drug and drinking behavior among youth. *Annual Review of Sociology 6,* 235–285.

Kandel, D. B. (1982). Epidemiological and psychosocial perspectives on adolescent drug use. *Journal of American Academic Clinical Psychiatry, 21,* 328–347.

Kandel, D. B. (1985). On processes of peer influences in adolescent drug use: A developmental perspective. *Advances in Alcohol and Substance Abuse, 4*(3–4), 139–163.

Kandel, D. B., & Andrews, K. (1987). Processes of adolescent socialization by parents and peers. *International Journal of Addictions, 22*(4), 319–342.

Kandel, D., Simch-Fagan, O., & Davies, M. (1986). Risk factors for delinquency and illicit drug use from adolescence to young adulthood. *Journal of Drug Issues, 16*(1), 67–90.

Kandel, D. B., & Yamaguchi, K. (1985). Developmental patterns of the use of legal, illegal, and medically prescribed psychotropic drugs from adolescence to young adulthood. In C. L. Jones & R. J. Battjes (Eds.), *Etiology of drug abuse: Implications for prevention* (Research Monograph 56) (pp. 193–235). Rockville, MD: National Institute on Drug Abuse.

Kaplan, H. B. (1975). Increasing self-rejection as a antecedent of deviant response. *Journal of Youth and Adolescence, 4,* 281–292.

Kaplan, H. B. (1980). Self-esteem and self-derogation theory of drug abuse. In D. J. Lettieri, M. Sayers, & H. W. Pearson (Eds.), *Theories on drug abuse: Selected contemporary perspectives* (Research Monograph 30). Rockville, MD: National Institute on Drug Abuse.

Kaplan, H. B. (1982). Self-attitudes and deviant behavior: New directions for theory and research. *Youth and Society, 14,* 185–211.

Kaplan, H. B., & Johnson, R. (1992) Relationships between circumstances surrounding initial illicit drug use and escalation of drug use: Moderating effects of gender and early adolescent experiences. In M. D. Glantz & R. Pickens (Eds.), *Vulnerability to drug abuse* (pp. 299–352). Washington, DC: American Psychological Association.

Keefe, K. (1994). Perceptions of normative social pressure and attitudes toward alcohol use: Changes during adolescence. *Journal of Studies on Alcohol, 55,* 46–54.

Kellam, S. G., Stevenson, D. L., & Rubin, B. R. (1982). How specific are the early predictors of teenage drug use? In L. S. Harris (Ed.), *Problems of drug dependence.* Rockville, MD: National Institute of Drug Abuse.

Kelly, R. M. (1985). The associative group analysis method and evaluation research. *Evaluation Research, 9,* 35–50.

Kelly, R. M., & Szalay, L. B. (1972). The impact of a foreign culture: South Koreans in America. In R. L. Merritt (Ed.), *Communications in international politics.* Urbana, IL: University of Illinois Press.

Klein, H. (1992). College students' attitudes toward the use of alcoholic beverages. *Journal of Alcohol and Drug Education, 37,* 35–52.

Klor de Alva, J. J. (1988). Telling Hispanics apart: Latin sociocultural diversity. In E. Acosta-Belen & B. R. Sjostrom (Eds.), *The Hispanic experience in the United States* (pp. 107–136). New York: Praeger.

Kluckhohn, C. (1959). *The scientific study of values.* In University of Toronto Installation Lectures. Toronto: University of Toronto Press.

Kluckhohn, F. R., & Strodtbeck, F. L. (1961). *Variations in value orientations.* Westport, CT.: Greenwood.

Konishi, M., Takahashi, T., Wagner, H., Sullivan, W. E., & Carr, C. E. (1988). Neurophysiological and anatomical substrates of sound localization in the owl. In G. Edelmen, W. Gall, & W. Cowan (Eds.), *Auditory function* (pp. 721–746). New York: John Wiley & Sons.

Kosslyn, S. M., Alpert, N. M., Thompson, W. L., Maljkovic, V., Weise, S. B., Chabris, C. F., Hamilton, S. E., Rauch, S. L., & Buonanno, F. S. (1993). Visual mental imagery activates topographically organized visual cortex: PET investigations. *Journal of Cognitive Neuroscience, 5,* 263–287.

Kuh, G. D., & Arnold., J. C. (1993). Liquid bonding: A cultural analysis of the role of alcohol in fraternity pledgeship. *Journal of College Student Development, 34,* 327–334.

Kumpfer, K. L. (1989). Prevention of alcohol and drug abuse: A critical review of risk factors and prevention strategies. In D. Shaffer, I. Philips, & N. B. Enzer (Eds.), *Prevention of mental disorders, alcohol and other drug use in children and adolescents* (Prevention Monograph 2) (pp. 309–371). Rockville, MD: Office for Substance Abuse Prevention.

Lettieri, D. J., Sayer, M., & Pearson, H. W. (Eds.; 1980). *Theories on drug abuse: Selected contemporary perspectives.* (Research Monongraph 30). Rockville, MD: National Institute of Drug Abuse.

Lewin, K. (1951). *Field theory in social science.* New York: Harper.

Lewis, O. (1966). *La vida.* New York: Vintage Books.

Lo, C. C., & Globetti, G. (1995). The facilitating and enhancing roles Greek associations play in college drinking. *International Journal of Addictions, 30,* 1311–1322.

Madianos, M. G., Gefou, M. D., Richardson, C., & Stefanis, C. N. (1995). Factors affecting illicit and licit drug use among adolescents and young adults in Greece. *Acta Psychiatrica Scandinavica, 91,* 258–264.

Maggs, J. L., Almeida, D. M, & Galambos, N. L. (1995). Risky business: The paradoxical meaning of problem behavior for young adolescents. Special section: Canadian research. *Journal of Early Adolescence, 15,* 344–362.

Malinowski, B. (1944). *A scientific theory of culture and other essays.* Chapel Hill, NC: University of North Carolina Press.

Maney, D. W. (1990). Predicting university students' use of alcoholic beverages. *Journal of College Student Development, 31*, 23–32.

Marlat, G. A. (1987). Alcohol, the magic elixir: Stress, expectancy, and the transformation of emotional states. In E. Gottheil, K. A. Druly, S. Pashko, & S. P. Weinstein (Eds.), *Stress and addiction* (pp. 302–322). New York: Brunner and Mazel.

Marshall, G. R., & Cofer, C. N. (1963). Associative indices as measures of word-relatedness: A summary and comparison of ten methods. *Journal of Verbal Learning and Verbal Behavior, 1*, 408–21.

Martin, E., & Sher1 K. J. (1994). Risk for alcoholism, alcohol use disorders, and the five-factor model of personality. *Journal of Studies on Alcohol, 55*, 81–90.

Martinez, J. L. (1977). *Chicano psychology.* New York: Academic Press.

Masson, M. (1995). A distributed memory model of semantic priming. *Journal of Experimental Psychology: Learning, Memory, and Cognition, 21*, 3–23.

Mausner, S., & Kramer, S. (1985). *Epidemiology: An introductory text.* Philadelphia: Saunders.

McGee, L., & Newcomb, M. D. (1992). General deviance syndrome: Expanded hierarchical evaluations at four ages from early adolescence to adulthood. *Journal Consultant of Clinical Psychology, 60*(5), 766–776.

McGue, M., (1994). Genes, environment, and the etiology of alcoholism. In R. Zucker, G. Boyd, & J. Howard (Eds.), *The development of alcohol problems: Exploring the biopsychosocial matrix of risk.* (Research Monograph 26) (pp. 1–40). Rockville, MD: National Institute on Alcohol Abuse and Alcoholism.

McHugh, M. C., Koeske, R. D., & Frieze, I. H. (1986). Issues to consider in conducting nonsexist psychological research: A guide for researchers. *American Psychologist, 41*, 879–890.

Mead, M. (1928). *Coming of age in Samoa.* New York: Morrow.

Mead, M. (1953). *Cultural patterns and technical change.* Paris: United Nations Educational, Scientific and Cultural Organizations.

Miller, W. (1977). *Manual for the description instruments used in a research project on the psychological aspects of fertility behavior in women.* Unpublished manuscript. Palo Alto, CA: American Institutes for Research-Transnational Family Research Institute.

Montgomery, R. L., Benedicto, J. A., & Haemmerlie, F. M. (1993). Personal vs. social motivations of undergraduates for using alcohol. *Psychological Reports, 73*, 960–962.

Negy, C., & Woods, D. J. (1992). The importance of acculturation in understanding research with Hispanic-Americans. *Hispanic Journal of Behavioral Sciences, 14*, 224–227.

Nelson, D. L., Schreiber, T. A., & McEvoy, C. L. (1992). Processing implicit and explicit representations. *Psychological Review, 99*, 322–348.

Newcomb, M. D., & Felix-Ortiz, M. (1992). Multiple protective and risk factors for drug use and abuse: Cross-sectional and prospective findings. *Journal of Personality and Social Psychology, 63*, 280–296.

Newlin, D. B. (1994). Alcohol challenge in high-risk individuals. In R. Zucker, G. Boyd, & J. Howard (Eds.), *The development of alcohol problems: Exploring the biopsychosocial matrix of risk.* (Research Monograph 26) (pp. 47–68). Rockville, MD: National Institute on Alcohol Abuse and Alcoholism.

Newlin, D. B., & Thomson, J. B. (1990). Alcohol challenge with sons of alcoholics: A critical review and analysis. *Psychological Bulletin, 108*, 383–402.

Nisbett, R. E., & Wilson, T. D. (1977). Telling more than we know: Verbal reports on mental processes. *Psychological Review, 84*, 231–259.

Noble, C. E. (1952). An analysis of meaning. *Psychology Review, 54*, 421–4401.

Novacek, J., Raskin, R., & Hogan, R. (1991). Why do adolescents use drugs? Age, sex, and use differences. *Journal of Youth Adolescence, 20*(5), 475–491.

Osgood, C. E., Suci, G. J., & Tannenbaum, P. H. (1957). *The measurement of meaning.* Urbana, IL: University of Illinois Press.

References

Padilla, A. M. (1980). The role of cultural awareness and ethnic loyalty in acculturation. In A.M. Padilla (Ed.), *Acculturation: Theory, models, and some new findings* (pp. 47–84). Boulder, CO: Westview Press.

Padilla, A. M., & Lindholm, K. J. (1983). Hispanic behavioral science research: Recommendations for future research. *Hispanic Journal of Behavioral Sciences, 6,* 13–32.

Patterson, G. R. (1982). *Coercive family process* Eugene, OR: Castalia.

Patterson, G. R. (1986). Performance models for antisocial boys. *American Psychologist, 41,* 432–444.

Pentz, M. A. (1994). Target populations and interventions in prevention research: What is high risk? In A. Cazares & L. A. Beatty (Eds.), *Scientific methods for prevention intervention research.* Rockville, MD: NIDA Research Monograph.

Perlstadt, H., Hembroff, L. A., & Zonia, S. C. (1991). Changes in status, attitude, and behavior toward alcohol and drugs on a university campus. *Family and Community Health, 14,* 44–62.

Petraitis, J., Flay, B. R., & Miller, T. Q. (1995). Reviewing theories of adolescent substance use: Organizing pieces in the puzzle. *Psychological Bulletin, 117,* 67–86.

Piavio, A. (1986). *Mental representations: A dual coding approach.* New York: Oxford University Press.

Pickens, R. W., & Svikis, D. S. (1991). Prevention of drug abuse: Targeting risk factors. In L. Donohew, H. E. Sypher, & W. J. Bukoski (Eds.), *Persuasive communication and drug abuse prevention* (pp. 35–49). Hillsdale. NJ: Lawrence Erlbaum Associates.

Ponterotto, J. G., & Casas, M. J. (1991). *Handbook of racial/ethnic minority counseling research.* Springfield, IL: Charles C. Thomas.

Posner, M. I., & Keele, S. W. (1968). On the genesis of abstract ideas. *Journal of Experimental Psychology, 77,* 353–363.

Raspberry, W. (1997, March 31). Music to my ears. *The Washington Post,* AI2.

Reber, A. S. (1993). *Implicit learning and tacit knowledge: An essay on the cognitive unconscious.* New York: Oxford University Press.

Robbins, L., & Regier, D. (Eds.; 1991). *Psychiatric disorders in America: The epidemiologic catchment area study.* New York: The Free Press.

Robles, R., Moscoso, M., Colon, H., *et al.* (1991). *El uso do drogas en los adolescentes escolores.* (Drug use in school adolescent). Rio Piedras, PR: Department of Addiction Services.

Roediger, H. L. (1990). Implicit memory: Retention without remembering. *American Psychologist, 45,* 1043–1056.

Rogler, L. H. (1994). International migrations: A framework for directing research *American Psychologist, 49*(8), 701–708.

Rooney, J. F. (1984). Sports and clean living: A useful myth? *Drug and Alcohol Dependence, 13,* 75–87.

Rotter, J. B. (1966). Generalized expectancies for internal versus external control of reinforcement. *Psychology Monograph, 80,* No. 1 (Whole No. 609).

Rotter, J. B. (1981). The psychological situation in learning theory. In D. Magnusson (Ed.), *Toward a psychology of situations: An interactional perspective.* Killsdale, NJ: Lawrence Erlbaum.

Schacter, D. L. (1987). Implicit memory: History and current status. *Journal of Experimental Psychology: Learning, Memory, and Cognition, 13,* 501–518.

Schlegel, R., & Sandborn, M. (1979). Religious affiliation and adolescent drinking. *Journal of Studies on Alcohol, 40,* 693–703.

Segal, B. (1977). Personality factors related to drug and alcohol use. In D. Lettieri (Ed.), *Predicting Adolescent Drug Abuse* (Research Issues Series 11). Rockville, MD: National Institute on Drug Abuse.

Segal, B., Huba, G. J., & Singer, J. L. (1980). Reasons for drug and alcohol use by college students. *International Journal of the Addictions, 15,* 489–498.

Shepard, R. M., & Cooper, L. A. (1982). *Mental images and their transformations.* Cambridge, MA: MIT Press.

Sher, K. (1994). Individual-level risk factors. In R. Zucker, G. Boyd, & J. Howard (Eds), *The development of alcohol problems: Exploring the biopsychosocial matrix of risk* (Research Monograph 26; pp. 77–108). Rockville, MD: National Institute on Drug Abuse.

Silverman, M. M. (1989). The integration of problem and prevention perspectives: Mental disorders associated with alcohol and drug use. In, D. Shaffer, I. Philips, & N. B. Enzer (Eds.), *Prevention of mental disorders, alcohol and other drug use in children and adolescents* (Prevention Monograph 2; pp. 1–22). Rockville, MD: Office for Substance Abuse Prevention.

Single, E., Kandel, D., & Faust, R. (1974). Patterns of multiple drug use in high school. *Journal of Health and Social Behavior, 15,* 344–357.

Slovic, P. (1987). Perception of risk. *Science, 236,* 280–285.

Slovic, P. (1992). Perception of risk: Reflections on the psychometric paradigm. In S. Krimsky & D. Golding (Eds.), *Social theories of risk* (pp. 117–152). New York: Praeger.

Slovic, P. (1993). Perceptions of environmental hazards: Psychological perspectives. In T. Garling, & R. G. Golledge (Eds.), *Behavior and environment: Psychological and geographical approaches* (Chapter 13, pp. 223–248). New York: Elsevier Science Publishers.

Slovic, P., Fischoff, B., & Lichenstein, S. (1979). Rating the risks. *Environment, 21*(3), 14–20, 36–39.

Slovic, P., Fischoff, B., & Lichenstein, S. (1984). Behavioral decision theory perspectives on risk and safety. *Acta Psychologica, 56,* 183–203.

Slovic, P., Flynn, L. H., & Layman, M. (1991). Perceived risk, trust, and the politics of nuclear waste. *Science, 254,* 1603–1608.

Slovic, P., Layman, M., & Flynn, J. H. (1990, September). *What comes to mind when you hear the word "Nuclear waste repository"? A study of 10,000 images* (Report No. NWPO-SE-028–90). Carson City, NV: Nevada Agency for Nuclear Projects.

Slovic, P., Layman, M., & Flynn, J. H. (1991). Risk perception, trust, and nuclear waste: Lessons from Yucca Mountain. *Environment, 33,* 6–11, 28–30.

Slovic, P., Layman, M., Klaus, N., Flynn, J., Chalmers, J., & Gesell, G. (1991). Perceived risks, stigma, and potential economic impacts of a high-level nuclear waste repository in Nevada. *Risk Analysis, 11,* 683–696.

Smart, J. F., & Smart, D. W. (1993). Acculturative stress of Hispanics: Loss and challenge. *Journal of Counseling and Development, 73,* 390–396.

Sokol-Katz, J. S., & Ulbrich, P. M. (1992). Family structure and adolescent risk-taking behavior: a comparison of Mexican, Cuban and Puerto Rican Americans. *International Journal of the Addictions, 27*(10) 1197–1209.

Spiwak, A. M. (1982). Child rearing attitudes and practices of Mexican-American parents: Effects of social class and acculturation. Unpublished doctoral dissertation. Los Angeles: California School of Professional Psychology.

Staats, A. W., & Staats, C. K. (1959). Meaning and memory: Correlated but separate. *Psychological Review, 66,* 136–144.

Stacy, A. W., Ames, S. L., Sussman, S., & Dent, C. W. (1996). Implicit cognition in adolescent drug use. *Psychology of Addictive Behaviors, 10,* 190–203.

Swisher, J. D., & Hu, T. W. (1983). Alternatives to drug abuse: Some are and some are not. *NIDA Research Monogrh Series, 47,* 141–153.

Szalay, L. B. (1990). *Evaluating the psycho-social impact of treatment.* Chevy Chase, MD: Rapport, Inc.

Szalay, L. B. (1994). Socialization into the T. C. culture. In G. De Leon & F. Tims (Eds.), *Therapeutic community research* (NIDA Research Monograph, pp. 54–79). Rockville, MD: National Institute on Drug Abuse.

Szalay, L. B., Bovasso, G., Vilov, S. K., & Williams, R. E. (1992). Assessing treatment effects through changes in perceptions and cognitive organization. *American Journal of Drugs and Alcohol Abuse, 18,* 407–428.

Szalay, L. B., & Brent, J. (1965). *Cultural meanings and values: A method of empirical assessment.* Washington, D.C.: The American University.

Szalay, L. B., & Brent, J. (1967). The analysis of cultural meanings through free verbal associations. *Journal of Social Psychology, 72,* 161–187.

Szalay, L.B., & Bryson, J.A. (1972). *Measurement of meaning through verbal association and other empirical methods.* Kensington, MD: American Institute for Research.

Szalay, L. B., & Bryson, J. (1973). Measurement of psychocultural distance: A comparison of American Blacks and Whites. *Journal of Personality and Social Psychology, 26,* 166–177.

Szalay, L. B., & Bryson, J. (1974). Psychological meaning: Comparative analyses and theoretical implications. *Journal of Personality and Social Psychology, 30,* 860–870.

Szalay, L. B., & Bryson, J. (1977). *Filipinos in the Navy: Service, interpersonal relations, and cultural adaptation.* Washington, DC: American Institutes for Research.

Szalay, L. B., & Canino, G. (1991). *Cultural influences and drug abuse: Psychological vulnerabilities of Puerto Ricans in the United States.* Chevy Chase, MD: Institute of Comparative Social and Cultural Studies.

Szalay, L. B., Canino, G., & Vilov, S. K. (1993). Vulnerabilities and culture change: Drug use among Puerto Rican adolescents in the United States. *International Journal of Addictions, 28,* 327–354.

Szalay, L. B., Carroll, J. F. X., & Tims, F. (1993). Rediscovering free associations for use in psychotherapy. *Psychotherapy 30,* 344–356.

Szalay, L. B., & Deese, J. (1978). *Subjective meaning and culture: An assessment through word associations.* Hillsdale, NJ: Lawrence Erlbaum-Wiley & Sons.

Szalay, L. B., & Diaz-Guerrero, R. (1985). Similarities and differences between subjective cultures: A comparison of Latin, Hispanic, and Anglo American. In R. Diaz-Guerrero (Ed.), *Cross cultural and national studies in social psychology.* Proceedings of the XXIII International Congress of Psychology.

Szalay, L. B., Diaz-Royo, A. T., Brena, M. N., & Vilov, S. K. (1984). *Hispanic American psychocultural dispositions relevant to personnel management.* Washington, DC: Institute of Comparative Social and Cultural Studies.

Szalay, L. B., Diaz-Royo, A. T., Miranda, M. R., Yudin, L. W., & Brena, M. T. (1983). *Comparative analysis of Mexican American, Puerto Rican, Cuban, and Anglo American psychocultural dispositions.* Washington, DC: Institute of Comparative Social and Cultural Studies.

Szalay, L. B., Inn, A., & Doherty, K. (1996). Social influences, their role in promoting substance abuse: The effects of the social environment. *Substance Use and Misuse,* 343–373.

Szalay, L. B., Inn, A., Strohl, J. B., & Wilson, L. C. (1993). Perceived harm, age, and drug use: Perceptual and motivational dispositions affecting drug use. *Journal of Drug Education, 23(4),* 333–356.

Szalay, L. B., & Kelly, R. M. (1982). Political ideology and subjective culture: Conceptualization and empirical assessment. *American Political Science Review, 76,* 585–602.

Szalay, L. B., & Lysne, D. A. (1970). Attitude measurement by free verbal associations. *Journal of Social Psychology, 82,* 43–45.

Szalay, L. B., Lysne, D. A., & Brent, J. E. (1970). *A study of American and Korean attitudes and values through associative group analysis.* Kensington, MD: Center for Research in Social Systems, American Institutes for Research.

Szalay, L. B., Lysne, D. A., & Bryson, J. A. (1972). Designing and testing cogent communication. *Journal of Cross-Cultural Psychology, 3,* 247–258.

Szalay, L. B., & Maday, B. C. (1983). Implicit culture and psychocultural distance. *American Anthropologist, 85(1),* 110–118.

Szalay, L. B., Ruiz, P., Lopez, R., Turbyville, L., & Strohl, J. B. (1978). *Hispanic American cultural frame of reference: A communication guide for use in mental health, education, and training.* Washington, DC: Institute of Comparative Social and Cultural Studies.

Szalay, L. B., Strohl, J. B., & Wilson, L. C. (1991). *Adolescent socialization: Changing views related to drug use: Comparison of elementary, junior high, and high school students.* Chevy Chase, MD: Rapport, Inc.

Szalay, L. B., Vasco, E. V., & Brena, M. N. (1982). *A Columbian–U.S. communication lexicon of images, meanings, cultural frames of reference.* Washington, DC: Institute of Comparative Social and Cultural Studies.

Szalay, L. B., Vilov, S. K., & Strohl, J. B. (1992). Charting the psychological correlates of drug abuse. In R. R. Watson (Ed.), *Alcohol and Drug Abuse Reviews, Vol. 4: Drug Abuse Treatment.* Totowa, NJ: Humana.

Szalay, L. B., & Windle, C. (1968). Relative influence of linguistic versus cultural factors on free verbal associations. *Psychological Reports, 12,* 43–51.

Szalay, L. B., Windle, C., & Lysne, D. A. (1970). Attitude measurement by free verbal associations. *Journal of Social Psychology, 82,* 43–55.

Szapocznik, J., Scopetta, M. A., Kurtines, W. M., & Aranalde, M. A. (1978). Theory and measurement of acculturation. *Interamerican Journal of Psychology, 12,* 113–130.

Tarter, R. E., & Vanyukov, M. M. (1994). Stepwise developmental model of alcoholism etiology. In R. Zucker, G. Boyd, & J. Howard (Eds), *The development of alcohol problems: Exploring the biopsychosocial matrix of risk* (pp. 303–330; NIDA Research Monograph). Rockville, MD: National Institute on Drug Abuse.

Thomas, B., & Hsiu, L. T. (1993). The role of selected risk factors in predicting adolescent drug use and its adverse consequences. *International Journal of Addictions, 28,* 1549.

Thompson, E. A., Smith-DiJulio, K., & Matthews, T. (1982). Social control theory: Evaluating a model for the study of adolescent alcohol and drug use. *Youth and Society, 13,* 303–326.

Tiffany, S. T. (1990). A cognitive model of drug urges and drug-use behavior: Role of automatic and nonautomatic processes. *Psychological Review, 97,* 147–168.

Tolman, E. C. (1932). *Purposive behavior in animals and men.* New York: Oxford University Press.

Tolman, E. D. (1948). Cognitive maps in rats and men. *Psychology Review. 55,* 189–208.

Tononi, G., Sporns, O., & Edelman, G. (1992). Reentry and the problem of integrating multiple cortical areas: Simulation of dynamic integration in the visual system. *Cerebral Cortex, 2,* 310–335.

Triandis, H. C. (1972). *The analysis of subjective culture.* New York: Wiley.

Triandis, H. C. (1990). Cross-cultural studies of individualism and collectivism. In J. Bergman (Ed.), *Nebraska symposium on motivation. 1989.* Lincoln, NE.: University of Nebraska.

Triandis, H. C. (1993). Recent research on individualism and collectivism. Paper in special issue on cross-cultural social psychology. In F. Neto (Ed.) *Les Cahiers Internationaux de Psychologie Sociale.*

Triandis, H. C. (1994). Culture and social behavior. Boston: McGraw-Hill.

Triandis, H. C., Marin, G., Betancourt, H., Lisansky, J., & Chang, B. (1982). *Dimensions of familism among Hispanic and mainstream Nary recruits* (Technical Report #14, Department of Psychology). Champaign, IL: University of Illinois.

Triandis, H. C., Vassiliou, V., & Nassiakou, M. (1968). Three cross-cultural studies of subjective culture. *Journal of Personality and Social Psychology (Monograph Supplement), 8*(4).

Tversky, A., & Kahneman, D. (1981). The framing of decisions and the psychology of choice. *Science, 211,* 453–458.

U.S. Bureau of Census. (1990). The Hispanic population in the United States: March 1989. *Current Population Reports,* Ser. P-20, No. 44. Washington, D.C.: US Govt. Print. Off.

Van Dijk, W. K. (1980). Biological, psychogenic, and sociogenic factors in drug dependence. In D. Lettieri, M. Sayers, and H. W. Pearson (Eds.), *Theories on drug abuse: Selected contemporary perspectives* (vol. 30, pp. 164–173). NIDA Research Monograph.

Vega, W. A., Gil, A. G., & Zimmerman, R. S. (1993). Patterns of drug use among Cuban-American, African American, and White Non-Hispanic boys. *Am I Public Health, 83*(2), 257–259.

Vilhjalmsson, R., & Thorlindsson, T. (1992). The integrative and physiological effects of sports participation: A study of adolescents. *Sociological Quarterly, 33,* 637–647.

Wallace, J. M., & Bachman, J. G. (1991). Explaining racial/ethnic differences in adolescent drug use: The impact of background and lifestyle. *Social Problems, 38,* 333–357.

Warheit, G. J., Biafora, F. A., Zimmerman, R. S., Gil, A. G., *et. al.* (1995). Self-rejection/derogation, peer factors, and alcohol, drug, and cigarette use among a sample of Hispanic, African-American, and White non-Hispanic adolescents. *International Journal of the Addictions, 30,* 97–116.

Weill, J., & Le Bourhis, B. (1994). Factors predictive of alcohol consumption in a representative sample of French male teenagers: a five-year prospective study. *Drug and Alcohol Dependence, 35,* 45–50.

Whorf, B. (1956). *Language, thought, and reality.* New York: Wiley.

Williams, J. G., & Smith, J. P. (1993). Alcohol and other drug use among adolescents: Family and peer influences. *Journal of Substance Abuse, 5,* 288–294.

Wilson, T. D., Hodges, S. D., & LaFleur, S. J. (1995). Effects of introspecting about reasons: Inferring attitudes from accessible thoughts. *Journal of Personality and Social Psychology, 69,* 16–28.

Wilson, T. D., & Schooler, J. W. (1991). Thinking too much: Introspection can reduce the quality of preferences and decisions. *Journal of Personality and Social Psychology, 60,* 181–192.

Wright, L. (1985). High school polydrug users and abusers. *Adolescence, 20,* 853–861.

Yamaguchi, K., & Kandel, D. (1984). Patterns of drug use from adolescence to young adulthood: predictors of progression. *American Journal of Public Health, 74,* 673–682.

Yee, A. H., Fairchild, H. H., Weizmann, F., & Wyatt, G. E. (1993). Addressing psychology's problems with race. *American Psychologist, 48,* 1132–1140.

Zeki, S. (1992). The visual image in mind and brain. *Scientific American, 267,* 68–76.

Zucker, R. A. (1994). Pathways to alcohol problems and alcoholism: A developmental account of the evidence for multiple alcoholisms and for contextual contributions to risk. In R. Zucker, G. Boyd, & J. Howard (Eds.), *The development of alcohol problems: Exploring the biopsychosocial matrix of risk.* (Research Monograph 26; pp. 255–290). Rockville, MD: National Institute on Alcohol Abuse and Alcoholism.

Index